Health and Cultural Values

Health and Cultural Values: Female Circumcision within the Context of HIV/AIDS in Cameroon

By

Ngambouk Vitalis Pemunta

CAMBRIDGE SCHOLARS

PUBLISHING

Health and Cultural Values:
Female Circumcision within the Context of HIV/AIDS in Cameroon,
by Ngambouk Vitalis Pemunta

This book first published 2011

Cambridge Scholars Publishing

12 Back Chapman Street, Newcastle upon Tyne, NE6 2XX, UK

British Library Cataloguing in Publication Data
A catalogue record for this book is available from the British Library

ISBN (10): 1-4438-2642-1, ISBN (13): 978-1-4438-2642-6

In memory of Mangi Martha Manga who first thought I could study culture and began teaching me informally and to my mum, Rikeh Juliana for foregoing her own education to take care of me. I hope she and Ngamboug Nkeme Alfred will find in the outcome of this scholarly venture ultimate satisfaction for their many sacrifices in my regard.

TABLE OF CONTENTS

LIST OF FIGURES

Maps

Illustrations

ACKNOWLEDGEMENTS

In attempting to transform my dim dream into reality, I received immeasurable assistance and cooperation from many individuals some of whom I must commend. I am particularly indebted to my doctoral thesis advisors, Drs Don Kalb and Ronnie Moore for their commitment, interest and intellectual enthusiasm in offering advice whenever I was going off track and for their kindness, friendliness and support from the conception to the realisation of this work. I must confess that I learned a lot from their intellectual experiences and they have since continued to be a source of inspiration for me.

I am indebted to my lecturers at the department of Sociology and Anthropology for their untiring efforts to point the path to inquiry, to Drs Ayse Caglar, Alexandra Kowalski, Balázs Vedres, Daniel Monterescu, Prem Kumar Rajaram, Dan Rabinowitz, Vlad Naumescu and Judit Bodnar for providing helpful suggestions and feedback on my work both individually and within the larger context of the departmental seminars. Anna Loufti apart from ultimate enthusiasm provided a useful 'touch down' point for me within the context of her course on the body for which I am immeasurably grateful. I am also grateful to Elissa Helms, John Harbord, Eszter Timar and to my colleagues for their individual critical feedback and to the departmental staff for their collaboration. I hope they find in this work the assurance that their help was both timely and duly valued.

My gratitude also goes to research participants and other individuals who provided invaluable information without which it would have been impossible to generate the data for this study. I am thinking particularly of members of the Otang family, (especially Nkoyo Emilia O. N)- who apart from recruiting potential and knowledgeable respondents, adopted me and served as a sound board for testing and clarifying information during their constant visits during my field stay in Ejagham land. Furthermore, their extended networks in various villages offered invaluable sources of information, collaboration and a congenial atmosphere. I also appreciate the efforts of Dr Mathiew Bonchuk of the History Department, University of Calabar, Nigeria for helping me locate relevant sources on the Ejaghams during my research stop over in August, 2006. I extend the same word of gratitude to Prof. Mbonji Edjenguele of the University of Yaounde1 for providing valuable sources.

I am most grateful and appreciative to George Soros' magnanimity and to the Central European University Corporation, Budapest, Hungary for awarding me a scholarship, for financial assistance towards the realisation of this project and for sponsoring my semester abroad stay at the School of Public Health Medicine and Population Studies, University College Dublin, Ireland where I became more acquainted with the role of the social sciences in medical education.

I extend particular gratitude to Awandem Mbecha, Kah Fossung Kingsley, Awung Ivo, Drs. Ndifor K. Tangie, Ntoko Jean-Marie and Tatah Peter Ntaimah, Tom Obara, Selmeci Zsófia, Lányi Weronka Judit, Njisuh Feka, Nforbin Charles, Mboni Johnston for their support, advice, kindness, conviviality and enthusiasm all through the gestation period of this work.

On behalf of CSP, I heartily wish to acknowledge Amanda Millar, Carol Koulikourdi and Soucin Yip-Sou (who prepares duct jackets) for their tireless efforts, time-consciousness and handwork. It was an immense pleasure working with them.

I heartily say thank you, merci, Méh yaka, oyé, köszönöm.

Ngambouk V. Pemunta, Ph.D
Budapest, November, 22, 2010.

PRELUDE

> These White peoples have put our vaginas on the internet for everyone to see while they hide those of their women. Now they say that if we cut women, they will contract AIDS. Circumcision instead protects the dignity of a woman and makes her a standard woman. Those who are not cut can easily be tempted for a man and can contract AIDS (George, 35 years old).

This study grew out of my doctoral thesis on the renegotiation of the ritual practice of female circumcision (herein after FC) as a larger process of socio-cultural changes in gender roles in general and changes in health, values and practices in particular, orchestrated by the moral paranoia that accompanied the advent of the HIV/AIDS pandemic among the Ejaghams of Cameroon. As an anthropologist, I was rather shocked and bewildered by the disdain that Bayang female students were treated with at the University of Yaounde1, Cameroon. Even though the Bayangs, immediate neighbours of the Ejaghams had given up female ritual circumcision in the 1950s, the stigma of ritual FC still haunt them in the popular imagination in present-day postcolonial Cameroon. They are often rumoured to have insatiable appetite for sex because of their presumed lack of clitorises resulting from the ritual cutting practice of FC. Then came the groundswell of Western media frenzy that greatly shaped my initial views on the ritual practice as a meaningless 'barbaric and dangerous' practice presupposing lack of autonomy, power and subservience to patriarchy, depicting participants as "barbaric and uncivilized", ''tradition-oriented'' and ''prisoners of ritual''. This colonization of the voices of "African women" has attracted the attention of African feminist scholars (Njambi, 2004, Oyewumi, 2004, Nnaemeka, 2005). Njambi (2004) rightly describes anti-FGM discourse as replete with conceptual oppositions: science/superstition, medical knowledge/tradition, civilized/barbaric healthy bodies/unhealthy bodies, normal/abnormal sexuality, expert/non-expert, educated/ignorant. This shows inequality in the power of cultural representations as the ultimate 'other' is negatively represented since the subaltern cannot speak. The representer through this process acquires an improved self-image. Oyewumi (2004) for instance, takes issue with Walker (1992) by noting that her tale of the horror of FC is couched in the Western/Non-Western binary opposition. Additionally, Alice Walker invents and presents a rather voyeuristic and groin-centered preoccupation with Africa, thereby making her book "... a veritable evangelical tale". In 1993, alongside Parmer, they exposed African women's genitalia as an anomaly in their film project *Warrior Marks*. This sexualization presents the African woman as being nothing other than hypo-sexual because of her presumed missing part (the clitoris[1]), "a collection of sexual parts". Whatever, the realities of Africa and African bodies they are liable to be paraded to suit the Western mind/body of its sexual predilections *du jour*. This mirrors the unequal cultural power and the Western tradition of employing stock images and ideas about Africa (2004:3). Alice pathologizes difference, as her vision is that society is a reflection of the physical bodies to be found in it. Phenotypical differences between Africans and Europeans has led to the pathology of difference and African women are consequently presented as the ultimate other. Oyewumi further notes that feminist purveyors of global sisterhood based on a common genitalia- are untenable because "*even apparently similar body parts have different histories and locations. It is similar histories and common interests, and not body parts, which should be the focus of alliances.*" Alice further homogenizes African women's lack of sexual pleasure despite the diversity of the ritual procedures (clitoridectomy, infibulation, excision etc), nations, cultures, and societies. This is a unalinealist view, or what Hountounji calls the "myth of Unanimism"- wherein it is believed that in "primitive" societies, there is universal agreement, no individual beliefs/opinions but only collective systems of belief exist (see also., Fanon.,1963). (cf Oyuwemi, 2004: 5), even when there is no consensus within a given culture, but rather contestation, disagreement, negotiation and renegotiation of cultural values and practices. In other words, view points even within the same cultural complex are never monologic but rather, polyphonic since even the concept of culture is characterized by contestation, negotiation, renegotiation and disagreement. Initiate's voices do not seem to bear Alice Walker and other activist scholars out[2]. Human rights studies that also use

[1] The clitoris seems to be a symbolism for women's political power since by lacking it, African women are said to lack agency and need to be saved. But as Abusharaf (2000, 2001) shows, women use their ''Bottom power'' (circumcision status) as a source of power by being able to resist sexual demands from their husbands and in the process to get them to do what they like. The Freudian concept of penis envy seems to be appropriate here.

[2] See Abusharaf (2000, 2001), and EL Dawla (1999) whose informants present the ritual as a symbol of their power. They are able to use their circumcision statuses to garner for resources from their husbands and to get their voices heard. Emic contextual personal accounts have equally been rendered by Kratz (1994), Ahmadou (2001), Njambi (2004) and others.

a biomedical model equally present FC using harmful effect as the unit of analysis. Within this framework, sexuality becomes a static object of enquiry, decontextualised from wider historical changes.

Simultaneously, the human rights discourse has paradoxically been appropriated against FC by some circumcised women. Two practical cases will illustrate this point of view. Ms Ayaan Hirsi Ali, originally from Somalia, has become an icon in championing the human rights of women in Islamic societies. Clitoridectomised at the tender age of five, she later escaped an arranged marriage by immigrating to the Netherlands in 1992 where she subsequently sought and received political asylum. She served as a member of the Dutch parliament from 2003 to 2006, during which time; she worked relentlessly on furthering the integration of non-Western migrants into Dutch society and on defending the rights of women in Dutch Muslim society. In 2004 alongside Theo van Gogh, she co-produced the film *Submission* about the oppression of women in Islamic cultures. The airing of the film on Dutch television led to the assassination of Van Gogh by an Islamic extremist, Mohammed Bouyeri because the film was alleged to have 'blasphemed' Islam. This murder horrified and sent shock waves across Holland, Europe and around the world. This story represents the clash of political Islam with western secularism, militant Islam and infidels and marks the very limits of tolerance within multiculturalism. The preservation of archaic values such as religious and male dominance are responsible for the oppression of Islamic women and the lack of individual rights, at the same time, it sustains the deeply entrenched poverty of Muslims within their communities and abroad. It is above all, a call for equality and the reformation of conservative religious pillars, a shift of values in modern Islamic societies. Hirsi Ali, as detailed in her memoir *Infidel*, shows that she became defiant of customary rules, rules that had shaped her habitus. She fled from a secret pre-arranged marriage to her cousin that endangered her family's honour so as to attend secretarial school and to work out of the private sphere of the household. Her personal transformation against her own culture offers an illuminatingly deep understanding and a promising message of resilience and renewal. As she points out "*We in the West would be wrong to prolong the pain of [a transition to the modern world] unnecessarily, by elevating cultures full of bigotry and hatred toward women to the stature of respectable alternative ways of life*". For detailed and elaborate accounts of the development of Hirsi Ali's habitus and the murder of Van Gogh, see Buruma (2006) and Hirsi (2007) among others.

The second case took place in the USA where the issue of FC is framed in terms of asylum law. The US passed anti-FC laws in 1996 partly prompted by the Kassinja case. Kassinja, 23 years old, of Togolese nationality had arrived the US under a false passport. She was duely arrested, subsequently detained and her application for asylum against 'mutilation' turned down. Upon appeal, she was given US citizenship as her lawyers argued her case on the basis of gender-based discrimination and "cultural punishment". This decision marked a precedence in US jurisprudence. The US thereafter passed federal anti-FC law in 1996[3] (Boyles & Preves 2000: 721) sponsored by Congress woman Patricia Schroeder who stated that "*Over 100 million girls and women in the World have undergone some form of FC*" and thereafter categorically stated that it is happening here (in the US). By focusing the searchlight of the Western media to Kassinja's fear of having an 'abnormal' genital should she set foot in Togo, Rosenthal, a New York Times columnist advised President Bill Clinton to resolve the 'genitalia plague' in these words:

> He called on President Bill Clinton to endorse a three –point plan, including designating $100 million of the American foreign aid budget for local campaigns against ritual mutilation, giving more aid to countries that actively work to eradicate female genital mutilation and less, or nothing to those that don't, and making the issue a top priority for American delegations to the United Nations (Gollagher, 2000:188).

Fears and media speculations thereafter mounted that African women will inundate America as an escape from the horrors of FC, as an alibi against poverty. This is partly how America came to link aid with FC eradication (as if it is a plague) in particular and human rights protection in general for most states where the ritual cuttings go on. Boyle & Preves (2000) however debunk this "responding to massive immigration argument" by conceding that despite massive migration to the US between 1955 and 1995, less than 4% of immigrants came from the FC-endemic zones of Africa[4]. And most immigrants are males with a probable western orientation. Certain US states such as California, Delaware, Illinois, Michigan, Minnesota, North Dakota, Rhode Island, Tennessee and Wisconsin, immigrant bastions had already outlawed FC well before the

[3] It appears in my view that since the national ban came only after the Kassinja incident, the aim of legislation was to stem the tides of immigration and asylum claims on gender-based claims of persecution from 'infected countries'.

[4] These are countries such as Ethiopia, Egypt, Liberia, Somalia and the Sudan where the invasive form of the procedure is visited on females.

Federal ban went into action (Dugger, 1996). Detailed and illuminating documentation of the Kassinja and other 'FC-flight' cases have been various provided by Njambi (2004), Kratz (2003) Egan (1994) and Dugger (1996) among others.

Both cases discussed above show the appropriation of human rights norms by individuals and the intersecting arena in which the issue of FC has become entangled. Here cultural actors are contesting their own culture showing lack of consensus over cultural norms. Feminist and human rights groups have always appropriated Western human rights concepts to make their case for the need to grant refugee status to 'victims' of FC. Furthermore, the human rights framework which most activist-scholars use evades cultural specificity or take the standards of one culture as universal when in reality, they are not. It also glorifies but the individual unlike the societal context in which the practices are visited on young females[5], which prioritizes but the group. In other words, initiates sacrifice their individual needs for that of the social group. Ironically, the practice is done for the very best of intentions, as a sign of motherly or self-love. Mackie (2001) compares FC to dentistry whereas Abdullahi (1999) maintains that it is like the Christian rites of "first Holy Communion and Baptism in the West". Among the Ejaghams, ''undergoing female circumcision is like graduating from a University with a degree" (MA Sophi, interview of 06/06/2006). Racialized representations contradict the lived experiences of the initiates who feel empowered, and proud that they have attained womanhood and are therefore exposed to the special knowledge, wisdom of elders and special treatment (Robertson, 1996: 21, see also Dellenborg, 2004, Ahmadou, 2000, Lori, 2000). These static representations suggest that ritual FC is cast in stone, is unchanging whereas practitioners are making procedural reforms all the time. When Green (2000) discussed the prospects for cultural resistance to male circumcision as protection against HIV/AIDS among non-circumcising groups with a South African healer, the latter observed that "When tradition and the health of our people are in conflict, it is tradition we must sacrifice."

[5] The adoption of FGC by girls among the Sara partly attracted by the feasting and pleasure they derive from it is an interesting case. They mobilize the necessary resources and recruit circumcisers by themselves and do it despite refusal by significant social others in their community and in the process declare their own self-autonomy by institutionalizing and bureaucratizing the procedures. (see Lori, 2000, see also Dellenborg, 2004.) They may be seen as vectors of 'negative change'.

Research has demonstrated that traditional healers are in line with sexually transmissible disease (STD) and HIV/AIDS prevention strategies from the logic of transmission and causation: limiting the number of sexual partners, wearing protective charms or tattoos, having "strong blood", using condoms to reduce the risk of "pollution", or undergoing a "traditional vaccination" consisting of introducing herbs in skin incisions (Green, 1992, Green et al., 1993, Nzima et al., 1996, Schoepf, 1992), as well as female and male circumcision. Some studies have reported that the spread of HIV/AIDS could be prevented by upholding traditional values regarding abstinence such as FC, observation of sex taboos and strengthening the roles of women's societies such as Anankungwi in Malawi, which plays a strong role in counselling girls to observe local traditions pertaining to respect of elders and dressing (Bowa et al. ND, see also Orubuloye et al. 1994). In most cases, condoms have become acceptable to traditional healers, especially when they dovetail with their belief system. For instance, many African healers consider semen an important nutritional element for the nourishment of a growing foetus, for the maintenance of the mother's health and beauty, but their concern for family and cultural survival can supersede this belief and allow them to promote condom use (Green et al., 1993, Schoepf, 1992). Traditional practices are neither impermeable to change nor incompatible with modern rational science- both can be harnessed and the outcome will be democratic.

My reaction as an African male anthropologist to the sensationalized and moralizing Western discourse that underpin and "influence Western media, law and feminist thought: ignorance and oversimplification of African history, cultures and religions and exaggerations of the extent and geographical distribution of the various female genital cutting procedures performed" (Stanlie and Robertson, 2005) as unchanging was to find out through local level ethnography from participants in Ejagham land what had changed over time in this ritual practice especially within the context of the moral panic generated by the HIV/AIDS pandemic. What are their diverse reactions and how are they responding to the huge mediatisation of the ritual practice? How are they negotiating change in the face of intercultural contact and opposition from local anti-FC NGOs and their external allies? But, above all, do participants really have any agency?

Despite my black skin, I was often seen as an agent of neocolonialism by virtue of studying in Europe. This is of course a reaction to Western criticisms of the ritual practice which often borders on hygiene and health. I was therefore caught up in "the chains of translations", in the cross-fire of this huge debate as a "Whiteman with black skin" (see Pemunta, 2009, 2010). I however remain deeply aware that the mere mention of FC in the

West attracts outrage, surprise glances and deep embarrassment. While in the field, I quickly came to the realization that this huge debate is based on nothing else- but on the conflation of several universalisms: particularly health and sexuality, even when these are dynamic, socially and culturally constituted realities (Foster and Anderson, 1978, Kleinman, 1980, Romanucci-Ross, Merman et al. 1991, Hahn, 1995). And even when local knowledge and modern science are not antithetical to each other-both can be harnessed together and the outcome will be both democratic and progressive. Ironically, FC has become part of the trope used both in wider political debates about an immutable and unchanging, famine-stricken, war-torn and AIDS-infested Africa and about the need to rescue and 'civilize' African women who are often described as having no agency of their own, as chattel imprisoned by ancient patriarchal customs. Regarding FC in particular and the politics underpinning political representation in general, Winter notes this misplaced priority and manipulation of women by feminists and sensationalists thus:

> as is often the case, the debate concerning these women is less about the women themselves than about the appropriation of women as political symbols. In other words, it is about the use of women as ammunitions in a polemic of central concern to their lives, but where the issue is not the women's own interests but rather the consolidation of the power of others to define those interests (1994:939).

The blatant failure to listen to "African women", take social change into account and to contextualize the practice of FC is reflected in most studies undertaken by activist-scholars (Walker, 1992, Walker and Parmar, 1993, Hosken, 1986, Daly, 1978). Paradoxically, although these activist-scholars have fuelled worldwide activism against FC, they have simultaneously, but inadvertently frustrated trans-cultural dialogue through their sensationalism, and have ironically become enemies to the very women they want to "save" through the benevolence of "civilization" because the needs of these 'victims' have been universalized and are being determined for them. Frank Hosken (1986) for instance, condemns female genital mutilation on one main count: the aim of genital mutilation is "to mutilate the sexual pleasure and satisfaction of women''. If women are already mutilated before their debut of sexual life, then they have no other sexual pleasure and satisfaction other than the one after circumcision. They have no prior experience of 'normal sexuality' on the basis of which to judge or compare their experiences after circumcision against. It is like telling somebody who has never eaten pork (devout Muslim) and will never eat it, about the pleasures of consuming it. Her Euro-American concept of sexual pleasure begs the question at best. From this premise, she then concedes that women's sexuality is controlled, as is their reproductive potentials. Contrary to her position, Boddy (1982) locates women as central and strategic actors and interprets FC and the covering or closure as symbolic acts that serve to foreground women's fertility by de-emphasizing their sexuality, and defining and creating women as potential mothers rather than as sex partners. FC becomes a barometer for assessing fitness and reproductive capacity. Nici Nelson (1987) has pointed out that among the Kikuyu; sexuality for women is not about sexual enjoyment. Rather, it has more to do with procreation than with pleasure and more specifically, social reproduction for the continuity of the patrilineage (see also Spaulding, 1992., Waly,1997, MacGaffey.,1996). Ritual FC therefore controls and channels female sexual desire towards social and biological reproduction. Hosken homogenizes male sexual politics in Africa and worldwide: 'to assure female dependence and subservience by all means' (1981: 3-24). Physical violence against women such as rape, sexual assault, excision, infibulation among others is perpetuated 'with an astonishing consensus among men in the World'. Here women are described as victims of patriarchal control- the sexually oppressed. Although male violence is a truism, defining women as archetypal victims reduces them into "objects-who-defend themselves" and every society into a binary opposition between powerless (women) and powerful (men), even when power is unevenly distributed within every given society. Abusharaf (2001) has argued that 'virtuous cuts', FC, is considered as an act of ritual empowerment by her respondents. The concept of patriarchy like power, should be seen as relational and dynamic, with spaces for the multiple deployment of power. Bordo (1993:23) has pointed out that dichotomies such as oppressed/oppressor, powerful/powerless are inadequate for capturing 'the social and historical complexities of the situations of men and women'. She cites the Pokot of Kenya among whom circumcision empowers women by equating them with men in terms of status. Patriarchy by demonizing men, she notes, fails to highlight the complexities of race, class and the sexual situations of both men and women who find themselves embedded in institutions that they neither created nor are in control. Male violence must be circumscribed, theorized and interpreted within specific societies so as to provide for both better understanding and to put in place effective mechanisms towards change (Mohanty, 1986., see also Chatterjee., 1993).

HIV/AIDS and the Politics of Exoticism

The advent of the HIV/AIDS pandemic and the continuous elusive search for a medical solution to the threat of this terminal disease has led to an increased focus on the social and cultural context of the disease, especially in Africa- the very epicentre of the scourge. A wide range of sex-related cultural and social practices including- but not limited to- wife exchange, widow inheritance, polygamy, dry sex, sexual cleansing and female genital mutilation have accordingly, come under the epidemiological microscope and attracted outrage. For a detailed analysis of cultural practices contributing to the transmission of HIV in Africa (see Hrdy, 1987, Piot et al, 1984, D'Costa et al, 1985). These practices simultaneously serve as a rallying point for blanket condemnation in the public health community- among policy makers, activists, academics and governmental and non-governmental actors- who are unanimously calling for the eradication of these practices because of their presumed incompatibility with the health, social well-being, human security and human rights of both women and children. Harmful myths from colonial times still maintain that all African women are circumcised and with the advent of AIDS, all Africans are HIV carriers. Following Stanlie and Robertson, popular Western perceptions reduce Africa and African women into "Three Rs":

> First, they reduce Africa's fifty-four countries and hundreds of cultures to one uncivilized, "traditional" place outside of history to be compared with the "modern" "West". Second, they reduce Africans and African women in particular, to the status of their genitals, to being malicious torturers or hapless victims. Finally, uniform depictions reduce all cutting of female genitals to the most severe practice-infibulation. The cumulative effect of these reductions is that all African women are represented as having been infibulated due to unreasoned adherence to tradition and/or malicious ignorance. (2005:5).

This reductionism actually conflates the myriad problems of "African women". As the Position Paper of the African Studies Association poignantly states "many African women need food for themselves and their children, greater control over the means of food production, access to clean water, a secure fuel supply, access to health care including family planning and ways to acquire cash income". *Heightened concern regarding clitoridectomy and infibulation as the sole obstacle to the achievement of the status of women may be a luxury that only the West can provide* (emphasis mine). The paper admonished benevolent humanitarian efforts to energetically support internal social change through collaborative research, discussion and dissemination of information about progress and technical support, instead of adopting a militant position that forbids aids to countries with FC practicing ethnicities. This was in the 1980s before AIDS came to add another burden to the problems of women and to re-energize colonial ideas and perceptions of, and demonization of Africa and Africans.

The advent of AIDS only came to re-ignite and re-enforce stereotypical images and representations of Africa and Africans since the authority of epidemiological statistics on AIDS in Africa has actually magnified because of what David Cohen (2004) calls an "epistemology of certainty" that affects the way ''Africa'' is studied. Simultaneously, ritual FC (a blanket term for a diverse set of polythetic social and cultural practices) continues to generate unending ideological debate because of its presumed association with the transmission of the human immuno-deficiency virus through the bloodletting that it entails. As pointed out by Hrdy (1987:112) FC might be an inadequate explanation for enhanced heterosexual AIDS transmission because "although the presence of lesion in the vagina may increase male-to-female transmission, it is unclear how female-to-male transmission would be enhanced in this situation". He further points to lack of correspondence of the distribution of AIDS and FC and although data are sketchy FC is not practiced in areas with the highest level of HIV seropositivity.

Representations of African women as powerless and unable to negotiate safer sex have also been correlated to their greater risk of HIV infection, even when the evidence base is shaky and speculative. Research has shown that there is wide variation in the relationship between HIV and income (Piot, Greener, Russell, 2007). Findings from surveys in eight African countries (Burkina Faso, Cameroon, Ghana, Kenya, Lesotho, Malawi, Uganda and then United Republic of Tanzania) demonstrate higher HIV prevalence among adults in the wealthiest quintile than among those in the poorest quintile (Mishra et al., 2007). Available survey data from five of six West African countries shows that women living in the wealthiest households have higher HIV prevalence than other socioeconomic groups of women, but the relationship between wealth and HIV is less clear for men in the sub region (Lowndes et al., 2008).

Female Circumcision, AIDS and Male Circumcision

Several researchers have been preoccupied with the relationship between AIDS and the presumed protective effects of male circumcision (Hirozawa, 2001, Bloemenkamp et al. 2000), as well as the medical complications resulting from FC (Althus 1997, Jones et al. 1995, Larsen et al. 2000, Obermeyer, 1999), partly because the ritual practice is hypothetically assumed among other harmful medical effects to be capable of transmitting AIDS, despite shaky and inconclusive biomedical evidence. On the basis of data from 28 studies conducted in eight African countries, Hirozawa (2001) concludes that circumcised men are only about half as likely to contract HIV as uncircumcised men, and that circumcision confers a protective effect on men at higher risk of HIV infection. He further reports that population-based representative cohort study undertaken in Southwestern Uganda found a lower incidence of HIV infection among circumcised than among uncircumcised men.

Bloemenkamp et al (2000) found a reduced risk of female-male transmission of HIV in circumcised men in high risk populations in Sub Saharan Africa, while Kirby and associates (1991), report more efficient male-to-female transmission of HIV than female-to-male because women have a higher risk of infection than their male partners-they are unable to negotiate safe sex-despite their lower risk behaviour. But Hunter et al.(1990) report that women with constant, uncircumcised sexual partners in Nairobi, Kenya had a statistically significant higher risk (OR of 3.7 (95 % CI 1.5-9.0) of seropositivity. Though surprising, nothing is said about the risk of infection per sexual episode. Seidlin et al (1992) through discordant partnership research found out that there does not appear to be a reduced risk of transmission from an infected, circumcised man to his female partner. Yet, a New York study of 142 women of HIV infected index cases showed that partner serostatus was unrelated to the circumcision status of index case. Studies from Brazil and Uganda respectively, show that lack of circumcision and a history of genital sores were significantly associated with HIV seropositivity in male sexual partners of HIV positive women but no association was found between male circumcision status and seropositivity of female partners. One key finding of the latter study is that viral load may affect the protectiveness of male circumcision when considering male to female transmission of HIV (Hellman, 1991, Seidlin, 1992). On the other hand, a few studies have investigated male-to-male transmission of HIV through receptive anal intercourse. Buckfinder et al (1998) for instance, found a relationship between lack of circumcision and seroconversion while Kreiss' (1992) cross sectional study in the same country found a significant association between seropositivity and being uncircumcised- a status, implying an increased risk of HIV infection in the insertive partner among men who have sex with other men. These studies suggest that the main problem with assessing infectiousness and susceptibility in relation to circumcision status in male sexual encounters is ascertaining the portal of the entry of infection.

However, this male-circumcision based intervention strategy to HIV/AIDS advocated for by the scholars mentioned above has been opposed. For instance, Bonner (2001) maintains that there are very diverse circumcision practices even among geographically proximate groups casting doubt on how much prepuce must be removed to confer immunity against HIV/AIDS. He further points to a loss of immunity at different ages and that there are different cultural and religious rationales for circumcision implying that there are religious and cultural barriers for implementing it as a public health intervention. To compound matters, circumcision, he points out, does not appear to have any impact on transmission from HIV positive men to their partners. Although research by Salamon (1999) shows attenuation in the protective effects of circumcision at later ages, Klouman et al (2005) did not find any positive association between female genital surgery, HIV infection, other STIs or infertility but rather, a positive, though non-significant association between female genital cutting and bacterial vaginosis was found with a crude odds ratio of 4.6. This however, warrants further investigation.

Studies that use a biomedical model equally present FC using harmful effect as the unit of analysis. These studies are replete with methodological problems, including, but not limited to-non-representative samples, lack of control groups, the infeasibility of conducting interdisciplinary large scale research at a population level, the diversity of FC practices and the perception that problems resulting from the ritual procedures is part of womanhood- factors that all compound rigorous research. For instance, through analysis of DHS data for the Central African Republic, Cote D'Ivoire, Egypt, Eritrea, Mali and Sudan respectively, it is not clear how frequently presumed harmful effects (medical complications) occur. And in societies in which almost every woman is circumcised, problems resulting from circumcision may well be perceived as natural and part of a woman's life cycle (Althus, 1997). However, a comparison of genital cutting practices in both Burkina Faso and Mali show a significant positive relationship between the severity of genital cuttings and the chances of a woman having both gynecological and obstetrical problems. They cite an unpublished report in Mali showing that women who have undergone FC are almost 7 times more likely than those who have not to experience complications at parturition (Jones et al. 1995). The study population was however limited only to women who had undergone FC. A comparison with women who had not undergone the ritual procedures would certainly have made the results more valid. A comparison of DHS data from the

Central African Republic, Cote D' Ivoire and Tanzania among other findings, concluded that circumcised women in Cote D'Ivoire and Tanzania had lower levels of childlessness, lower infertility rates by age and higher total fertility rates than uncut women. A reverse pattern prevailed in the Central African Republic. There was however, no statistically discernible impact on women's ability to reproduce. A further finding was that knowledge of complications are based on observations of clinical cases and that no studies have been undertaken at the level of a population with the aim of documenting complications (Larsen et al. 2000). There is, for instance, no comparison of uncut women for their study and they relied on self-reports without any comparison with medical examination.

A meticulous review of publications dealing with the so-called harmful effects of FC by Obermeyer (1999), shows that the evidence base is shaky. According to her, original reports are replete with numerous methodological errors (small or unrepresentative samples, lack of control group and vague descriptions of supposed medical complications). Only 8 studies lived up to standard epidemiological control criteria for scientifically validating evidence. She concludes that medical complications are the exceptions and not the rule, and "that female genital surgeries are not incompatible with sexual enjoyment". Research has also been undertaken on presumed male sexual complications resulting from FC. Almroth et al (2001) for instance, report penetration difficulties, exposure to wounds and infections on the penis as well as psychological problems when having intercourse with circumcised women by men in the Gezira scheme along the Nile Valley in the Sudan. Furthermore, more young men showed the willingness to accept a woman who had not undergone FC as a spouse and 55% of young men preferred marriage to a woman without FC, unlike 13% of grand fathers. However, by not capturing women's voices and perspectives, they failed to produce a balanced account.

A hypothetical association exists between FC and HIV/AIDS: the ritual cutting practice can facilitate HIV/AIDS transmission because pharoanic circumcision narrows the vagina and in an attempt to penetrate, men are likely to be wounded and therefore to be exposed to HIV/AIDS transmission (Kun, 1997). He points to the use of the same instrument for 5 to 10 females simultaneously during a circumcision session. He rather seems to hold a hardened view of culture as unchanging since practicing societies are increasingly making procedural and hygienic changes such as: the use of a fresh blade for each initiate in the wake of the incurable HIV/AIDS pandemic. Curiously enough, there is no scientifically established correlationship between HIV endemic zones and circumcising societies in Africa. This is, however, not to downplay the fact that FC can fuel the spread of HIV transmission and is a likely risk factor.

In reaction to the perceived risk of FC, particularly its ability to transmit AIDS, Shell-Duncan (2001), while perceiving a double standard in the condonment of male circumcision and medically unnecessary cosmetic surgeries by the same institution prohibiting FC while simultaneously indulging in male circumcision and unnecessary surgeries as hypocrisy, advocates for medicalisation as the way forward towards effective eradication. However, opponents of a harm reduction strategy mention lack of consent from the initiate, reject both sanitation and medicalisation of the procedures on grounds that it is performed on minors who are unable to grant "informed consent" (see among others, Price 1997, Bartow, 1999, Mason, 2001). Mason in particular takes issue with criminalization because it clashes with consent and capacity and yet, male surgery is not forbidden. She attributes the prevailing situation to a "legal gender bias", the very outcome, in her viewpoint, of a liberal conception of "tolerance" and the limits of consent in Australia. Any act of circumcision (male or female) is an unnecessary act of violence, is 'non-therapeutic' and circumcision lacks consent since rights reside in children with parents acting only as custodians and executors (Price (1997). These scholars however underlook the fact that in some societies like among the Ejaghams who are the focus of this study, there are several categories of initiates among which are mature women. Furthermore, the whole notion of rights is relative: human rights have a Western constituency. Women will rather choose community membership through circumcision than to exercise their human rights at the risk of their gendered personhood and marriage. Ironically, there are few cultures the world over in which only girl's genitals are modified. There also exists kinship, religion, economy, family life and ceremonial differences among African ethnic groups that practice circumcision for both sexes. Some of these groups are matrilineal, some Islamic, some puritanical. Shweder accuses the West of using its own anatomical folk concepts about proper female bodies and aesthetics in presenting African mothers as torturers (Schweder, 2005).

It seems safe to maintain that the effect of circumcision seen in high risk population is not generalisable, cannot be extrapolated to other groups and that the protective effects of male circumcision varies. Furthermore, complications resulting from FC are the exceptions since they depend among other things, on the type of circumcision undergone. This calls on us to recommend risk reduction strategies of proven efficacy against HIV/AIDS such as condom use and hygienic environments for the performance of both male and female circumcision since potential morbidity and mortality and the calculation of risk are some of the most serious considerations in developing countries where the prevalence of complications is patchy and anecdoctal unlike in the developed world.

Ironically, despite mounting epidemiological evidence suggesting that male circumcision provides some modicum of protection against STD and HIV infection especially in resource poor countries with predominantly heterosexual transmission (Halperin and Bailey, 1999, Bradley 1998, Moses et al, 1994), public health officials have been ambivalent and have failed to promote male circumcision as a harm reduction strategy despite the rush for male circumcision in traditionally non-circumcising societies as protection against HIV infection. Mundhenk (2000, cf Green, 2000) reports that:

> There seem to be a variety of motivations given when I ask people why they are getting circumcised. Apparently boys from the areas where circumcision is practiced have been boasting about the values of circumcision, mentioning two in particular. First, they claim that women get a lot more pleasure sleeping with a circumcised person than with an uncircumcised one. Second, they say that being circumcised helps to prevent you from getting various diseases, including venereal diseases and AIDS, so that after being circumcised one can sleep around with confidence.

Green (2000) has outlined six obstacles for this skepticism in public health programmes.

1. In resource constrained country settings, circumcision often takes place in non-medical settings, under conditions conducive to sepsis. If men in non-circumcising societies were to opt for circumcision, this might increase the chances of health problems as a result of dangerous surgical practices by poorly trained or untrained practitioners.
2. Circumcision might give men and their partners a false sense of security from HIV infection. They may consequently engage in riskier sexual behaviour (cf. Richens et al., 2000).
3. There is insufficient evidence that later circumcision in adulthood would protect men from STDs including HIV infection. In fact, the evidence suggests that the earlier the age of circumcision, the greater degree of protection against STDs and HIV (Kelly et al. 1999).
4. There is an anti-circumcision movement in the USA which equates male circumcision to useless genital mutilation, thereby indirectly linking this with the female genital mutilation issue in Africa.

5. Finally, some HIV/AIDS workers are simply unfamiliar with epidemiological findings related to AIDS and MC, or they are familiar with the evidence but they don't believe it.

Integrated HIV/AIDS and Anti-FC Programmes

The emergence of FC in the global discourse on HIV/AIDS multiplied and led to a flood of integrated anti-HIV/AIDS and FC eradication programmes. These efforts are however misplaced because they focus on health alone, see local knowledge as antithetical to rational science and are based on a static notion of culture in FC practicing societies, even when culture is dynamic. They de-emphasize the fact that the ritual practice is open to modernization, sanitization and rationalization. These interventions by both state and civil society actors and their allies are therefore underpinned by dominant perspectives, the influence of material hegemony, and dichotomous ideological debates: local/global knowledge, culture/human rights, and tradition/law, primitive/civilized and inferior/superior among others. Circumcised females are represented as victims of a universal patriarchy, as casualties of male chauvinism whereas, patriarchy does not preclude both resistance and agency. These representations became increasingly prevalent in the decades of the 1990s as activist scholars diffused images of infibulated women through the mass media, thereby giving these diverse practices a new and transnational coherence, but simultaneously triggered a backlash of resistance in practicing societies who saw them as merely out to eradicate not only the practices but their social selves and cultural well-being.

While FC practicing societies vary in social structure-some are matrilineal, others are patrilineal, anti-AIDS and -FC activism has continued to scape-goat patriarchy and to place a high premium on health alone whereas, these are recognized social, economic, development and human rights issues. Influenced by sensational popular and academic texts that portray circumcised women as victims in need of rescue by the more 'civilized' world, individual activists have fuelled national and international activism with one aim- eradication, as if it is an epidemic, and not sanitization.

Yet, cultural insiders perceive eradication as imperialism and cultural corruption, especially within the medical and institutional context of the HIV/AIDS pandemic in which the concept of health risk has paradoxically been doubly appropriated among the Ejaghams (see Pemunta, 2007). The pandemic has instead provided a platform for both resistance and simultaneous practice of FC as children are increasingly being circumcised at tender ages so as to forestall contestation at maturity under the influence of the "Whiteman". Hardliners are arguing for the tightening of control over women through FC, whereas progressives point to the bloodletting that the ritual procedure entails as capable of spreading diseases with HIV/AIDS inclusive among participants. Simultaneously, sensationalized, fetishized and unitary representations which often times underpin eradication initiatives and materials have instead stonewalled benevolent eradication campaigns, thereby reinforcing resistance to change in the name of cultural authenticity among hardliners.

It is important to acknowledge that FC is an act of gender-based violence, but the tropes of male power and Western dominance in the debates as well as the monolingual construction of the different realities of FC have silenced, erased the voices of and demonized participants- who are in fact, their own change agents. In the same light, dichotomous models of power permeate AIDS prevention discourses- that is the colonized/colonizer binary of nationalist discourse as well as feminist discourses of masculine oppression and female subordination- re-inscribing stereotypical images of African women as downtrodden, passive and sexually exploited victims. It might be argued that the images of circumcised women in the minds of public health/social care experts, activists, and bureaucrats has more to do with anti-colonial and feminist politics than with the life world of FC.

But for a few anthropological studies that have provided detailed, perceptive and nuanced accounts of FC (Hayes, 1975, Boddy, 1982, Gruenbaum, 1982, Abusharaf, 2000, 2001), it is most often the case that participants are demonized, pathologized and spoken for. This calls for the need to wear 'native spectacles', to listen empathetically to these subalterns in both analysis and intervention research on this thorny and controversial issue. Although I do not claim spokesman status, it is possible to interrogate why the voices of these subalterns are silenced- unequal power to construct social reality about FC.

This study is based on nine months of multi-locale ethnography among Ejagham tribes in Southwest Cameroon. It provides an insider perspective on the series of intergenerational conflicts over cultural values and practices resulting from the moral panic engendered by the advent of the HIV/AIDS pandemic. It further documents transformations in the institution of FC orchestrated by the changing medical and institutional context of the HIV/AIDS pandemic and the implications for understanding the agency of participants. Their stories contrasts sharply with the simplicity of homogenizing representations and demonization discourses used to describe them, and ground an understanding of FC in the place it matters most- life world of participants. It emphasizes the need for a nuanced 'transnational feminist standpoint'- to engage women inside, outside and *beyond* representations of a victim identity and to see them as constructing their world through an empathetic understanding that lays bare the fluidity and paradoxes of women's subjectivity *insitu (*See Law, 2000, Kempadoo, 2004). The overall lesson is that we should avoid representations that portray FC participants as having no agency (even when agency is structured). There is the need to avoid reductionism and to ground an understanding of FC in the lives of its participants, while simultaneously being aware that it is a multifunctional phenomenon calling for a multi-pronged development approach.

As a polythetic cultural complex, FC is intertwined with the whole cultural political economy of the Ejaghams, providing a social security network and gendered power to participants and not merely a health issue. By reducing the complexity and nuances of the ritual cutting to health alone, anti-FC activism has instead produced a backlash marked by simultaneous contestation and practice. Furthermore, the anti-FC campaigns have resulted in the privatization of FC on increasingly younger girls. However, the recent waiving of the ritual cutting as a precondition for membership into the Moninkim cult partly because of the ageing of the initial initiates, the health risk of the HIV/AIDS pandemic and anti-FC advocacy campaigns by local NGOs shows that change is underway. Simultaneously, inter-tribal marriages with members of non-circumcising tribes and romantic love relationships beyond the purview of the traditional patriarchal orbit have led younger lovers to be increasingly seeking mutually satisfying love relationships for which FC, a 'virtuous cut', becomes an obstacle.

This study argues for the need to tailor health education and social change initiatives with and not against the beneficiaries. Rather, change should be in the interest of the target population and not against them. Theoretically, I call attention to the need to look at local level processes and to trace resistance from below through an analysis of actor's multiple positioning, resources and their linkages to and alliances with other actors. Local processes are rooted in wider fields of power and are affected by forces at various scales calling for the need to look at the entanglement between local and global, economic, social, political and historical processes in the study of health and other cultural issues.

Scope of Study

In line with the power-oriented vision of culture adopted for this study, in chapter one, I examine the concept of culture, power, agency, gender in the construction of the reality of FC. The penultimate section examines the methodological approach used in the data elicitation process.

Chapter two addresses the political economy of the Ejagham region. I highlight their historic place and embeddedness in the regional economy and explore the impact of larger global economic processes and the changes it caused with particular reference to women and youths, a situation that has generated unending conflicts between generations and the sexes. I factor in the analysis the dynamics of the traditional sexual organization of the Ejaghams while capturing the impact of patriarchy on women's bodies and their sexuality. I make note of, and account for changes in the institution of marriage and in the pattern of female socialization over time.

Chapter three examines the relationship between various male and female institutions among the Ejaghams and the conflict of authority between traditional and modern systems of rule given the present postcolonial context in which the people find themselves. It further examines the dynamics of Moninkimhood and the FC process as an instantiation of local patriarchy. The Moninkim cult is the centre of all the conflicts going on about FC among various loose segments of Ejagham society.

Chapter four examines how the moral panic generated by the advent of the HIV/AIDS pandemic became an ambivalent framework for support, resistance and contestation of FC. This contest pits western rational science represented by NGOs and the state against local culture and knowledge system represented by various loose actors in Ejagham community. Both knowledge systems, I argue, can be harnessed and the outcome will be both democratic and progressive. In line with my power-oriented vision of culture as contestation, I examine state and NGO initiatives geared towards change in the practice of FC and the position of local stakeholders such as Traditional Birth Attendants (TBAs), the medical corps, local community leaders and members of the Moninkim cult- the very source of all the conflicts going on among generations and sexes in the community.

Chapter five looks at the people's attitude towards FC and the factors militating both for and against change in the ritual procedures. Generally, their attitudes may be segmented into a fluid, tripolar but interwoven continuum- resistance and acceptance of the necessity for change and oscillating mute voices both for and against FC especially in the wake of the HIV/AIDS crisis.

Lastly, chapter six draws the curtains on this study. In it, I critically look back at my own findings and make some recommendations that will eventually lead to change in the practice of FC in the study area and simultaneously identify gaps for future research.

CHAPTER ONE

NOTIONS OF CULTURE, POWER AND THE DEBATE ON FEMALE CIRCUMCISION IN CAMEROON

This study represents the first attempt to provide a novel understanding of the current practice of 'Female Circumcision', also called 'Female Genital Mutilation' within the context of the HIV/AIDS pandemic among Ejagham clans in contemporary Southwest Cameroon, Africa. I analyze the transformations that the Moninkim cult whose precondition for membership was female circumcision recently underwent in a changing medical and institutional context set in motion by the ravaging AIDS pandemic. Against the functionalist idea that "tradition" resists change unless it is destroyed by institutional modernization, I show how the advent of the HIV/AIDS pandemic set up institutional dynamics that triggered new debates between partisans and opponents of ritual female mutilation, causing certain segments of the practicing communities to reconsider and modify the modalities and function of the practice.One evidence of social and cultural change is the recent waiving of the criterion of circumcision and the subsequent extension of membership to some uncircumcised women who are variously called 'social Moninkims' and 'modern Moninkims' in contrast to their traditional counterparts.

This new development, calls for an investigation of various changes in the institution of FC. I use the Moninkim ritual society as a useful prism through which to investigate these changes. This exclusively female socialization institution whose values are publicly enacted and re-enacted through the dancing of the "NKIM" dance is believed to be the repository of gendered knowledge and feminine personhood. For centuries, Moninkimhood was the preserve of Ejagham upper class families who also exclusively owned male secret societies while excluding so-called 'slave families' who gradually came to adopt the institution for purposes of identification with the mainstream. While the meaning of the performance has transformed over time from ritual to spectacle, its meaning as a marker of gendered feminine personhood has remained salient since not only the initiates but also, their families and members of their extended kinship network achieved social prominence due to their association with the initiate. While most of the elderly generation still wants continuation with the past, the younger generations are submitting everything to intense questioning because there are other avenues at their disposal for the attainment of status and prominence such as western education and modern jobs. Most members of the former generation still consider the ritual as salient, a marker of feminine personhood and ethnic identity, a mechanism to control the younger generation's presumed frivolous attitude to sex unlike the latter who are more preoccupied with bodily autonomy and freedom. This has pitted both generations at conflict with each other, a conflict that is epitomized by the debate over FC. Despite its transformation from a ritual to a spectacle and from chastity to commercialism both within and beyond the Ejagham locale, it has remained an icon of both individual and collective identity and a source of livelihood. During important national days and the visits of government officials, the Moninkim dancers can be seen providing entertainment and garnering financial resources for themselves. These female dancers like the men associated with them, enjoy high prestige and represent traditional womanhood. Today, this instantiation of traditional patriarchy is at the centre of the debates between partisans and opponents of F C, between tradition and modernity, local and global knowledge, science, modern medicine and tradition. This association, the very source of endless debates and conflicts between the old and younger generations and between internal and external stakeholders with different amounts of resources, provides a useful window through which to enter and study FC and the interaction of multiple stakeholders occupying different interconnected power fields within the context of the HIV/AIDS pandemic. At the same time that various actors and their allies among the Ejaghams are debating the continuous relevance of the ritual cutting of F C, external actors are naming it differently and taking different positions against it, showing unequal power to construct social reality. To name a social reality, I suggest, is to take a position towards that reality.

1.1 The discursive politics of defining Female Circumcision as a power field

The United Nations Organization (UN) and the United Nations Children Emergency Fund (UNICEF), jointly defined 'FGM' to mean: "all procedures involving the partial or total [amputation] of the external female genitalia or other injury to the female genital organs whether for cultural or other non-therapeutic reason" (WHO, 1998). Various expressions such as "Female Genital Mutilation" (FGM), "Female Genital Castration", "Female Genital Surgery", "Female Circumcision" have been used among others to designate the ritual practices in the anti-FGM advocacy literature. However, any of these expressions seems to be suggestive of an ideological position, an ideological dichotomy, Western/Non-Western, superior/inferior, primitive/civilized. This has therefore led to the use of any of the above expressions being politically contested. "FGM" for instance, present initiates as "mutilated", which to them is vituperative. "FC" although it immediately announces the gender of the initiate, however equates the ritual procedures with male circumcision which feminists hold is less severe as compared to the operation performed on girls and women. Ironically too, it suggests that male circumcision is acceptable and normal, whereas groups like Attorneys for the Rights of the Child want all forms of circumcisions/ bodily modification practices to be totally outlawed. On the other hand, the use of the expression "Female Genital Castration" conjures an image of rendering initiates infertile whereas the people under consideration here, the Ejaghams partly believe that it prepares women among other things, towards motherhood.

The above-mentioned terminological debate shows different framings of the issue and multiple conceptions of health. From a human/health security and reproductive rights perspective, "mutilation" reinforces the view that it is a violation of women's rights and a form of culturally endorsed child abuse that lacks "informed consent". At the same time however, it helps in promoting both national and international advocacy towards its abandonment. In 1999, the United Nations in reaction to this terminological divide and the conflict it engenders, appealed for tact and patience regarding activities in this area and drew attention to the risk of "demonizing" certain cultures, religions and communities. Thereafter, "cutting" has been increasingly used to avoid alienating practicing communities since parents most often resent the suggestion that they are mutilating their daughters. The World Health Organization (WHO) and UNICEF (1998) have gone even further to classify genital cuttings into four overlapping categories. Type I is called excision of the prepuce, with(out) excision of part of the clitoris. Type II is the excision of the clitoris with the total or partial excision of the libia minora. Type III includes the excision of part or all of the external genitalia and stitching/narrowing of the vaginal opening (infibulation). Type IV is unclassified and includes pricking, piercing, stretching, burning, scraping and any other procedure inclusive of the above.

Ironically, the WHO describes genital operations as 'unnecessary' but curiously enough, does not include male circumcision and elective surgeries in the category of 'unnecessary' practices. This is despite the fact that they equally lead to 'unnecessary pain' and irreversible changes to the human physiognomy. However, the above definition and categories are problematic in several respects. First and foremost, they presuppose the universality of the concept of "health". Conceptions of health, however, greatly vary across time and space. Health is more adequately conceived of as a socially and culturally constructed reality (see among others, Foster & Anderson 1978, Kleinman, 1980, Romanucci-Ross, Moerman et al, 1991 and Hahn 1995). I am not a relativist when it comes to knowledge. I recognize the fact that biomedical knowledge has strong truth claims based on positivism but I am talking much more about social and cultural practices and institutions, in which case, I argue that the opposition against modern health concepts is not based on the capacity of different institutions to adapt and incorporate knowledge of modern medicine and science. Local knowledge and modern science are not antithetical to each other, both can be harnessed together.

While the WHO does recognize the existence of alternative medicines and by implication, local therapeutic knowledge systems, it seems to consistently privilege the Western biomedical health model over local health concepts in its language and policy recommendations (WHO, 1998) thereby relegating to the background alternative health practices and the communities that practice them. Secondly, the WHO's definition homogenizes many different practices by subsuming them under the heading of "circumcision" even when no two societies practice the ritual cuttings alike or for the same reasons. The practices reflect different local nomenclatures and are based on different social and cultural logics, which tend to be erased in the literature under all-encompassing concepts like culture, religion, and aesthetics (Njambi, 2004) thereby negating specificity, breadth and the prospects for historical and processual change.

For the purpose of my study, I concur with Tangwa (1999) that circumcision is "*any surgical intervention on the genitals of a human being for cultural, religious or purely secular and profane reasons*," because this definition takes into account a broader range of realities encompassed by "circumcision". However, the expression "Female Circumcision" (herein henceforth FC) provided a common discursive ground with my informants and I will use it all through this book despite its shortcomings.

In what follows, I examine the geography of FC and current analysis of the ritual procedures, the research questions, the empirical and theoretical justification for selecting the Ejaghams as case study, the theoretical background and contribution and lastly, the rationale and methods used in the data elicitation process.

1.2 Geography of Female Circumcision and Current Analysis

It is estimated that over 130 million girls and women have had their genitalia subjected to some form of modification and another 2 million are circumcised annually in about 40 countries the world over (WHO, 2005, Mbacke et al,1998, Adongo et al, 1998). The real extent of the existence of the practice in most of these countries is not known. However, governmental reports, anecdotal evidence and limited surveys with non-representative samples estimate that prevalence rates range from between 5 to 98 percent. It is now included in DHS in most countries. The practice is reported in 28 African countries concentrated in a band crossing the continent from the Horn of Africa to Senegal and Mauritania on the Atlantic Coast (Effiom, 2001). Cameroon is one of the countries where FC is practiced and the focus of this study.

In Cameroon, FC is practiced in several communities with different cultures and religions. There is neither a legal nor a religious prescription prohibiting or sanctioning FC in Cameroon. It is however, very likely that in case of prosecution, general assault laws will be invoked and applied. WHO (1998) estimates that there is a 100% prevalence rate among Muslims and 63.6% among Christians in practicing societies all over the world. In Cameroon, there exists no publication on the prevalence rate at the national level. However, approximately 20% of females in zones where FC is practiced (the South West, the Extreme North and the Eastern Provinces), have undergone the ritual cutting (Miscouna 1999, C.I.A.F 1994). The practice is rooted in the social, political, cultural and economic structures of the communities that have adopted it. Although there is no one clear justification for it, it is attributed considerable socio-cultural value in these groups (Government of Cameroon, 1998:6), which include the Ejagham community.

Western/Northern research curiosity has tended to focus on the most drastic form of the ritual operations, infibulation in the Sudan (see among others, Hayes 1975, Boddy 1982 and Gruenbaum 1982), and channelling interest mostly toward the Islamic context. Most of these studies have ended up with the use of a functionalist analytical framework. "Islam" is then used as the unit of analysis, thereby subsuming the practice under the dogmatic aspects of religion. "Islam", in fact, is a symbolic and relational power field and therefore highly dynamic over time. Arnold Van Gennep (1960) was one of the earliest front-liners to interpret rituals in psycho-analytical terms as meant essentially for the fulfilment of psychological needs, the desires and impulses of individual actors: "to modify the personality of the individual in a manner visible to all" (Ibid,1960:71). Although he brought important insights to the analysis of rituals, particularly his tripolar theory of nothingness, liminality and aggregation, he however de-emphasized the corporal and historical aspects of ritual practices, framing it merely as an instrumental process and therefore not subjected to social change. Along the same theoretical path, Goldman (1997) analyses the relationship between circumcision trauma and life course occurrences and the skyrocketing divorce rate in the USA and suggests that circumcision is undertaken as a mechanism for the transmission of gender identity, in which case a child is circumcised so that s/he might identify with the genital status of his or her parents. However, he does not contextualize the cultural meaning of pain, as is the case with the human rights oriented studies.

Socio-structural and symbolic interpretations only provide insights into FC at a particular moment in time, suggesting an overemphasis on the present, on confined groups and on presumed cultural consensus rather than on contestation and change over time. In the present research, I go beyond this by exploring transformations over time and look at the situated agency of individuals and groups alike.

Contrary to the studies cited above, I believe that a historically based account might provide alternative understanding about the ritual practice and the institution of Moninkim. One of the aims of this book is to identify and analyze some available pathways for internal institutional change through an analysis of different positions in a complex, contested debate involving local, national, regional and international actors occupying different and shifting power fields. This is possible as evidenced by the recent waiving of the obligation of circumcision for some members of the Moninkim cult (see above).

I will therefore further expose the various relationships among the different stakeholders involved in either the contestation or change of the ritual procedures. Such a historical, processual analysis will contribute to the critical feminist scholarship on FC and to the theory of critical anthropology of health in Cameroon in particular and the Central African region at large.

In contrast to the usual policy-led or demographic approaches to issues of circumcision, culture and health (see among others, Althus, 1997 and Larsen et al. 2000), my work is grounded in historical processual analysis and local level ethnography. Based on a nine month's extended case study of the Ejaghams of Southwest Cameroon, my study highlights contestation and resistance about FC among local inhabitants with diverse and shifting attitudes. This reflects the notion of culture as a constantly contested and renegotiated field of practice and praxis among internal cultural stakeholders and between them and outside activists, occupying different interconnected power fields: governmental agencies and NGOs both at the local, national, regional and international scales. My argument is that culture is not a universe of consensual meanings and practices but rather, a contested field of meanings, practices and power (see among others, Wolf, 2001, Gupta & Ferguson, 2001, Appadurai, 2004). Stated otherwise, there are stark disagreements about FC and modern medicine, tradition and culture on the one hand and modernity, local and scientific knowledge on the other. In the face of the ensuing ferocious confrontation between these two centrifugal forces: Western rational science and African cultural practices, scientific modernity and local cultural practices, my message is contextual dialogue, the need for modernization with and not against the people, dialogue among and between local societies and global organized NGOs.

My point of entry into this debate is the search for openings that allow for an alliance of local cultural practices/processes and modern medicine to emerge through the dialogic balancing of local and international interests. In other words, modernization should not be the imposition of another power or "the sublimation of traditional culture into a global way of thinking" (Wissner, 1988:51). Gausset (2001) has demonstrated that the eradication of the exotic aspects of African systems of sexuality and kinship (polygamy, wife sharing/exchange, adultery, dry sex and sexual cleansing among others) are not antithetical to the fight against AIDS in Africa. These practices are constantly changing so as to avoid spreading the HIV. Along the same lines, Green (1999) argues that the suppression of indigenous health beliefs and practices (polygyny, bride payments, initiation rites) as anti-HIV/AIDS and other sexually transmissible disease strategies instead backfired and the practices went underground in Mozambique. Both scholars articulate a fluid and dynamic view of culture and the need to identify and graft local concepts with their biomedical parallels in change initiatives and not imposition. This approach showed first that *siki* (syphilis, gonorrhoea and chancroid) for instance, had a correlationship with the "germ" medical model of sexually transmissible diseases (STDs). Secondly, healers' prevention of sexually transmissible infections (STI) was biomedically sound: avoiding adultery, and intercourse with 'strangers', avoiding intercourse during menstruation, refraining from intercourse and alcohol consumption until *siki* was cured, healers locating and treating recent sexual partners of patients. Other parallels include the recognition that STIs can infect newborn infants and that STI symptoms can become latent, and the fact that untreated STDs can lead to infertility. Stated otherwise, local medical systems, local knowledge systems are not incompatible with biomedicine, with scientific knowledge.

It is my view that if health education is to succeed, it must be with the local people in mind, rather than against them. Stated otherwise, there is the need for a more fluid and dynamic notion of culture, one that focuses on disagreements, contradictions among people, but not on local and parochial consensus. In calling for an ethnography beyond ''cultures'', for instance, Gupta and Ferguson (2001:3) characterize culture as 'polyphonic', not 'monophonic' because it is more fragmented than bounded and there are a multiplicity of voices within every given culture. Knowledge is simultaneously local and global (Moore 1996) meaning that both the so-called indigenous and scientific knowledges appropriate and refine each other and are therefore not incompatible. There is the need to search for compromise that will bridge local and modern knowledge. Knowledge is never exclusively local. It interacts with science and the practices of development and is the outcome of complex negotiation practices linked to knowledge interfaces (Pottier, 2003:5), and the production of knowledge is embedded in social and cultural processes, power, authority, legitimacy, social struggle, conflict and negotiation (see among others Scoones and Thompson, 1994, Sillitoe, 2002, Pottier, 2003 and Kalb, 2006). As global rational knowledge confronts local cultures, there is permanent syncretism and a dynamic debate depending on actor's position and resources and the power field they are occupying. Modernity remains a negotiated process. Local institutions, habits, relationships can be appropriated by the process and project of modernity and the overall outcome might be democratic. My aim is to bring some inputs to this debate by contributing to the critical brand of studies on FC that has increasingly put into question the validity and pertinence of official discourses and policies about this ritual practice. In the next section, I state the puzzle that this study seeks to resolve.

1.3 Research questions

Excision is presumed from the standpoint of biomedicine to lead to medical complications that can range from haemorrhage and infection with HIV/AIDS to shock and death. Despite these severe consequences and campaigns by governments, national NGOs and transnational organizations alike to eradicate the practice, excision persists in Cameroon and is taking place among increasingly younger girls. Indigenous societies all over the world have their reproductive health practices. From an emic perspective, they hold that these practices enhance health, even though in biomedicine, they are termed “harmful traditional practices”. This expression announces the international health agenda that recommends the eradication of such practices, rather than modification. It further suggests that local cultural practices are obstacles to change.

To complicate matters and give FC practicing communities only one option, eradication, the WHO (1998) warns health professionals against medicalization of the procedures because it might lead to the perpetuation of “this heinous practice”. The dominant view among many biomedical advocates conceives of ‘culture as a barrier’ and presumes that culture is unchanging and homogeneous. As Gausset (2001) shows, these views have marred the campaign against HIV/AIDS as drug addicts, gays and lesbians in Europe are being told to use clean syringes, needles and condoms whereas Africans are being told to eradicate whole cultural institutions such as widow inheritance, polygyny, wife exchange among other practices. Following Gausset’s (2001) suggestion, I suggest that the aim should be to make behaviour and practices safer rather than launching an all-out attack on local cultures and local societies. Women’s health advocates, pressure groups, national governments, common initiative groups have been educating and raising awareness on the negative health consequences of FC, whereas some segments of local communities have continued to argue that their practices enhance health and uphold sexual morality particularly in this era of HIV/AIDS and are therefore functional. Voices have been raised for and against this practice both within these societies and beyond, thereby making this local cultural practice a global issue. My contribution to this debate will consist in analyzing, through empirical and historical research, the paths that have led to or may lead to internal institutional change.

One fact supporting the view that internal socio-cultural change is actually happening is the history of the Moninkim cult among the Ejaghams. Female circumcision used to be a prerequisite for membership but has partly transformed today into the symbolic type of circumcision called “social Moninkims”. Some individuals (mostly wealthy and powerful women, but also skilful uncircumcised dancers) have acquired membership without undergoing the actual physical ritual procedures.

A central question for me is thus the following: how to explain the changing rules of membership into this dancing and female socialization institution over time. What explains the fact that the obligation of circumcision was waived for some and not others? What explains the simultaneous persistence of the ritual procedure in these other cases? This research will accordingly inquire into the changes in this female institution and in the practice of FC over time, the forces contributing to the present state of acceptance and practice. It will particularly focus on why particular individuals and groups are advocating the maintenance of the *status quo* or the eradication of the ritual procedures. How are actors renegotiating the practice of FC in the face of inter-cultural contact, cultural change and social transformations? In other words, how is this renegotiation process affected by local, national, regional, and international power relations?

By empirically comparing and contrasting the trajectories of different clans with particular focus on the Ekwe, among whom change has been most radical, can operationalize this question. Why the continuous resilience of the ritual practice of FC when circumcision is no longer the criterion for membership into the Moninkim society among the Ekwe?

Secondary empirical questions deriving from this main problem include the following:

1) What changes have taken place in the institution of Moninkim and FC over time, where and why?
2) What factors are contributing to the present state of acceptance and contestations of FC by particular individuals and groups among the Ejaghams?
3) How do various people and groups within Ejagham society renegotiate the ritual practice of FC when confronted with cultural difference and opposition?
4) What alliances have the people been drawn into at the local, national, regional, and international contexts given the multiplicity of actors at various scales and how are these alliances/forces shaping both the present state of acceptance and contestations of the ritual practice of FC?

1.4 Empirical case and theoretical justification

My choice of the Ejaghams as an empirical case study is dictated by theoretical concerns and the people's historic connections with outside groups by virtue of their strategic location within a "culture contact zone" (Bizzell, 1997) with multiple actors. The Ejagham people are today found astride the Cameroon-Nigeria border region having been divided, like other African ethnic groups between these two countries during the colonial partition of the 19th century. My focus is however on those in Southwest Cameroon, more specifically, those in Eyumojock Sub Division. Historically, the area has been characterized by multiple flows. This exposes the people to mobile actors such as traders, border guards, the Cameroonian and Nigerian military, the police and the gendarmes, reputed high risk groups with regards to HIV/AIDS transmission. Their peri-urban location further exposes the Ejaghams to powerful actors who are at work at various scales in the fight against FC and HIV/AIDS-despite the poor road network in the entire region. These stakeholders include the Cameroonian state and a dense network of local, national, regional and international NGOs. At the same time, there are divergent views among the Ejaghams themselves (see chapter five). Larger processes of economic change at the global scale have led to deep social transformations at the local level. This has generated fierce intergenerational conflicts as well as heightened concern over the commodification of female sexuality.

The Ejaghams of Southwest Cameroon are made up of three clans—Ekwe, Obang and Keakas. Three reasons make the Ekwe, Ejaghams a fascinating anthropological case study. The first is the fact that they are the most 'urbanized' among the three clans and therefore provide a point of convergence for the confrontation between western science and local cultures. Their crossroad 'peri-urban' location exposes them to multiple actors. This particular characteristic of the area equally impacts on the spatial geography of intervention against FC and fuels the spread of the AIDS virus as people are always passing into and out of the region, spreading both new ideas and diseases in the process. Secondly, although in the present context political developments have been kept constant, FC practices are continuing. Even more interesting is the diversity and functions of the forms of this violent ritual practice among the three clans, a diversity of functions that provides for a comparative case study and the generation of different sets of data.

Until the 1980s, the circumcision ritual as practiced among the Ejaghams produced four distinct categories of "initiates" (circumcised women). One group of initiates, predominantly found among the Ekwe and Obang clans, underwent the ritual initiation at birth or at puberty. Another type of circumcisions, practiced in the three clans, was and still is believed to be a cure against infertility. A third category of circumcisions practiced by the Keaka and the Ekwe is the first part of a status-granting ritual that includes a period of confinement and a graduation ceremony formally conferring membership into the Moninkim cult. The fourth and last category is, as in three, a step in the process of accession of some women to the title of Moninkim, but it is essentially a symbolic representation of ritual circumcision without actual physical mutilation: mere confinement and fattening are substituted for the cutting.

Actors variously call this practice "social Moninkim", "modern Moninkim" to differentiate it from the previous type. It is practiced on women whose high socio-economic status enabled them to buy their title and membership into the Moninkim cult, or who were included in the group because of their ability to dance the "Nkim" dance. "Social Moninkims" were traditionally granted only among the Obang but they have progressively diffused today among the Ekwe and the Keaka—a result, I argue, of the ageing of the previous generation of initiates, of formal education, but also, most importantly, of a broader process of social change that followed anti-HIV/AIDS campaigns.

Until the late 1980s, FC, accompanied by confinement, fattening and the outdooring ceremony was a precondition for becoming a Moninkim. As the central ritual of patriarchy, it conferred on its initiates and their husbands and other close associates, social prominence and pride. This women's oriented institution charged with feminine personhood has now become commercialized into a dancing group and a spectacle. The uninitiated, variously called 'Social Moninkims', 'modern Moninkims' have joined the group over time performing both within and beyond the village locale for money.

As part of an institutionalized patriarchal complex, this female institution is intertwined with male institutions such as Ekpe (Ngbe), also called the Leopard society and entangled with the Ejagham political economy of sexuality. Ekpe provided protection to the initiate during her confinement in return for jugs of palm wine marking both her entry and exit from the fattening house system (RÖschenthaler,1998:40) where intensive indoctrination and tutoring in secret gendered knowledge had taken place. During seclusion, elderly Moninkim women schooled the initiate(s) in gendered feminine knowledge, in the secrets of man-woman relationships and taught her dancing skills in preparation for her outdooring ceremony in front of the Ekpe hall for her publicly certified role of entertainer in society. Members of the NKanda, a junior grade of Ekpe performed the opening of the dancing floor while the Ngbe 'roared' in the background. Her caretakers received presents from every visitor before granting access while Moninkim entertained her visitors by performing dances under their supervision. On graduation day, she received a staff of authority certifying that she had been transformed and her needs as an individual suppressed in favour of the needs, survival and continuity of her kinship group and community. The economics of confinement reflect the thrift and loan aspect of ritual FC- one bone of contention in the debate.

A conglomerate of factors has led to the dynamism of the Moninkim cult and the institution of FC over time. These factors include but are not limited to- the advent of formal educational institutions, the ageing of the initial initiates and the need to replace them with agile and energetic dancers- but more importantly, a wider process of social and cultural change resulting from intercultural contact. One key factor for change is the advent of the HIV/AIDS pandemic with its accompanying moral and sexual panic which orchestrated endless emotional debates between partisans and opponents of ritual FC. I argue that the persistence of the Moninkim cult and FC over time can only be understood within the larger context of the complex social, economic, power and authority structure of patriarchal Ejagham society. As we saw above, Moninkim was conferred with the staff of authority by Ekpe certifying her ritual power but above all, old Moninkims became privileged, honorary members of Ngbe, an exclusively male society. This shows the fluidity, dynamics and relational nature of gender and gender relations in African societies. As a social construct, gender regulates daily social life between the sexes and between culturally defined norms of femininity and masculinity while age mediates gender, making relationships more dynamic and fluid over time. Patriarchy as a power field should therefore be conceptualized as fluid and dynamic, offering spaces for both individual and collective agency, permitting while simultaneously disallowing certain behavioural patterns.

The three Ejagham clans thus show different patterns and historical trajectories, the investigation of which, in the context of the HIV/AIDS pandemic, promises to deliver illuminating insights. The spread of HIV/AIDS sparked off and reinvigorated intense debates between pro- and anti-female circumcision advocates. Partisans of circumcision argued for increased control over women's bodies and their sexuality as a useful 'native' therapeutic model with which to confront the pandemic. Opponents pointed to the dangers and harmful health effects of 'female ritual mutilation'. Women's bodies, together with their children's and their own welfare, became a battlefield for these conflicting partisan debates in which the contestation of, and change in, the ritual procedures is at play. They are literally under fires from many directions: they are caught up between two contradictory modernities and multiple actors with different, often conflicting agendas. In the Cameroonian context, in which no particular law criminalizes 'female circumcision', the state leaves it up to national and international NGOs to frame the terms of the debate, while various actors of local civil society, confronted with intercultural contact, changing practices and the threats of the HIV/AIDS pandemic, negotiate changes. Analysis of my data shows the coexistence of mute or vacillating voices, 'hard-liner' and 'soft-liner' attitudes towards change—a balance of forces which I assess more precisely in chapter six of this study by suggesting the pathways for institutional change.

In fact, two main conflicting hegemonies (and modernities) are competing to frame the issue of FC in Cameroon. On the one hand, the state, in alliance with NGOs and the international community, is calling for the eradication of this 'violent ritual' because of its harmful health effects. On the other, some members of the community defend a version of "traditional modernity" by articulating a static, a historical notion of tradition to justify the continuation of the *status quo*. The argument of the latter is that customary rule provides a moral check on women's sexuality and can be an effective "native" tool with which to stem the tides of the AIDS scourge. Previous research thus suggests that anti-female circumcision advocacy (see among others, Hosken, 1979, and Gruenbaum, 2000), as it is currently framed, is a double-edged sword that tends to generate strong resistance to change. Whatever the arguments and counter-arguments of the various camps, what is at stake remains patriarchal control over women's bodies, their sexuality and the compromise of their welfare.

Since the late 1980s, NGOs in the Ejagham region have been training "Traditional Birth Attendants" (TBAs) and circumcisers through workshops. They also actively lobby local communities, opinion and political party leaders, both at the local and national level, focusing their efforts on legal arrangements. All these actors are therefore involved in either the maintenance or change of the procedures and regulations. It is partly the impact of the different relationships and alliances between these actors and groups that I document and theorise in my research of the Ekwe (with an extension to the two other Ejagham clans). What degree of agency do women hold as a group or as individuals in these conditions, and what are the prospects for both cultural and institutional change over time? My analysis reveals that NGO efforts have instead led to a backlash over the past twenty years. The ties of these organizations with international finance capital, together with the universalizing health concepts they promote lead them to be perceived as agents of a form of neo-colonialism, thus reinforcing the position of circumcision advocates. Furthermore, the grassroots activists are disunited; their campaigns are fragmented and sporadic owing to the limited budgets on which they operate and to the alarming state of roads between their urban headquarters and areas of intervention. They are therefore active only on a seasonal basis.

The Ejagham people's "culture contact zone"(Bizzell,1997) location places them within a multitude of interconnected power fields with powerful ambivalent actors. There is, first and foremost, the local- global nexus in which the state alongside national, regional and international NGOs is in alliance against the ritual cutting of women's genitals. Secondly, there is wide division among the people themselves. Some segments of the population are subscribing to the alliance between the state and its allies (modernity) while others are against, yet others are in a limbo when faced with the HIV/AIDS threat. This group of loose actors maintains a somewhat "double discourse" as tradition is at times contested in response to modern pressures and at other times, modernity is appropriated. Outcomes therefore shift in response to power fields through time. Patriarchy should be seen here not as an abstract concept but rather, as a specifically structured field of power. It locates power within the household in fathers and at the local community level in men though not so much in men as a group because there are inequalities even among men themselves. But even within patriarchy, women create some space for their own agency through "strategic and structural power" within the "several operating units" (Adams, 1966, 1975, quoted in Wolf, 2001) given the multiple capillaries and ways of subverting power through resistance. Structural power following Wolf (2001) shapes the social field of action. It is political and takes clout to set up, maintain and defend, and wielding this clout is a target for competition among actors, alliance building, resistance or accommodation to the practice of FC. In this light, structural power includes cultural processes that demand attention for competition, alliance building, resistance and accommodation. It encourages particular types of behaviour while discouraging others, and allocating different quantities and sorts of resources to some and not to others. It is this particularly fluid and contestation-oriented vision of culture that I want to apply to the study of FC. To reiterate, my study sets a power and contestation driven concept against a consensual and traditionalist (functionalist-glue) concept of culture. The power-laden field in which the Ejaghams formulate their responses to contestation of anti-FC campaigns is even more complicated than suggested so far because it still needs to be situated in local context. In other words, there is the need to situate resistance from below.

The interplay between various segments of the local population with national, regional, international NGOs and the state must be understood in this light with regards to the contestation and acceptance of the ritual cuttings. This brings me on to methodological contingency and to cultural relativism given that identifiable fields of social power include the local-global network of transnational actors, regional and national state(s) and the Moninkim society. This calls for an analysis of local power fields and structures surrounding responses to external incentives. As a result of the local-global power fields, which get shaped through responses, people have stakes in the Moninkim, a marker of Ejagham women's ethnic identity which has become an ambivalent platform for both modernity and tradition, manifested through resistance or contestation of FC. The power-laden field of contestation in which the Ejaghams formulate their various responses to anti-FC campaigns is even more complicated as reflected by the 'double discourse' phenomenon that they maintain with themselves and with outsiders. This shows the 'polyphonic' as opposed to a 'monophonic', unitary, unilineal notion of culture and the existence of multiple versions of modernity. Interaction between various loose segments of the population and outside activists has thus set several complex processes in motion and the very complexity of power fields creates contestation and dynamism, a process, which is worthy of ethnographic exploration given the situational properties of the region.

Some of the important situational properties of the Ejagham region include its crossroad location, constant migration into and out of the region, the implantation of plantation agriculture and the diffusion of Nigerian film contents (properties which have integrated the Ejaghams into a Nigerian public sphere characterized by money, crime and sex). The people's strategic historical location made them middlemen in the transatlantic slave trade economy between the Cameroon hinterlands, the coast and Nigeria. The area has always remained an important crossroad junction and trade outpost between Cameroon and Nigeria and the West and Central African regions. The area is characterized by multiple flows. There is a lot of traffic coming into and going out of the region. Such crossroads areas, as studies demonstrate, have a high incidence of AIDS. The principal mobile actors are traders, military officers and truckers, all of whom are generally reputed as carrying high incidences of HIV and other sexually transmissible diseases (STDs). Considerable evidence suggests (Orubuloye et al 1994:87, Tierney 1990) that in Africa such border regions present their contiguous countries with huge risks of further HIV transmission even while most of the interior regions remain uninfected. Drivers as a high risk group for instance, are relatively well-off despite their meager salaries. They often take other goods for direct payment on their way and truck driving attracts adventurous men who are more likely than others to take risks and to hire prostitutes. Various studies have concluded that the military and police forces too are high risk groups (National Intelligence Council 2002, Garrett 2005), partly due to the mobile nature of their jobs. A comparison of Cameroon's civil and military infection rates for 1993 showed that the infection rate was 6.2% for soldiers versus 2% of the general population (Civil Military Alliance Newsletter 1996:2). A Nigerian military survey showed that the rate of HIV infection among soldiers based near their wives and homes mirrors that of society- about 5%, while rates among those deployed elsewhere on peacekeeping operations in Africa are up to three times higher. Forty-three percent of the surge in military mortality in Nigeria is ascribed to HIV (Garrett 2005).

Apart from constant mobility into and out of the area, the establishment of plantation agriculture in the coast led to an influx of people, "strangers", the monetization of the economy, urbanization, deep social transformations and changes in values. Patriarchy waged war because the advent of plantation agriculture led to additional income opportunities which initially expanded but later relaxed its scope over the younger generation. On the one hand, parents tried to lay hands on the income of their children because of kinship networks. At the same time, the rise of plantation agriculture relaxed patriarchy and increased the price for patriarchy as it created generational conflicts. The recent depression of the plantation has subsequently led to the relaxation of or to tensions within patriarchy because of migration to the city and unemployment. The unemployed are a proletariat that cannot be easily integrated into the patriarchal network. The depressive phase of plantation agriculture has created tensions within patriarchy as the youths are contesting patriarchal authority and making choices for themselves. Tensions have increased within households and there has been the dispossession of children within patriarchal networks, the urbanization of unemployment and underemployment. The younger generations have as a result been exposed to high mobility and prostitution.

Some of the consequences of the ensuing social dislocation include changes in the people's traditional economy and value system as elders are increasingly finding their authority like tradition, the very source of this authority, contested and challenged by the younger generation. On the one hand, elders no longer have control over the land as their ancestors did, neither can they command the labour of the younger generation. On the other, members of the younger generation are increasingly migrating to urban areas where anonymity is the rule and where they are out of the purview of elders and patriarchy. My argument here is that plantation agriculture as a form of modernity led to collapse as it afforded young men and women an opportunity to escape from the authority and control of their elders. I develop this argument in chapter three of this work.

There is a whole series of profound conflicts going on between the elderly and the younger generation over money, consumption and female sexuality. In the face of these generational conflicts, there is a sharp decline in the prestige of elders whose role of cultural custodians is now under contestation. Multiple crashes and shifts in the world's economy and in the economy of the region, and its negative impact on the youths in general and women in particular have been further bad news for the elders. Various contractions on the cash crop economy at the global scale for instance, have led to a deep social crisis between the countryside and the city and between tradition and modernity. This rural-urban migration has given rise to the weakening of control over youths and women and to the subsequent commodification of female bodies. At the same time, the value of agricultural land is on the decline and the prestige of parents that depended on agric labour too is waning. On the one hand, they are unable either to command the labour of the youths nor to compete with them and other mobile actors such as traders who are constantly moving through the region. On the other, the elders are unable to stop the youths from watching Nigerian movies whose central themes are love, sex and crime. Stated otherwise, the economic, cultural and symbolic values of older society that dictated blind obedience from the youths are being contested and are fast declining alongside the prestige of elders who are unable to compete in the new socio-economic dispensation because they lack the requisite social capital.

The various situated historical and material processes mentioned above all impinge on patriarchy and there are on-going conflicts and renegotiation of a generational nature. The Ejagham people's crossroads location suggest a focus on female sexuality, patriarchal concern and focus on FC as a less explicit way to control female sexuality and gender. I discuss the theoretical background and contribution and then the rationale and scope of this study below.

1.5 Theoretical background and contribution

My focus in this study is on an important contemporary socio-cultural and health issue: the heightened debate around FC in Cameroon in the context of the HIV/AIDS pandemic and the global anti-AIDS interventions. These interventions are often based on the notion of culture as static, on local cultural practices as unchanging "risk factors", on culture as an obstacle to change, on the blaming and demonization of culture, on the view that the 'traditional man' is a prisoner of culture, on local communities as *tabula rasas*, on "the fallacy of the empty vessel" and on the view that so-called "traditional societies" are static. Appadurai (2004) has rightly pointed out that culture remains a warehouse for embedding and nurturing future and past ideas and that culture should be seen as a source of hope, as a resource for development, not as an obstacle to progress. In fact, local people have the capacity to aspire and to take risks through experimentation. In this light, Douglas (2004) disparages the idea that 'traditional culture' is an obstacle to development and instead attributes the failure of development projects in most parts of the world to people's unwillingness to take risks and to a culture of apathy induced by helplessness.

I argue that the problems of rural development do not reside in the 'traditional cultures' of underdeveloped people, they are rather the bases of any effective development (Pottier et al. 2003). There is the need for what Marsden has eloquently described as 'a negotiated situation-specific approach' (1990:267) through a dialogic model that combines western scientific rationality and local knowledge, that conceptualizes 'development as a set of practices and relationships'(Pottier et al. 2003:10). The two knowledge systems, I argue, are not incommensurate with each other. Rather, they can be harnessed, incorporated and appropriated by change agents because by its very nature culture is dynamic, marked by contestation and constant renegotiation over time. Traditional ideas and practices are not necessarily obstacles to progress, neither are local people ignoramuses. This calls for accommodation, the necessity to avoid the pitfalls of intellectual and material hegemony and to engage in an 'actor-oriented approach', not one that privileges only western 'scientific rationality' but one that harnesses and incorporates both local and global knowledges and gives 'voice' to 'beneficiaries'. Ironically, change initiatives based on dominant perceptions, on the notion of culture as cast in stone, on local knowledge as 'irrational', as superstition, are critical of so-called local 'harmful traditional practices' such as FC even when these practices are being constantly rethought and modified by cultural stakeholders in function of their preoccupations and through interaction with other knowledge systems and societies.

There are two competing visions of culture among scholars. The first takes culture as an obstacle to change whereas the second conceives culture as dynamic, fluid and open to change. I adopt an integrated, relational power-based vision of culture which sees social and cultural institutions as dynamic, paving the way for the integration of local people into development as dialogic partners. I do not subscribe to an either/or position but to one that integrates the dynamism of local and global knowledge systems. This vision sees culture as a potential and necessary resource for development, as subjected to change in the light of the changing and shifting preoccupations of stakeholders, as a contested and constantly renegotiated process and power field. In the wake of the HIV/AIDS policy debate, the obligation of circumcision was recently waived for some members of the Ejagham (Moninkim cult, see above). This fact suggests that radical social change does happen within so-called traditional practices. How do the Ejaghams as a group, negotiate the ritual practice of FC in the face of external criticisms? And how do powerful groups among the Ejaghams, negotiate contestation or resistance from within? In order to identify the combination of local, national, regional, and international forces that provided a pathway for change in the practice of the ritual cuttings, I analyze the various forms of interaction between participants involved in either the maintenance or the change of the procedures of FC. Such an institutional, process-oriented account provides a new, alternative understanding of the ritual practice and institution of Moninkim, one that integrates the contributions of the socio-historical scholarship of post-colonial contexts, but also those of critical feminist scholarship.

While I seek to account for women's agency, I remain deeply aware that agency is structured (Giddens 1982, Sewell 1992) by systematic inequalities and social power. My research is inspired by theories of patriarchy (Learner 1986, Walby 1990, Paterman 1991, Nkiru 2002), governmentality (Foucault 1979, Rose, Rose and Miller, 1992) and/or hegemony (Gramsci,1971, Guha,1999), the analyses of critical medical anthropology (CMA) (Baer 1982, Singer 1986, Morgan, 1987) and of the anthropology of the body (Foucault 1979, Foucault 1991, Barkty 1990, Wolf 1991, Turner 1992) which emphasize in different but complementary ways the impact of multiple fields of power (Wolf, 2001). The critical medical anthropology (CMA) approach captures particularly well the impact of power on health and cultural issues (Singer 1986), usefully suggesting that the contestation and defence of 'female genital cuttings' turns women's bodies into a site of struggle between two hegemonic representations: "modernity" on the one hand, represented by the Cameroonian state and its "ideological state apparatuses" (Althusser, 1971) of schools and NGOs, and "tradition" on the other, represented by dominant segments of the local population. I have chosen to use the expressions "soft-liners", "hard-liners", "double discourse", and "group think phenomena" to describe the various shifting positions among the people. Although everyday resistance is the main characteristic of these loose groups, its members vary in terms of class, gender and status. They are those challenging the Cameroonian state's "monopoly of symbolic violence" (Bourdieu, 1992) and its governmental power.

These combined frames are further instrumental in identifying the various alliances, programmatic approaches and concepts used by actors at different scales in the process of discussing the practice, contesting or resisting changes to the ritual bodily cuttings. They will further permit me to combine thick local ethnography of deep generational conflicts and disagreements with an analysis of the global health field and its local NGO initiatives, generalized risk represented by HIV/AIDS and global medicine. In the following sections, I state the rationale, ethics governing the data elicitation process, problems encountered in the field and scope of my study.

1.6 Rationale

My contribution to the global anti-HIV/AIDS and anti-FC debate is that global insights and the activities of NGOs can find bridging points of contact through the local point of view, through contextualism. Culture is not static but rather contested, renegotiated. The focus is on disagreements, contradictions among people as stakeholders, not local parochial consensus or a unilineal point of view. Global rational knowledge confronts local cultures and there is a dynamic debate and dialogue. Local knowledge, culture as tradition argument is not part of the problem as postulated by the modernization approach. There can be a fruitful synergy between local and global rationalities. I therefore propose a dynamic notion of culture, one in which contestation is embedded within shifting fields of power.

This study seeks to provide novel understanding about the fight against FC in an era of AIDS, and transformations in the institution of Moninkim over time among the Ejaghams. One of the aims is to identify the prospects for internal institutional change and the agency of women and for the prospects for dialogue between local and scientific knowledge. To achieve these aims, I adopt a power-driven vision of culture as a process of constant contestation and renegotiation among stakeholders.

This extended case study of the dynamics of the Moninkim cult and FC in an era of HIV/AIDS among the Ejaghams was undertaken during nine months of fieldwork between February and October, 2006. I had made initial contacts with key stakeholders through conference participation and work in the study area as far back as 2001. I selected the Ekwe, Ejaghams because of the 'gatekeeper's' willingness to take part in the study and easy access unlike Northern Cameroon where FC is also practiced but where the language of communication is fufulde. The fact that most of the people speak both the English language and pidgin English greatly facilitated communication. To achieve the aims of this study, I combined various qualitative data gathering techniques: individual in-depth interviews, focus group discussion sessions, informal interviews, case studies and case histories, passive and active participant observation. Through these combined methods, I successfully and voluntarily elicited data from a total of 273 individuals in various Ejagham villages. I also inspected relevant documents on the status and well-being of women and children with specific relevance to the objectives of my study.

In consonance with standard social science practice, the concept of voluntarily informed consent is at the very centre of this study. Despite my initial rapport and familiarity with the stakeholders and the community, certain problems that served as ethnographic 'eye openers' still cropped up. The first of these problems was my identity as an international student. By virtue of this, I was often seen as conspiring with the anti-FC camp (the Western world) and as having been given money with which to buy information about FC. To aggravate matters, local NGOs who most often rely on foreign funding usually provide food and drinks as a mechanism to lure people to come out in great numbers and take part in their campaigns thereby providing them with graphic pictures with which to attract more funding. Through this strategy, they have come to monetize FC and partly, to reduce it to the fight against poverty as conditionality (whereas, it is a polythetic cultural category). At the same time, everything about FC in these communities is about money. Since it is common knowledge that these NGOs are funded by the 'Whiteman' and I am his friend, therefore I am also funded by the same 'Whiteman' and should generously share the money I have been given as an agent of neo-colonialism, like these NGOs. Apart from pointing out that Hungary where I am schooling is at the periphery of the world's economy, I sometimes had to maintain a juggled identity and present myself merely as a 'student'. This worked in most instances because university students have been coming and going. But in other instances, they accused me that like other researchers, I will finish my fieldwork and go forever while they will remain poor. I constantly had to plead that I will not behave in the same way. My most important strategy to counter the problems generated by my returned immigrant status was my 'failure' to behave as all other returned immigrants- who usually dress lavishly and indulge in ostentatious consumption- (signs of coming from the West in the local imagination), by- dressing moderately, hanging out and sharing palm wine with whoever was willing indiscriminate of age and status. The second obstacle was the great distance separating various villages within the study area. This has impacted seriously on the spatial geography of the anti-FC and HIV/AIDS campaigns. With poor access, NGOs conduct sensitization only seasonally, hardly going into the hinterlands where there are still strong sentiments in favour of the ritual procedures of FC. For me, this entailed trekking for several hours, a situation that attracted both sympathy and collaboration from participants in the hinterland villages who were glad that I had come to hear their own side of the story on FC.

Despite the above-mentioned obstacles, tape-recorded interviews were transcribed as soon as possible and usually within 48 hours. I simultaneously kept extensive field notes. Qualitative data analysis involved both individual and cross case analysis which generated comparative data.

Having pointed out that the existing literature is unable to account for social and cultural change and that it negates the agency of women as an important group of actors, I discuss the methodology that I used to generate the data to fill this research gap through a historical processual analysis of the ritual practice of FC and of the pattern of interactions among stakeholders at various scales in the Ejagham communities of Southwest Cameroon in the next section.

1.7 Research Methodology

In this section, I will set out the main features of my research strategy, the study design adopted, sampling procedures, data gathering instruments and procedures, access into research settings, ethical issues raised by the study and data analysis techniques used to investigate the anti-FC and anti-HIV/AIDS fight among Ejagham clans in Southwest Cameroon and the interaction of various stakeholders involved in either change or contestation of the ritual procedures of FC. I take on relevant issues of practicality, ethics and research politics as they crop up. I will however start with a critical overview of the paradigm informing the study.

The main research question under investigation is exploratory and this has determined the choice of a qualitative research method. This will permit access to changes in the Moninkim cult over time and its impact on the persistence of FC. It will accordingly, give a feel of the natural environment and the socio-cultural realities ('ecological validity') (Vulliamy et al (1990:12, see also Tangie, 2004) of the setting under investigation. I strongly believe that it is only through the researcher's presence in the natural setting and direct contact with respondents that information about people's 'lived experiences' and realities can be fully elicited. Although I have adopted a qualitative research strategy, I nevertheless include tables and statistics wherever necessary to summarize my findings in keeping with the method of statistical documentation as postulated by Malinowski (1922). However, to implement this ethnographic study, I needed access into the research sites.

Initial contacts had been made well in advance through workshops, work and during a pre-field visit. For instance, I met and exchanged views with five excisers at the April 18-20th, 2001 workshop organized by the Yaounde based local chapter of the Inter-African Committee for the Fight Against Harmful Traditional Practices (IAC). I further contacted members of the Ejagham Cultural and Development Association. This organisation brings together elites, influential government officials, Presidents of various associations in the study area and students. I undertook a pre-field visit to the area between 12-19th May 2002. I had equally worked among the people between 1999-2003 as an HIV/AIDS educator for the NGO, Noble Social Group. Through these opportunities for contact, I met gate-keepers and asked questions of them which partly guided the focus of this study and exposed the gulf between local traditional practices such as FC and modern medicine. During these informal meetings, women who had undergone the ritual expressed their willingness to provide important relevant information about it. The thrust of their argument was that the traditional education of the girl child produced better housewives and mothers than the formal education of today. They mentioned that it instilled in them a sense of communal living, societal norms and values through socialization, conjugal roles, and social relationships.

I therefore selected the Ekwe, Ejaghams partly because of the 'gatekeeper's hospitality and expressed willingness to co-operate in the study and its geographic locale. It is within reach (easy access as compared to Northern Cameroon where the language of communication is largely Fufulde). Almost everybody in the area understands and speaks Cameroon Pidgin English and English. This facilitated communication with the respondents. These were the languages of enquiry. Furthermore, the people's peri-urban and strategic location exposes them to multiple flows. As pointed out in chapter one, the Ejaghams are located on the Cameroon-Nigeria border. They were middlemen during the transatlantic slave trade, and the coastal plantations are located around them. Today, they are still on the regional trade route between Cameroon and Nigeria on the one hand and the West and Central African region on the other. This implies that people have always been passing into and out of the region for trade spreading both new ideas and diseases in the process. Mobile actors here include the Cameroonian and Nigerian border guards and police forces. In addition to this, most NGO actors because of the poor and seasonal access road network hardly go into the hinterlands. They are therefore better exposed to the outside world than their co-ethnics in the hinterlands.

I arrived Cameroon from Budapest, Hungary on February 11th 2006 and three days later, I left for Eyumojock in Ejagham land where I set up my fieldwork base but constantly moving from there into the hinterland villages and back, spending weeks talking to people and observing events until October 15th 2006 when I left after a nine month's stay. The success or otherwise of the data generation process partly depends very much on our entry point into the field. It can either facilitate or hamper the research process. Despite my initial contacts with the people partly through elites out of the village, my own former students and previous work experience in the region, I still had to re-enter through the village gatekeepers as my new role demanded and in keeping with anthropological conventions.

Since I was doing an 'extended case study', I was constantly shuttling across various locations within the three Ejagham clans. I did multi-sited ethnography. This implied looking at the phenomenon under investigation as a whole on each occasion and at each location- throwing a large net since I am conscious that cultural elements are bound up with each other. Following Clifford (1997), who has appropriated the concept of 'multilocale' ethnography from Marcus and Fischer (1986), intensive habitation in one village was usually replaced by repeated visitations, since I had to shuttle between various locations where informants were based and where important social events were taking place. Given the discrete nature of the field, the field in my case was wherever I met informants within and beyond the study site. I was involved in a "travel encounter" in Clifford's (1997) words, going and coming, moving forward and backward and talking to people, following up information and events and making note of all these simultaneously.

Below, I explain my research design, sampling procedures in terms of institutions and the selection of participants for the data generation process. Lastly, I discuss the data analysis process and reflexivity respectively.

1.8 Research strategy: the extended case study method

The 'extended case study' method of enquiry implies that the researcher seeks evidence to describe, understand and explain the case(s) under investigation, rather than to test a hypothesis. Also called 'situational analysis' (Gluckman, 1940, Cocks, 2001), "extending out" from the field means looking beyond native claims as to what "natives" are doing and recording what they are actually doing, diarising 'accounts of real events, struggles, and dramas that [take] place over space and time' (Buroway, 1999:5). As Buroway, rightly notes, this approach is capable of highlighting the discrepancies between normative prescriptions and everyday practices- discrepancies that can be traced to internal contradictions 'but also to the intrusion of colonialism'(Buroway,1995:5). This strategy permitted me to move from the "micro" to the "macro" and 'to connect the present to the past' (Buraway, 1999:5). Furthermore, to incorporate the wider context by taking local, national, regional and international politics, economic context and to uphold Dorothy Smith's (1987) feminist injunction to ground lived experience within its extra-local determinations[1] with specific reference to FC among the Ejaghams. This implies taking cognizance of social and economic changes at the national, regional and global scales and their impact on intergenerational relations, on women and their sexuality but above all, on cultural change. Following Wolf (1982), we need to trace the causes of the present in the past since humans construct their culture in interaction with others and not in isolation. Rather than opting for a single case study to answer my research questions, I conducted a multiple case study involving one clan, the Ekwe but extending out to two others (the Keaka and Obang) so as to give more latitude and provide more context for the study while at the same time providing for a much more nuanced approach. By so doing, I am still operating within the same research strategy. Yin (1994:44) notes that 'the difference between single and multiple –case study designs are variants that 'operate within the same case study strategy'.

1.8.1 Research design and sampling

I adopted an 'embedded multiple-case study design' (Yin, 1994:51) involving members of the Moninkim cult who gained membership by undergoing the ritual cutting of FC, those who gained membership without undergoing this ritual cutting, community leaders, health workers, NGOs working in the various research sites, men and women in general so as to explore the various dynamics going on in this society as a result of the

[1] Smith takes issue with abstract, decontextualised, and universalistic sociology as the ideology of ruling men and takes the experience of women as the point of departure. In this case, the microstructures of everyday life, which is under women's control, constitute the foundation and invisible premise for microstructures controlled by men.

HIV/AIDS pandemic and the campaign against FC. I considered it appropriate to contact initiates and non-initiates alike, as well as those fighting against the procedures so as to elicit their attitudes. Travel limitations, time constraints and insufficient funds prevented me from covering the other two clans in detail. However, FC practices among the three clans have changed over time and are essentially the same today probably due to the anti-HIV/AIDS and anti-FC campaigns which have partly given rise to the increasing circumcision of female children at tender ages for fear they will grow up and eventually start contesting circumcision now that "the whiteman has come and told them that circumcision is not good" (Ndifon Abang, interview of 18/06/06). Although findings from multiple-case studies are more compelling as mentioned earlier, it is however appropriate to exhaustively deal with one clan while talking about the others in passing. Following Gomme et al (2000:1) 'other things being equal, the fewer the cases investigated, the more information that can be collected about each one of them'.

The selection of the Ekwe clan was purposive. They are the most 'urbanised' of the three clans and are largely accessible considering the poor state of the roads in most of Cameroon. I had worked among them as an HIV/AIDS educator for the NGO Noble Social Group, and I was therefore familiar with some of the 'gatekeepers' and key informants who had demonstrated their willingness to be part of the study. Purposive sampling, following Burns (2000:465) is useful if it 'serves the real purpose and objectives of the researcher by enabling him to discover, gain insight and understanding into a particular phenomenon'.

However, to a limited extent the selection of the Ekwe clan was based on the 'sampling logic' or 'those that are representative of the total population of similar cases' (Yin, 1994:47). Although many have taken issue with this latter sampling method in case study research on grounds that such research is no more concerned with generalization through representative sampling as with the generation of theoretical insights, (see for example, Yin,1989,1994, Gomme et al, 2000), I believe that an attempt be made in qualitative studies to consider the extent to, and conditions under which findings from a given number of cases studied can resonant on the smaller, if not wider population of cases from which the samples were drawn. In this regard, I opted to work in one clan, the Ekwe, which meets the criteria of familiarity, proximity and willingness. I however extended out to the other two clans, the Keaka and Obangs, where I did a limited case study for purposes of comparison. This is partly because the people's history is intertwined and the same local, national, regional and global processes are affecting the three clans despite differences owing to location: the Ekwes are more exposed given their 'peri-urban' location.

Before allowing my respondents to share their experiences with us, I need to say something with regards to the ethics governing this study, the data analysis process which is the next task after the data gathering process as well as on reflexivity.

1.8.2 Ethical issues in the study

In keeping with standard social science research practice, ethical considerations guided my actions in the implementation of this ethnographic study. An example is the principle of access given the sensitive nature of the topic under discussion. As a former health educator in the community, I had attended conferences and workshops on reproductive health during which I had the good fortune to meet and make contacts with circumcisers, initiates and traditional birth attendants. They agreed to provide relevant inside information to me in strict confidence. My kinship ties to the people (my cousin is married from within this group and I too went ''native'' following my adoption in the course of the ethnographic encounter), knowledge of the local lingua franca, Pidgin English and the English language gave me access that I would not have had if I was a complete stranger in the community.

Respondents were on each occasion before the conduct of an interview or a focus group discussion session informed of their right to freely participate or not to participate. In fact, the concept of voluntary informed consent is at the very centre of research ethics in the social sciences. The subjects of research according to this notion, are entitled to know the nature, purposes and implications of research and to autonomously choose whether to take part in it or not (McNamee and Bridges, 2002, Homan, 2002).In this light, when one woman insisted she would not participate, I allowed her, only for her to later on learn from others what my mission was and to return to me insisting I should interview her, which I did. The principle to respect the terms of negotiations with participants (Reynolds,1982) underpins this research. This basically has to do with issues related to trust, anonymity of persons, places and confidentiality, issues that are of utmost importance in this research initiative.

At each stage in the research, though against the expectations of some informants as some strongly expressed the zeal and enthusiasm to be quoted word verbatim, research participants were given assurance that the information collected will be reported in anonymized form. Finally, disengagement from the research site proved to be difficult especially from some of my key informants because of my prolonged presence in their midst and the intimate relationship we had developed from frequent impromptu visits to their homes. They feared I would be going for good like other researchers who have often come and gone forever. I have since had to keep one foot in the community, partly by calling some people over the phone and through email from time to time and extending greetings to others who cannot be reached, while at the same time, clarifying doubts over some of the issues I recorded during my field stay.

Using the wide array of methods exposed above, data was successfully elicited from a total of 273 voluntary respondents: 190 women and 83 men respectively. Most of the women, 165 were initiates whereas 25 were not. Twenty co-interviews and numerous informal discussion sessions were held with members of the community during which I raised and discussed issues of pertinence to the study. All these constitute the data for this enquiry, but below I describe how this data was analyzed and reported.

1.9 Data analysis and reflexivity

After obtaining the necessary data, the next task is how to analyze them. The information tape-recorded was transcribed as soon as possible in the field and usually within 48 hours. In keeping with my case study strategy, I identify themes, patterns and processes, commonalities and differences. Following Edwards and Talbot (1994:45), such an analysis 'takes us beyond the notion of the case study as illustrative' and allows us to look for 'common themes and patterns to be elicited, hypotheses generated and theory generated'. This was the general framework for analysis although data from specific information sources such as observations, interviews, focus group discussion sessions, documents, etc) were analyzed either qualitatively or quantitatively. Data will then be presented in prose and in frequency tables and interpreted by percentages where and whenever appropriate. I however agree that making sense of lessons learned is shaped by my experiences and background (Lincoln and Guba, 1985, 1994, Miles and Huberman, 1994:9).Generally, analysis was carried out at two levels: 'individual-case' analysis and 'cross case analysis' (Stake,1995). At the former level, I identified patterns, consistencies and differences in what was observed, obtained from subject interviews, focus group discussion sessions with gender and status within the social structure as important variables. In the latter stage, individual cases were compared; similarities and differences of opinion identified and possible explanations were generated.

Conscious that my identity, values and beliefs can bias my interpretations, I allow room for alternative interpretations by allowing the facts to speak for themselves (verbatim quotations). The information obtained from the informants will be reported word verbatim wherever necessary. This, following Clifford (1988), is one way of conferring co-authorship and authorial authority, by allowing the informants to speak through the text, allowing their voices to be heard. In writing up the final research report, I am conscious, as Clifford (1988) rightly notes, that ethnographic texts are multivocal exchanges and that subjectivities are produced in politically charged situations. This implies incorporating dissenting voices into the piece because culture remains a contested domain since respondents are multiply located within their own culture and unanimity is always difficult to reach. Culture, following Caglar (1997) among others, is not a homogenous and bounded entity, neither is anthropology the study of "the little community" as was the case in the past. I do not presume the existence of an *apriori* spatialised community nor do I naturalise this community in keeping with Caglar's (1997) cautious note. The people of course find themselves within multiple scales- local, regional, national and international- which shapes their idea and reactions about FC as well as their entire socio-cultural life.

Conclusion

Previous research on FC negates socio-cultural change, specificity and women's agency. This process-oriented study aims at bridging the chasm between local and global knowledge and carving out a path for dialogue among different internal stakeholders so that health education be with and not against the people. I have further shown how the research tools were designed to collect the data for this investigation and how this data will be interpreted and reported in subsequent chapters. In the next chapter, I will locate the study area so as to give my findings, social context and 'ecological validity' and thereafter reporting and discussing my research findings will be the focus.

CHAPTER TWO

THE POLITICAL ECONOMY OF GENDER AND SEXUALITY

In this chapter I examine the political economy of the Ejagham region and the dynamics of the sexual political economy of Ejagham society through an analysis of the intersection of various historical processes that have led to social and cultural change among the people. This implies an examination of how processes such as colonialism, the implantation of plantation agriculture, urbanization and structural economic changes in the region and beyond have impacted on their values and practices, orchestrated conflicts between generations and sexes and with outside groups living among them. I argue that patriarchy is the linking moment between capitalism and kin- ordered modes of production ushered in by the advent of plantation agriculture. There is a link between these two modes of production leading to conflict and the creation of contestation as parents struggle to maintain control over land and the labour resources of their children. Capitalism never destroyed but rather worked through the kin-ordered mode of production using patriarchy. I further look at the impact of the Ejagham's strategic location on the historic trade route between the Cross River region (CRR) and Cameroon. An examination of the dynamics of the people's sexual political economy shows a shift from parents and other close relatives in the match-making process to the prospective spouses themselves and an increase in eroticized relationships. The advent of the HIV/AIDS pandemic reinvigorated debates over female sexuality and the need for control- a debate that led to increased tension over the institutions of Moninkim and FC became, within the present context of the HIV/AIDS pandemic a ''native'' therapeutic model against inordinate sexuality among partisans.

In what follows, I will first locate the people and their economy, before documenting the social impact of colonialism, particularly the implantation of plantation agriculture and the contradictions of the traditional social organization in terms of the duality of traditional and modern authority systems, what Mamdani (1991) calls "decentralized despotism". Both systems magnify men's power at the detriment of young men and women. Secondly, I will look at the effects on women of various twists in the global and regional economy and on the sexual political economy of the people. My main focus here is on the development of prostitution and various changes in value system and social structure orchestrated by the implantation of plantation agriculture and by various global and regional economic shifts. This will provide a useful backdrop against which to understand social and cultural changes and conflicts between generations and sexes in this region.

2.1 Historical background

This study is a case-based, historical processual analysis of changes in the institutions of FC and Moninkim in the wake of the HIV/AIDS pandemic among the Ekwe, Ejaghams, but with an extension to their Keaka and Obang co-ethnics. The Ejagham groups under study are the present day occupants of Eyumojock Sub Division, in Manyu Division of Southwest Cameroon. For detailed history of the Ejagham people see among others Abasiattai (1990) and Sandy (1992). They are located between latitudes 4.5 to 6.5 North of the equator and longitude 8.15 to 9.3 East of the Greenwich meridian on the African continent. They are flanked in the North by the Cross River State of Nigeria, where the majority of the Ejagham population is found. In the South they are bounded by Ndian division, East by their Bayangi neighbours (a former FC practising group which abandoned FC in the 1950s) and West by the Federal Republic of Nigeria.

The Ejagham people of today's Southwest Cameroon are part of the larger Ejagham nation that used to be found astride the Cameroon-Nigeria border area. During the colonial partition of the early 19th century, the Ejaghams like other African ethnic groups that came under different colonial masters, were portioned out between Cameroon and Nigeria by Great Britain. Her Majesty's government for purposes of easy administration brought together British Southern Cameroons and administered it alongside Eastern Nigeria and Northern Cameroon alongside Northern Nigeria. One remarkable cultural dislocation of the colonial era was of course, the splitting up of native areas and communities. This is instanced in the case of the Ejaghams and Boki groups of Manyu Division who were divided between Nigeria and Cameroon into Ejagham Nigeria and Ejagham Cameroon, Boki Nigeria and Boki, Cameroon (Niger-Thomas, 2001). The divisions were in consonance with the boundary demarcation of 1912-1913 by the German

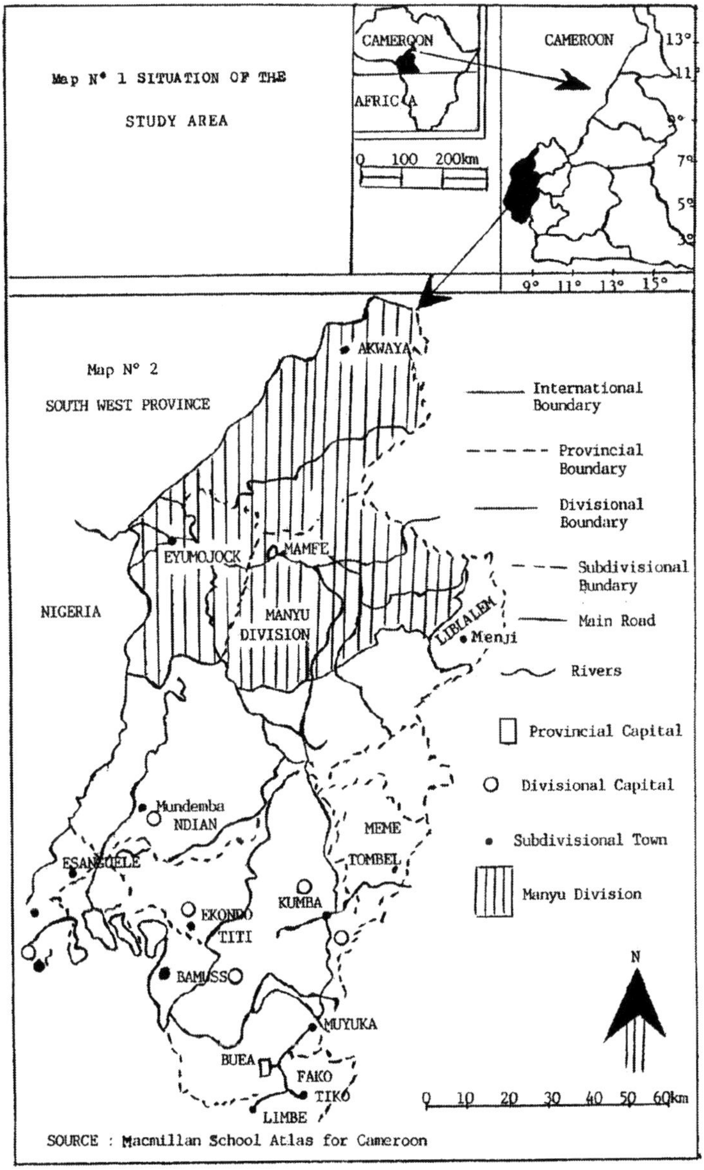

Fig. 1 Map of Cameroon showing neighbourig countries and Provincial headquarters

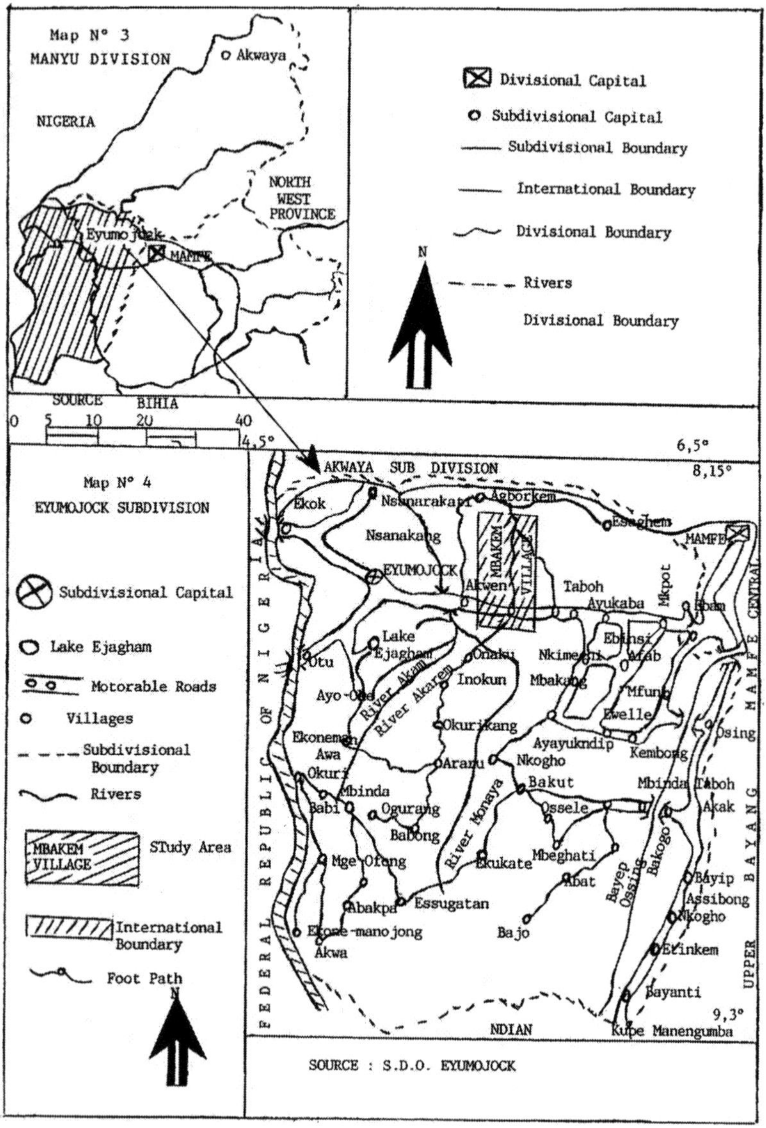

Fig. 2 Map of Eyumojock Sub Division

and British colonial masters. Trade restrictions were instituted and this affected free trade between the Efik traders of Calabar, Nigeria and the Ejaghams as middlemen in Mamfe, Cameroon.

The Ejagham people served as middlemen during the transatlantic slave trade linking the CRR and the Western Grassfield region of Cameroon. Furthermore, the colonial plantations which attracted other people into this region are located in the fertile coastal plains of Southwest Cameroon. Their strategic location on a trade route within a "culture contact zone" (Bizzell, 1997) on the Cameroon-Nigeria border has given rise to multiple flows of ideas and fashions in and out of the region fuelling the spread of HIV and other sexually transmissible diseases. It is also an impediment to the fight against FC since the people can cross the border, circumcise their daughters and return. Simultaneously, various shifts in the world, regional and national economy have led to profound transformations in their values, social structure and forms of life. An analysis of local historical processes within the region will foreground local ethnography within the extra-local context of larger historical processes and multiple flows. This will lead us towards a 'critical junctions" perspective in health and culture focusing on:

> the connections in space (and in and out of a place/in and out of a group), the relations through time, the internal and external relations of power and dependency, and what Wolf has called "the interstitial relations" between apparently separate institutional domains" (Kalb and Tak, 2005: preface).

In line with this theoretical path, my focus in this chapter is two fold. First I document the impact of local, national, regional and global forces and flows on the people's lives with a specific focus on women and youths, secondly I explore issues of intergenerational conflicts over land and in their interaction with outside groups.

In Cameroon, the Ejagham people are found in present-day Manyu Division of the Southwest province and in Nigeria in the Cross River region. In the East, they are bounded by their Bayangi neighbours who until the 1950s practiced FC and the West by the Federal Republic of Nigeria. The Ejagham people studied here are comprised of three clans: the Lower and Upper Ekwes (Ejagham Njemaya) found in Eyumojock Sub Dvision and who are the main focus of this study, but with an extension to the other two groups: the Keakas (Ejagham Ngunaya) and the Ejagham Obang who are in the minority. They are characterized by a lineal settlement pattern. Spread out in 46 hamlets, there are over 200,000 of them (ABEMO, 2002:5) in Southwest Cameroon. Most live in thatched houses while a small number have constructed their houses using cement blocks and corrugated iron sheets. The area has towns such as Mamfe, Kembong and Eyumojock with administrative functions such as military camps and offices. These towns have bars, night clubs, markets, schools, cybercafés and money transfer outlets. In the cybercafés in Mamfe, young men and women can most often be observed dating and searching for spouses abroad. Almost every village has a primary school but only the main towns have secondary schools which have partly entailed migration from the rural countryside to the cities. Upon completing school, most of the youths remain in the cities only visiting their villages from time to time, while others even drop out of school and remain in the city. They do not see themselves taking up farming and choose to remain in town because of the existence of social amenities such as electricity, pipe-borne water and employment opportunities. In Eyumojock, electricity is rationed and people have electricity only from 12 am to 8 pm but in the hinterland village, people depend on bush lamps. There are two hospitals in the region: the Provincial hospital in Mamfe and the Divisional hospital in Eyumojock but some individuals prefer to cross the border and seek medical care in Nigeria. It is a medically pluralistic society. Patients shuttle between modern and traditional medicines. Eyumojock Sub Division has a modern health care facility, the Eyumojock District hospital as well as traditional healers and birth attendants (TBAs) who cater for the health needs of the population. Individuals equally resort to auto-medication with herbs or over the counter drugs. The biomedical health care facility here is bedecked by lack of logistics as most medical equipment is obsolete and it has few and demotivated personnel who are on the most part, volunteers. The health care outlets in the region are located far away, are often without essential drugs and suffer from lack of personnel. Further, they are generally inaccessible in terms of physical distance given the enclaved nature of the area and the rural population suffers from abject poverty. Though there is a road network linking some of the villages, there is no regular means of transportation but for motor bikes which transport people at cut throat prices by local standards. Partly because of distance from the available modern health care facility, illiteracy and poverty, there is high attendance at antenatal clinics but low rate of child delivery at the various hospitals. Most births are still taken care of by TBAs who also perform circumcisions for both sexes.

The equatorial forest area in which the people live as well as some of their social habits seem to be strongly incompatible with good health. It is the habitat of the anopheles mosquitoes, the vector for the malaria parasite, which is the most common ailment in this area. The "black fly" bites equally without mercy, transmitting filaria in the process. The people's social habits further provide clues to their health status. The people squat in the forest and bushes and at times, excreta by children and adults alike can be found littered around households. Flies hover over human waste and most of the time, settle on food meant for human consumption. Apart from malaria and filaria, other common diseases in the area include diarrhoea, typhoid and gastritis, which are nutrition related.

In addition to the lack of toilet facilities, potable water is non-existent. In fact, clean potable water is still a luxury. ABEMO (2002:5) has observed that *"Everyone (here) gets sick of malaria at least 3 to 4 times a year and due to lack of safe drinking water and poor hygiene, water borne diseases are common in the region*". Children, men and women alike can be seen early in the morning and in the evening covering long distances to fetch water from streams and springs for domestic use. Curiously enough, this water is never boiled to kill germs. They bath and do their laundry in these streams and springs. At times, men are bathing up whereas women are bathing downstream. Apart from the divisional hospital, only a few individuals in Eyumojock have bored holes from which they fetch potable water. Eyumojock has some taps but water has never flown from them since they were constructed because the local council and the government, which provided these tapes are still divided over who should take responsibility for their maintenance. The former is of the opinion that the taps be privatized and that any individual who wins the tender will provide electric power to permit the water to be flowing constantly and will supply to the community at a moderate price per litre. The latter wants the former to shoulder the burden of maintenance and the deadlock has persisted at the detriment of the health of the local population.

Despite the colonial partition, both Ejagham groups in Nigeria and Cameroon still form a cultural continuum as they maintain strong kinship ties and their cultural institutions have remained relatively stable until recently. What is of utmost importance here is the fact that the people's location astride the Cameroon-Nigeria frontier and their kinship ties to groups in Nigeria has an impact on efforts to eradicate FC. This is the case because they can cross the loose borders either way, circumcise their daughters and return. But most important is the fact that areas characterized by multiple flows and mobility show high rates of HIV/AIDS transmission.

The principal mobile actors are traders, military officers and truckers. These mobile areas are generally reputed to have a high rate of AIDS and other STDs. Orubuloye et al (1994:87) point out that in Africa, such regions with their contiguous countries, huge unrestricted geographical borders present even uninfected areas with the greatest threat of the AIDS pandemic (See also Tierney, 1990, Von Ryne, 1990). Drivers are a high risk group, for instance, they are relatively well-off despite their meagre salaries because they often take other goods for direct payment on their way and truck driving as reported by Orubuloye et al (1994) attracts adventurous men who are more likely than others to take risk. Various studies have concluded that the military and police forces, too, are a high risk group (National Intelligence Council, 2002, Garrett, 2005), partly due to the mobile nature of their jobs. In fact, mobile men are everywhere the largest of concerns about AIDS.

A comparison of the infection rate between Cameroon's civil and military populations for 1993 showed 6.2% for soldiers compared to 2% of the general Cameroonian population (Civil Military Alliance Newsletter, 1996:2). A Nigerian military survey shows that the rate of HIV infection among soldiers based near their wives and homes mirrors that of society-about 5%, while rates among those deployed elsewhere on peacekeeping operations in Africa are up to three times higher. The forty-three percent of the surge in military mortality in Nigeria is ascribed to HIV (Garrett, 2005).

2.2 The economy

The Ejaghams are occupants of the mosquito and 'black fly' infested equatorial rain forest where tree species like mahogany, iroko, and ebony are under the threat of deforestation from both individuals and commercial logging companies alike. Poaching for "bush meat" is another environmental threat. The area has few roads and during the rainy season, spanning from March to November, the roads are like the fighting grounds of elephants. The roads are only passable during the extreme dry season from November to March. They do slash and burn farming in the forest and on the banks of the rivers Akarem and Monaya with all its inherent negative environmental impacts. They clear the forest using hand tools such as cutlasses and burn the grass thereby polluting the environment in the process. Respiratory tract diseases are common in the area partly due to the pollution of the atmosphere in the course of cultivating the soil using fire. After clearing the forest, they then make mounds using hoes and plant varied food crops. This small scale farming is gendered. Perhaps because of the intensive labour required for clearing the virgin forest, packing, burning, hoeing and weeding, only men plant cocoa and coffee as cash crops. This implies that these crops are male preserves, leaving women with autonomy only over food crop production. Both genders however encounter the impact of various economic shifts in varying degrees with women more affected than men.

Most women concentrate on the cultivation of coco yams, melon seeds, maize, plantains, ground nuts, cassava which is used for their highly starchy staple food of *water fufu*, eaten with *eru*. But women are however still required to give their husbands a helping hand in the cultivation of cocoa usually during the harvesting season. They equally plant fruit trees such as oranges and plums, both for household consumption and for sale. However, given the seasonal nature of the roads and the fact that almost everybody owns a farm, seasonal poverty is the order of the day as there are almost no buyers for the surplus foodstuffs. During the cocoa season in particular, most of the people live lavishly and thereafter, they fall back into the poverty cycle as they start borrowing in advance from the so called 'cocoa merchants' hoping to pay back during the next cocoa season. Some even receive money well in advance for yet to be produced cocoa without thinking of the possible prospects of better prices in the future or even the outright failure of the cocoa harvest. It might be stated that the 'cocoa merchants' seek to indebt farmers in order to exclusively lay claim and to prevent competition among themselves at the time of the harvest.

Cocao is at the root of some conflicts in this society. Apart from reliance on family labour, some cocoa farmers contract labour and take chemicals on credit to be paid for when they harvest their crop. At other times, some of the farms are rented out in exchange for a given quantity of cocoa. Some are contracts for the extension of cocoa farms. Some farmers practice share cropping. They give out particular sections of their farms usually for a given period of time in return for a specific quantity of the annual yields. In any case, once one of the parties to the agreement fails to live up to expectations, there is conflict and the need for traditional justice. For instance the "work man" might steal some of the yields just as the farm owner might refuse to settle him on any flimsy pretext such as poor harvest. A fall in harvest might attract violent reactions but most often, peaceful negotiation is the norm. Cocoa traders as a group of powerful actors both from within and out of the region often hold down prices in their favour, making the farmers poorer. These elites and wealthy individuals often mention the poor state of the road as the main reason for offering low prices. These traders and middlemen buy up cocoa and provide credits and are very much interested in extending these credits during the dead season. One effect of the people's dependence on cocoa for cash is seasonal poverty as traders create monopoly claims on future produce through credits and low prices. Seasonal poverty alternates with periods of plenty and often leads to migration into and out of the area. The youths usually return to the area during and leave once the cocoa season is over. Women usually come in to the region to benefit from the temporary boom. In fact, the gender division of labour involved in the entire production cycle leads to the locking of women into kin-based mode of production, and the imposition of power and prestige by men who own and control the cash while women remain workers. There is increased serial monogamy, popularly called "cocoa season concubines","cocoa season marriages'' and polygyny as some men usually take more wives after selling their produce. This hypersexuality of the cocoa season leaves numerous young girls pregnant while the rate of sexually transmissible diseases multiplies by leaps and bounds.

My focus on the people's present-day economy is important because it partly explains the general culture of seasonal poverty in which most of the people find themselves. Almost everybody owns a farm and food crops have minimal economic value except the "mole'' cash crop of cocoa. It further gives us a feel for their physical environment and its impact on their lives and on gender relations given the existence of gendered food taboos as a symbolism of patriarchal power. Furthermore, this poverty and dependence partly explain the fall in the "moral economy" of the people as epitomized by rampant youth pregnancy, an issue which I take up later. Some of the mobile actors in this area apart from 'cocoa merchants' include trans-border traders, military men, policemen, gendarmes, border guards and drivers who are always passing in and out of the region spreading both new fashions, ideas and diseases in the process.

2.3 Colonialisms, Plantations and Company towns

The establishment of plantation agriculture by the colonial German administration all over Cameroon created a large plantation complex which was exceptional in West Africa for its size and intensity of cultivation (Konings 1993: 219). When Germany was ousted from Cameroon in 1916 by a joint Franco-British force, the French and British took over plantation farming. Everywhere, colonialism relied on forcefully appropriating the labour of native populations for public work infrastructures. Natives were alienated from their land as the colonial administration expropriated most of the fertile lands for plantation agriculture to produce raw materials such as rubber, banana, tea, and cocoa for the metropolitan economy while confining the latter on particular spaces. German, French and British colonialism in Cameroon was similar in several respects. One point of convergence was the confiscation of native lands by these colonial authorities under the pretext of land reforms.

In the particular case of Germany, lands were declared "vacant and ownerless" and proclaimed property of the German colonial state by the Crowns Land Act of 15th July 1896 (Njoh, 2000, 2002). Zoning was informed by the principle of racial segregation, the fear of contamination and the maintenance of racial purity. The spatial segregation that was partly concretized through zoning set aside large tracts of land for colonial agricultural development as native populations were herded into "native reserves". This policy for instance, freed up large portions of land at the foot of Mount Cameroon for the establishment of German plantation farming (Fisiy,1992, Fanso, 1989). Africans further paid rents for land use to the colonial administration and to ensure the success of this policy, the colonial administration set high artificial land prices in urban areas so as to discourage most natives from settling in the colonial cities (Simons,1992) and from acquiring these lands. Several towns because of their economic or strategic importance to the colonial enterprise were singled out for the implantation of colonial rule. Three towns best illustrate this in the case of Cameroon.

The port city of Douala had strong ties to the colonial era and administration. It served as the entry point of the Germans into the territory and as an outlet for the shipping of raw materials from the plantations. However, the local Douala population, following Eyongetah and Brian (nd), put up stiff resistance to the German appropriation of their lands in particular and to German hegemony in general as the former refused to serve as porters to the latter. They further refused to pay German imposed land taxes, and were against German expropriation and sale of land around the Wouri estuary to Europeans at astronomical prices.

Yaounde was the site of the German colonial government station. The town's strategic location served as "the launching pad for further expeditions to various parts of the territory" (Njoh, 2000). It was a major trade centre and to develop it, the German colonial administration depended on forced participation in several public work projects, particularly road construction. Large numbers of young men from the western Grassfields were herded to the coast to serve as labourers in the newly created German plantations. Even when the British took over from the Germans as of 1916, the pattern of forced recruitment continued unabated as evidenced by the forceful enlistment of labour and other inputs.

The third town, Buea served as the German and British colonial headquarters and for strategic reason, the German colonial station was built here so as to be able to monitor events in Douala. Like elsewhere in Cameroon, the Germans built meandering footpath access roads leading up to the steep slopes. During the apogee of German plantation agriculture in Cameroon, a number of different schemes were tried out including the confinement of the local population so as to freeze up more land for the latter purposes. Surrounding areas like Tiko emerged as colonial agro towns in 1892. It was the site of private German plantations such as the African Fruit Company and Holforth Company. By 1914, as much as 264,000 acres of land in Victoria and Kumba Divisions (present-day Fako, Meme, and Ndian Divisions) were under the monopoly and control of German farmers while a large portion of the rest was held as Crown Lands (Njoh, 2000, Arderner, 1996, Rudin, 1958).

Paradoxically, by the close of the Second World War and immediately after independence in 1960, European companies continued to maintain overwhelming monopoly and hegemony over most of the land in Tiko. The Likomba Estate owned by Messrs Elders and Fyffes Ltd and the German plantation firm, the Likomba Company, jointly owned as much as 15,584 acres of freehold estate while the rubber plantations were owned and operated by the British-based Commonwealth Development Corporation which later became the Cameroon Development Corporation, the CDC (see Njoh, 2000). The advent of plantation agriculture led to urbanization with attendant consequences on both local social structures and on family relationships.

2.4 Plantation agriculture and urbanization

The establishment of plantation agriculture in the fertile coastal areas of Cameroon led to forced labour conscription and to an unprecedented upsurge in the population of these areas, particularly Meme and Fako Divisions in present-day Southwest Cameroon. This upsurge of largely single males came mostly from the hinterlands of the Western Grassfields region as well as from neighbouring Nigeria. Plantation agriculture therefore led to an unprecedented wave of rural-urban migration as well as to movement out of the patriarchal orbit. Young men were brought to the coast in large numbers to supply labour. This separated them from their families and spouses. It further gave rise to changes and dislocations in local social structures, and simultaneously afforded them to escape from tradition and patriarchy as a power field. European plantation landlords established company towns to accommodate their workers. Concomitantly, the authorities paid no heed to the population increments experienced by the "native settlements" in response to the ever growing need for goods and services orchestrated by plantation agricultural activities. This led to a drastic decline in sanitation, living standards and related conditions in the native settlements. Since these were populated by single men, there was an acute shortage of women. This is the exact point at which large scale prostitution enters the scene. One elder told me that the few available women "sold like hot cakes". Other social consequences for families, following Arderner (1996), included a sharp increase in divorce rates and prostitution as families became unstable. Some men are reported to have appropriated the sexuality of their wives for professional mobility in the colonial plantation civil service. My informants told me that some seniour African officials slept with the wives of their junior colleagues and even threatened to sack them from work if they made any noise about it. In other instances, today some men with their wives' connivance, use the latter's sexuality to lobby for advancement in the plantation labour force. On the other hand, others emphasize their ethnic and tribal belonging both to gain access to the low end plantation jobs and for advancement within its ethnicized hierarchies. The subsequent expansion of the plantation led to more coercive and intensive recruitment of young men from the hinterlands. These men were compelled, as is usually the case with migrant labourers, to migrate to the coastal areas without their spouses or families. Back in their villages, some of the men were dispossessed of their wives during their protracted absences by their love rivals.

Plantation agriculture has other disadvantages, such as the external economic dependence of plantation towns and the discouragement of entrepreneurship. First and foremost, it is characterized by the economic dependence of the town on external economic forces. The primary production of the town serves as raw materials for 'real' production elsewhere. To compound matters, the prices of the raw materials are dictated from outside, by powerful supranational institutions and core countries. Workers in production have virtually no control over their agricultural produce as these products are meant for the export market. Njoh (2001:412) has ably pointed out that the impact of the economic crisis, and by extension, the Structural Adjustment Programmes (SAPs) of the 1980s, "magnified on townships such as Tiko, Limbe, and Kumba", traditional plantation towns in Cameroon.

Plantation agriculture further poses a challenge to tradition and culture in terms of land ownership, particularly between local communities and the state. This is instanced by the ongoing suit brought against the Cameroonian government by the Bakweri Land Claims Committee (BLCC) at the African Commission for Indigenous People's Rights in Banjul, the Gambia. The former is claiming ownership over the land it gave the German and later the British colonial administration for plantation agricultural development. In the wake of privatization, the government sold the plantations alongside the land but the Bakweris on whose lands the plantations are found are insisting that the new owners of the agro-industrial complex bought only the plantation and not the land on which these plantations are found. They want compensation from the new plantation management. For a detailed ethnographic analysis of the trajectory of this conflict, see Pemunta and Fonmboh, 2010).

Furthermore, the low wages paid out to plantation labourers kill the spirit for personal entrepreneurial initiatives. A combination of low-wages for these dead-end jobs and subsequent benefits such as "free company housing" in the plantation camps are the main motivations. In these camp houses, there is virtually no privacy as adults and children are crammed together and the latter learn about sex at rather very tender ages, leading to a high rate of unwanted pregnancies. Apart from total reliance on their meager salaries, the tedious nature of plantation labour and lengthy hours of work accentuate social problems such as excessive drinking, teenage pregnancies, lack of privacy between parents and children in the camp houses, high rate of school dropout and juvenile delinquency.

By seizing and expropriating native lands, the colonial masters introduced changes in the traditional relationship between native people and land as these people were dispossessed ourightly with no compensation. Elders as custodians of culture were the most affected. Land creates links between the worlds of the living, the dead and the yet to be born (Mbiti, 1965). When the postcolonial state took over, this pattern continued as all land became the property of the modernizing state, unless it was "effectively occupied". The colonial land reform measures led to the commodification of land. Unlike in the past land could now be bought and sold in the open market. This is in sharp contravention of the concept of land within the framework of African cultures and traditions. Njoh, (2000:244) quotes a Nigerian Chief as commenting that "land belongs to a vast family of which many are dead, few are living and countless members are still unborn". This has led to conflicts over ownership of land between individuals and between the state and local communities. As I intimated above, in the face of privatization for instance, the Cameroonian state sold off the CDC industrial complex, alongside the land.

This commodification has further given rise to stiff prices and competition for land in the coastal regions of Cameroon. Members of local communities were first disenfranchised by the colonial and then by the postcolonial state, which transferred rights to plantation farmers and corporations. In the actual sense, land belonged to members of a given community. Many Africans believe that they are only custodians or trustees and have no power to alienate land. In the dual political system and dispensation put in place first by colonialism and sustained by the postcolonial state, lineage and family heads own family land while the Chief is de facto owner of all the land in the village. At the supreme level is the state which claims ownership over all parcels of land. Following Mamdani (1991:139- 146) there is no contradiction in the notion of communal ownership of land, as corporate and individual land rights co-exist explaining why the colonial notion of "private property" was a unilineal reductionism of community rights based on the universal European concept of legal tenure. And as Elizabeth Colson (1969:196-97) states "they assumed that the full range of land rights covered by the principle of proprietary ownership must exist in Africa as in Europe". Stated otherwise, rights in the European sense had to be exclusive with no possibility for multiple and overlapping ownership. The second distortion was the conflation of ritual offices with proprietary rights over land whereas they were only concerned with ritual activities and not with the allocation of land. Thirdly, there was the conflation of community with tribe. 'Strangers' were seen as having no traditional access to land whereas in most of pre-colonial Africa, strangers were welcomed as wives, clients, 'blood brothers', settlers or disciples thus enhancing the prestige and labour force of a household, kin group or community (Mamdani, 1991: 139-146).

The colonial notion of land tenure revolved around the above stated three distortionist pivots: community as proprietor of land, community leaders as wielders and executors of that proprietorship right and tribal affinity as defining access to community land. Following this logic, all owners of land had to be identified and protected against exploitation by being denied the right to freely dispose of their interests and land became a sole community ownership, what Colson,(1969) calls 'customary but untraditional'.

One area of perennial conflict over land brought about by the advent of plantation agriculture is between native populations and settler groups. Migrant labourers in Southwest Cameroon, mostly from the Western Grassfields region who worked in the plantation came to obtain land for cultivation via borrowing, inheritance, leasing and pledging, core features of indigenous tenure systems. Most eventually settled on this land. In the face of state-sponsored ethnicity, they are being told by the new generation of South westerners "to go home". They are being further excluded from political participation, thanks to the enshrinement of ethnicity in Cameroon's 1996 Constitution as a smokescreen to protect minority rights. In keeping with the institutionalized politics of ethnicity in Cameroon, local politicians and elites alike constantly pit these 'slave strangers' (in their own country) against the indigenous population by fanning flames of animosity for their own political gains and interests. They always tell their co-ethnics that the stranger population will always prefer to vote for parties from their own regions of the country. This implies that by 'sanctioning', voting against the government, they will incriminate the native population to the government as political enemies implying the loss of development projects meant for them since these resources are usually shared on the basis of political clientelism[1] and patronage. Most of the time, these 'strangers'[2] have been outrightly disenfranchised during the usually 'ethnically' discriminatory voter registration process and later on victimized for the victory of the opposition in some neighbourhoods in the area during electoral contests. In its 1996 constitution, the Yaoundé regime in the wake of the presently stalled democratization process in the country redefined citizenship and equated political participation with ethnicity in the guise of protecting minority rights using the concepts of 'authocthones' and 'allogenes'. The former, in Cameroonian political parlance, implies that an individual can put up his candidature for an electoral post only in his village or region of origin. This policy fosters ethnic political participation and "ethnic citizenship". On the other hand, the latter present 'non-natives' (citizens of the same country) as foreigners and bar them from political participation out of their regions of origin. In line with the politics of ethnicity, people's political affiliations are subjectively defined in terms of their regions of origin. This conflict is in fact, one of the fall outs of and part of the effort to contain, the perverse legitimacy-effects of imposed SAPs of the 1980s, a process that led to devolution, instead of democratization in the real sense of the word in most Third World countries.

The Ejagham area is also the hub of inter-regional and inter-country trade linking the West and Central African regions on the one hand and Cameroon and Nigeria on the other. The region's trade road location informs us about various flows leading to the adoption of new fashions, lifestyles, values and STDs with HIV/AIDS inclusive by various mobile actors who are constantly passing in and out of the region. It is to this important feature that I shall now turn my attention.

---

[1] In the Cameroonian postcolonial state system, development resources are usually attributed only to regions with their sons and daughters in juicy, strategic positions within the centralized administrative set up. Political appointments are in this light subjectively equated with development projects, in which case, those appointed usually end up developing only 'their stomachs' (enriching themselves) and those of their family members. In this weird notion of development, appointment is equal to development.

2.5 Trade and mobility

The Ejagham area is well known for its cross-road facilities which have always encouraged diverse trading activities between Nigeria and Cameroon in particular and the Central and West African region in general. The Cross river track in the Old Calabar region in Nigeria with its large basins has at all times been instrumental for communication between Cameroon and Nigeria and the West and Central African regions. In fact, these people are not localized; there is a lot of generational movement around, both into and out of the region. The Ejagham acted as middlemen between the Cameroon Grassfields and the hinterland during the slave trade and the colonial times due to their strategic culture "contact zone" (Bizzel, 1997) location. Röschenthaler (2007) has brought an interesting and informative twist to the slave trade economy and to processes of cultural transfer in this region. She observes that many people who were uprooted from their homes with varied cultural capital and knowledge of secret societies which they later disseminated, remained slaves on the continent as they were never sold to Europeans and therefore never reached the Atlantic ports. Rigid social hierarchies existed between 'free-born' and slave families in terms of ownership of secret societies and the level of an individual's participation in these associations. This segregation has continued to affect patterns of social interaction especially marriage and political participation in the region between 'free-born' and so called slave lineages. This gives us some historical clues that partly explain women's presumed lack of marriage opportunities which some attribute to their close kin relationship. Most young men attribute it to women's failure to respect the discrete "moral economy" of sexuality as the commodification of women's sexuality for social networking has become the order of the day in the face of global and regional economic changes.

By 1914, the British took over this area as part of the Franco-British agreement that partitioned Cameroon between France and Britain following the First World War. The British named their area of occupation the Southern Cameroon and merged it with Eastern Nigeria for purposes of easy administration. After independence, the British zone was divided into the Northwest and Southwest provinces. Simultaneously, the British administrators opened the border between Nigeria and Cameroon, so "that Cameroon could draw upon the financial and economic resources of Nigeria" (Chiabi, 1986). This led to the influx of Nigerians into Cameroon and vice versa. This trend continued with the opening of the road between Mamfe and Ikom in 1945. During this period, there were no custom barriers at the Cross River, which alongside the porous Cameroon-Nigeria border formed the axis of trade. Oral accounts maintain that until the 1970s, there were no limitations on women's cross-border activities but there were more restrictions and cross-border checks on men.

After 1945, there was the opening of the road from Mamfe to Ikom but this did not limit river traffic. The road infrastructure remains poor to the present-day, making the Cross river highway, known in Cameroon as the Manyu river still a major route into Nigeria particularly in the rainy season. The poor state of the road network negatively affects the geography of anti-HIV/AIDS and anti-FC mobilization as intervening NGOs and health personnel, most often do not reach the hinterlands.

The 1970s oil boom in Nigeria led to a decline in agricultural and food production in the country. When the prices plummeted in the world market, the government of Nigeria instituted austerity measures and basic necessities were in short supply. Cross-border black marketeering for both sexes became rampant. Some combined this trans-border trade with prostitution. Certain women, including Moninkims, came to earn the title of "Ikom Line Women" because they were trading between Ikom in Nigeria and Mamfe in Cameroon. In Mamfe, they owned a group of shelves where they sold various products from Nigeria. These entrepreneurs were mostly unmarried women and even today over 75% are either single, divorced or widowed. Niger-Thomas, (2001) who studied women's black marketeering in this region observes that they carved out:

> ...an unorthordox economic survival strategy for themselves and their families. Some got involved because they disliked farming or could not find farm land in the village. In the 1980s, women's smuggling activities reached its apogee in the area. At this time, mostly prostitutes were involved in this trade, including a group of women called "Kaduna Come Down" (Niger-Thomas, 2001)

I examine the ''Kaduna Come Down'' and another group, "The Bush Lamp Women", groups which included some Moninkims below in greater details. This pattern of illicit trans-border trading continued until the 1990s when the economic meltdown set in and the government of Cameroon adopted the structural adjustment plan. In 1994, Cameroon together with fourteen other African countries within the franc zone devalued their currency. In Cameroon, a 65% salary cut was imposed on civil servants. Unemployment skyrocketed and there was a general fall in living standards since the government is the major formal employer. Informal economic activities such as cross-border trade by both men and women increased dramatically as an alternative avenue for accumulation. Though lucrative, as it generates "fast cash", it has its constraints. One of these obstacles is the open solicitation of cash bribes and female body commodification by those in positions of state control and authority along the Cameroon-Nigeria border. One of Niger-Thomas' respondents observed that:

> We try to avoid customs control by all means, sometimes we succeed, and sometimes we don't. But when we happen to fall into their trap, all we do is negotiated and settle them (Ibid :43).

Young women entrepreneurs are often targets of sexual harassment as in some cases even their "settlements[3]" are turned down in preference for sex. Niger-Thomas (Ibid:60) has noted that:

> although the most prevalent form of settlement involves a cash transaction,... it can also take the form of sexual harassment. Certainly, female entrepreneurs have been known to flirt with officers on duty with the aim of establishing familiarity in order to evade cash payments. On the other hand, officers have been known to demand sex from female entrepreneurs (Niger-Thomas, Ibid:60).

Most of this illegal money as I observed during my field stay in the area goes into the maintenance of multiple concubines and lavish evening entertainment at Ekok, the last border town between Cameroon and Nigeria. Although most of the officers are married, they do not often come along with their wives and families. I was told by most residents that these officers have a minimum of three girlfriends each. They pay the rents for some of their concubines, while others come into this cross-border town to see them only on appointment. I witnessed frequent fist fighting and quarrels among women over particular officers in the bars in Ekok. Most often, the Nigerian and Cameroonian border guards and police officers compete with each other over free women in the area.

---

[3] It is a form of bribery, called "egunje" in the Yoruba language or "family support" in the English language. This euphemism is widely used by officers on the Nigeria-Cameroon frontier for interaction with entrepreneurs and passers-by. I overheard an officer on September 25th, 2006 telling an entrepreneur that "We have seen your papers, but settle us. We do not eat papers. Settle us." It is also called 'nyare' on the Mamfe beach.

2.6 Colonial capitalism, Patriarchy, "Prostitution" and Women's agency

Sex work as conceptualized here is an all encompassing concept that involves the sale of sex and the creation of eroticized relationships for material accumulation. Some of the sexual encounters are temporal; others last long and eventually lead to marriage. In fact, women's lives are complex. Whereas some are full time, others are part time sex workers, but they also have other statuses. Some are students, maids or traders. (For a detailed discussion of the fuzzy boundary between commercial sex work and intimate relationships, see among others, Kalb, 2004 and Demirdirek &Whitehead, 2004). As a blanket term, sex work is characterized by a fuzzy boundary between gift and commodity, desire and economic calculation and 'sexuality becomes part of a series of partly commodified and partly gift-like encounters' (Demirdirek &Whitehead, 2004:9).

Naaneen (1991: 61-62) dates the advent of prostitution in the Cross River basin as a profession to British colonial rule between 1888 and 1909. She points out that this ever flourishing trade was linked to the integration of the area into the global economic and social network through colonialism and the consequent structural changes in the existing economic and value system. According to her, this development was facilitated by the presence of "stranger elements", meaning the intrusion of non-agrarian forces such as sedentary or migrant labour and modern commerce. These exogenous forces were largely absent in pre-colonial Cross River society. Apart from economic forces, the high degree of political decentralization ensured that the political structure did not transcend the village level (Ford, 1939, 1950b, 1964), and the coming together of "mutually antagonistic ethno-linguistic groups combined to hinder the free movement of people and the development of those social forces that are integral to the growth of prostitution"(Ford,1964).

Talbot (1969:227-228) recorded that various small tribes in the Cross River region engaged in traffic with their immediate neighbours, which often led to frequent strife, quarrels and into war. This situation, following him, was ameliorated by the British conquest of the area between 1888 and 1909. The demand for forced labour for the putting in place of colonial government infrastructures led to male emigration during the colonial process. In addition to this, enhanced security and the growth of merchant capital all gave rise to changes in sexual relationships.

During my field research, elders frequently placed the presumed fall in moral standards as evidenced by youth sexuality on "the Coming of the Whiteman". This implies that the forces of Western civilization in general, but especially its demoralizing gadgets (television, newspapers, pornographic films etc) are held responsible for the presumed fall in moral values. This dovetails with Naaneen's (1991:62) view that even in colonial days, elders put the upsurge in sex work in this area at the doorstep of the "Whiteman". According to her, a colonial official interviewed the elders and discovered that forced labour during the early stages of colonial rule was an important contributory factor for the growth and proliferation of prostitution in the area. Young men, she points out, escaped from forced labour by fleeing to other areas where colonial rule was firmly established and forced labour was gradually waning. By so doing, they left behind "surplus women". On the other hand, those who remained behind coerced and cajoled these women into having intercourse with them. The establishment of export trade in cocoa further fuelled sex work as the opening of trade stations brought African staff from the hinterlands to the coast, some of whom took the local women as paid concubines and mistresses. When the factories closed down, the men left for their tribal homes whereas the women moved to the coastal towns to render sexual services. She identifies Ediba and Bansara as commercial centres and sexscapes on the Upper Cross River basin where most ''prostitutes'' opted to remain.

It seems that with colonial and modern expansion, sex work was simply reinforced by the structure of the colonial political economy, especially the pattern of the regional divisions of labour and the resultant regional inequality. In Cameroon, the Southwest and Centre provinces were well incorporated into the world economy through slave trade and thereafter to the colonial economy through the production of cocoa, rubber and banana. This is thanks to the former's coastal and the latter's location as the political capital of French Cameroon. While the local population has remained poor, there was and still is gendered division of labour and power in the production cycle. This has contributed tremendously to greater poverty among women than men. Men derive most of their cash income from the sale of coffee and cocoa, which are traditionally branded as men's crops. Women, on the other hand, receive their meagre revenue only from the sale of excess foodstuff, which sells at the lower end of the market since "almost everybody is a farmer"(Nkoyo, interview of 16/04/2006). With slim opportunities towards self-improvement, women had to gravitate towards economic opportunities elsewhere, partly encouraged by colonial imperatives such as the accelerated monetization of the economy, the creation of new tastes, values and status symbols which the indigenous economy could not sustain.

One unanswered puzzle that however arises is whether sex work was/is the only available avenue to these women. It seems that women in other parts of Cameroon unlike those in this region have accepted their traditional status as "dependent" housewives as defined by the traditional sexual division of labour. What seems clear is that sex work is certainly more profitable (despite the risk of infection with venereal diseases and today, HIV/AIDS) than peasant occupations. Compared to other kinds of businesses, it takes fewer resources to set up and to maintain. In fact, it does not require a heavy start up capital except for a healthy body and the ability to engage in emotionally detached sexual intercourse. What is observable among women from this region of Cameroon is that upon their arrival in the city, they most often stay with relatives or with other women from the same area. They may be sharing a flat or room that they contribute to pay the bills and use in turn with their sexual partners. Some are brought into the urban sphere to work in "secuires"(brothels) as 'maids', 'servants', usually under a mistress. Some begin as short term holiday-maker-prostitutes so as to make money for their school needs. Some however end up eventually dropping out of school and take up sex work full time. The Madam, usually an older woman, acts as a pimp, collects their earnings and pays them at the end of every day, week, or month as the terms of the arrangement might be. This trend might continue until when these young novices become independent or fall out with their Madams. In the former situation some, after amassing enough money, eventually opt to move out of the brothel and rent a room/ flat of their own. They then set up their own free sole proprietorship enterprise and are no longer under the control and supervision of anybody. In the latter situation, conflicts sometimes occur out of jealousy or when some men go out with the Madam and with one of the girls or with two girls at the same time. In the case of a Madam, she might drive away the girl in question so as to keep the man to herself. It is common practice that while the girls are at everyone's disposal in the brothel, some men still keep them as permanent, paid concubines, "titulaire". The men have unlimited access to them at anytime that they want. However, while these men are away, they secretly have "fun for money'' with whoever is capable of paying, usually on a short term basis ('coup pressé'). Most urban brothels are staffed by young females from this region of Cameroon. They can be recognized both from their facial marks and from their language. Most are primary or secondary school drop outs who have chosen to work as commercial sex workers.

Therefore, it can be stated here that patriarchal control over land, kin and cash has apparently made sex work for some women an attractive venture. The income from sex work makes some women "itinerant gold mines"(Naaneen 1988). Some of these women are visibly rich and influential and sex work has probably become one of the most important sources of accumulation in the area. Their parents and other relatives within their extended kinship networks rely on them for cash support and status. Although there are no hard statistics on remittances entering the region, some of the sex workers have been able to give their children and relatives university level education. Some have constructed houses and most are reported to send remittances back home through both formal and informal channels such as visiting relatives and through various money transfer outfits that have sprouted up in the area. The implication is that families benefit from sex work while the state does not since the practice is informal in Cameroon.

Sex work in this region further seems to have been accentuated by the cultural pattern of "free unions". These are situations in which couples are merely co-habiting. That is without the man having paid the culturally laid down bride price. Naaneen (1991:65) has noted that the area was characterized by "generous sexual attitudes" and that marital customs and sexual attitudes had reminiscences to those of the Ikom Division where one study demonstrated that "as long as anyone can remember, marriage ties with free women have been rather fragile". Many marriages with free women allowed the women to have lovers (Harris, 1972:13, cf, Naaneen, 1991:65).

According to rumours and stereotypes in Cameroon, coastal women in general and Bayang women in particular are reputed for their ability to captivate, dominate and mesmerize men using charms. They, alongside Bakweri women, further have a reputation for never staying in marriage. Moreover, dangerous perceptions about their presumed wanton sexuality and divorce instincts linger on to this day. Coastal women in general and Bayang women in particular are said to have raised quite a stir in the coastal plantation towns in the 1950s. Combined with their presumed tendency to seek independent lives, ideas about the presumed danger these women posed fed rumours about Bayang and coastal women. It is widely alleged that Bayangi women in particular are dangerous and have an insatiable appetite for sex because of their lack of clitorises due to circumcision, which until the 1950s was a general culture trait in this region. In most of urban Cameroon, Bayang sex workers dominate the profession, though women from other tribes do become sex workers as well.

The practice of outward migration by females from this region to sell illicit sex all over Cameroon and beyond has a long history. Historians and anthropologists have made references to this pattern. Ardener, Ardener and Warmington (1960: 236:37) in their discussion of plantation and village life in Cameroon for instance estimated that in 1953 in Tali, about 25-30 women left for the southern plantation towns to earn money as an outcome of disaffection with their husband, or members of the kin-group into which they had got married. Ruel (1969:263-274) in his study of constitutionalism among the Bayang discusses the Ndifaw Union's abortive move to end sex work by repatriating all women from the area in coastal towns back home. Recently, ABEMO (2002) in its anti- FC advocacy campaign recognizes the fact that sex work has been a long time female activity in this region. Colonial capitalism and particularly the development of plantation agriculture in Cameroon like in Southern and Central Africa led to the growth of both migrant and sedentary labour while simultaneously freezing legitimate cash earning opportunities for women (Van Onselen,1982, Cutrifelli,1983:29-35). The German colonial government began plantation agriculture in Southwest Cameroon. This economic venture was exceptional in West Africa for its size and the sheer intensity of cultivation (Konings 1993:219). With the creation of plantations, there was the need for labour and young energetic men from other tribes all over Cameroon and beyond. This development further led to significant changes in village social structures as in particular the Grasslanders, some of whom eventually settled in the Southwest and are today referred to as "strangers" in their own country, took along with them their traditional reputation as hard workers. (See Warnier, 2007 on the transfer of this work ethos among slaves from the Western Grassfields region). One unfettered effect of the male-controlled monetization of the economy by the advent of plantation agriculture was urbanization, which in turn led to a split in relationships as parents could no longer mobilize the labour of their offspring. A further outcome was the challenge of parental and elder's authority as they lost control over the youths and their labour, leading to a decline in kin-ordered mode of production. Simultaneously, 'free women' asserted their agency by migrating to the plantation towns where they commodified their sexuality and challenged patriarchy. I will illustrate this point with three specific case studies. In what follows, I will draw heavily from the accounts provided by Ruel (1956) and Ardener, Ardener and Warmington (1960) complemented by reconstructive memories from elders.

2.6.1 The Ndifaw Village Group and "Wicked women"

I borrow the expression "wicked women" from Hodgson and McCurdy (2001) to capture the wrangling between 'free women' from the Mamfe area and the largely abortive efforts of the Ndifaw Village Group to repatriate them from the towns of the south in the 1950s. Broadly conceptualized, the expression "wicked women" refers to women who challenge patriarchal rules of conduct based on tradition, and assert their individual and collective agency, usually by appropriating (colonial) modern concepts like self-autonomy and sexual liberty.

The Ndifaw modern association was formed among others to forge clanic unity partly by prohibiting adultery between a member and another's wife and as a political platform to confront the colonial administration with their problems. Although marked by disagreements on various constitutional issues, one issue that received overwhelming agreement and support was the cultural problem of female prostitution. Ruel (1965: 266) delineates this group of women:

> migrant women who had left the village group for the plantations and urban areas of the south and who in doing so had walked out of the complex set of rights and monetary arrangements that depended upon their fulfilment of their roles as wives and daughters(Ruel,1965:266).

A close reading of the above cited quotation shows that in a patriarchal society, the elopement of these women from those to whom they were socially married had several repercussions on the prestige and authority of the elders. First and foremost, it entailed the loss of bridal wealth for the elders as they would be hard pressed to refund whatever they had already consumed on behalf of those women who were already married. These women further served as bad examples to young, unmarried women who might be tempted to follow in their footsteps and get engaged in sex work, meaning the loss of future bride prices to the elders. Secondly, their action further entailed the loss of kinship gifts and labour and engendered conflicts between their various families and the lineages into which they had been married. Marriage in African societies is a union of families and lineages and bridal wealth payments continue for decades, and even for life across generations. In addition to the foregoing, Ruel (1969) notes that the elders were bitter because "they were diminishing the future numbers of children that could be born into the home society". This implies that they were diminishing the future labour that the birth of more children would have brought to them and on which the elder's authority partly depended.

Against this backdrop, women who came back home for various social and cultural obligations such as for visits and the celebration of second burials for their dead relatives were restrained from going back to the city. They were further excluded from performing any cultural obligations such as participation in the clan's Union functions, including the dance which went alongside the general meeting. Their sexy dress codes, the carrying of umbrellas, the wearing of trousers and the putting of make-up were forbidden and they were debarred from celebrating funerals. In league with the Bayang Native Council Authority, five village elders from different village groups went down south and temporarily brought back about two hundred women (Ruel,1969). Back at home, their own kinsmen were to be in charge of them and to be responsible for their behaviour. Some however returned to their matrimonial homes upon return to the village despite the stigma of their former status.

The colonial administration was initially amenable to the village leaders' war against 'prostitutes' and against women who had appropriated the new modernity. Both were "protecting" women. However, the former later became ambivalent pointing out that the campaign was a violation of basic liberties showing a clash between human rights and culture, modernity and tradition. This further shows that women's bodies and their sexuality became the site of struggle and contradictory partisan debates between the colonial masters and the village elders. On the one hand, native men representing patriarchy claimed to be protecting ethnic identity by inscribing sexual morality on the bodies of women. On the other, the colonial administration was upholding the women's liberty by insisting that they be allowed to enjoy their liberty. This situation challenges notions of the reproduction of the colonial labour force noted elsewhere in Africa. Unlike in other parts of the continent, colonial administrators were worried about women's fertility to ensure the colonial labour force such as through the introduction of Western medicine and obsession with African women's bodies (see for instance, Allman et al, 2002:6, Jeater, 1993 on Southern Rhodesia, McCurdy, 2001:211-223 on Manyema women in Tanganyika). Jeater (1993) for instance, deals with marriage relationships and the regulation of sexuality in terms of both the political and the production systems and offers insightful insights into the nature of gender relationships before and during the colonial period in Southern Rhodesia.

The fight over the control of women's body here has historical reminiscences to the long drawn out conflict and deadlock between the Islamic fundamentalists and the Egyptian government over FC, in which the former wants continuation of the ritual cuttings, while the latter is against. And to the confrontation in colonial Kenya between the British administration and the Gikuyus over clitoridectomy, in which case the British wanted to eradicate the ritual cuttings while the anti-colonial movement under the Mau Mau appropriated it for their fight against British colonialism (see Kenyetta, 1937, Paderson, 1991).

I was told that some of these returned "wicked" women hoodwinked the clan union and obtained permission to go back to the coast so as to settle their affairs such as collecting monies they had saved in various thrift and loan societies and parking their belongings back home. However, most of these women failed to return home for good. The Union undertook another expedition that recorded only limited success as its representatives met with stiff resistance. They were constantly jeered and booed at in various towns. Ruel (1965: 268) affirms for instance that in Douala, the delegation in a widespread campaign recorded only partial success. Some members of the delegation are even said to have failed to bring back home their own erring relatives. Other members of the delegation were alleged to have been bribed with money by the prostitutes. He further observes that some of those who had been forcefully repatriated to the villages escaped back to the cities between 1954 and 1955. And some are even reported to have been smuggled across the frontier into French Cameroon. They eventually settled in the port city of Douala. They were clearly eager to escape the policing gaze of patriarchy at home. Ruel (1965:274) accounts for the failure of the anti-urban prostitution campaign in terms of two main reasons. The first is the duality of legal systems and clash of authority between the village Union and the colonial administration. This was particularly the case due to the fact that the village group overstretched its authority into the urban sphere of the colonial administration, which in protest, withdrew its support from them. The second was the need for overall consensus among the villages over other issues apart from the war against prostitution like the award of educational scholarships and the digging of pit –latrines. This, alongside other competing interests and divisions eventually led to the foundering of the campaigns. It was probably this anti-prostitution movement that, instead, led to the migration of Bayang prostitutes all over Cameroon and beyond today. Some of these prostitutes combine commercial sex with long distance trade. It is to two of these groups that I now turn my attention.

2.6.2 "The Bush Lamp Women" and "Kaduna Come Down Women"

The expressions "The Bush Lamp Women" and "Kaduna Come Down Women" are metaphors for two distinct but interrelated groups of Bayang sex workers. The former expression denotes free women from this area who can be observed in most urban centres in Cameroon sitting beside their doorposts with their lanterns waiting for commercial sex partners at night. On the other hand, "Kaduna Come Down Women" were Bayang sex workers who had migrated to Nigeria and who were among aliens forced to leave the country in 1984. This measure was adopted as a retaliatory move to the repatriation of Nigerians from Ghana in the 1980s. The covert anti-Ghanian campaign in Nigeria was termed "Ghana must Go". Niger-Thomas (2001) in her study of women entrepreneurs in the Mamfe region of Southwest Cameroon suggests a historical connection between smuggling and sex work. Following her, most of the female entrepreneurs of the 1980s in the region were former "professional prostitutes". Some officers along the Cameroon-Nigeria border still believe that most women doing inter-country business are sex workers., reason why they often harass them "to get their own share of the national cake". This expression is a euphemism that compares women's sexuality to the government treasury which never lacks money-implying that every part of the country, like every individual, should have its/his due. Applied to sexuality, it means that anybody who is financially capable should be able to sleep with a woman because her genitals like state finance never gets finished. In other words, a woman should maximise her beauty and femininity to the maximum. Other similar metaphors compare women to "bush meat', and to "elephant meat". Here the forest, meaning abundance is invoked.

They often prefer settlement in bed rather than collecting illicit cash from these women. One of my key informants, a spinster, Eliza, told me she abandoned trading in jewellery along the Cameroon-Nigeria border region in the late 1990s because of perpetual sexual harassment from officers on duty. After initially pretending to be giving in so as to establish familiarity, one day however, one officer seized her national identity card. He then insisted that she must go to his house to collect it. When she turned up with a delegation of three male relatives, the officer was furious and threw it at her. After this incident, she abandoned the trade.

Some of the female entrepreneurs, who have today instituted an occupational shift, are retired sex workers who are used to a lavish and sumptuous lifestyle. This needs money to maintain: nice clothes, good food and drink, make-up and other forms of luxury. It is common knowledge in the area that most of these female entrepreneurs, like their male counterparts in a bid to cut down on cost and to maximize more profit, often have sex partners on the trade route from Cameroon to Nigeria and vice versa. They spend the nights with their concubines (an inclusive category for regular partners of the opposite sex) and avoid paying hotel bills. One interesting case is that of a woman, Mami Bessong in her fifties, who trades in second hand clothes between Cameroon and

Nigeria. She told me how a polygynist, a wealthy Alhaji, introduced her to his two wives as their prospective co-spouse. This gave her the freedom to come and go as she likes. Each time she stops by to spend the night, the man's wives would prepare her food, give her water for a bath and arrange the bed for her and their husband. Before she goes off on most occasions, the man will ask his family members to select whatever they want from her wares and he will pay generously. Another female entrepreneur, Etah, 34 years old, in expressing disaffection with her gendarmerie concubine for not being generous to her pointed out that she has her "real friend"("correct massa") across the border in Nigeria. She stays there each time she goes on her business venture and not in a hotel like other women. She pointed out that unlike the law enforcement officer mentioned above; the man in Nigeria is more caring. She went on to intimate that this is the reason why she is always on 'trans-border business'. These are clearly instances in which sex work is combined and used as a marketing strategy, all with the aim of cutting down on cost and at the same time, making more money. It is clear that 'sex work' does not do justice to the complexity of these women's lives. Unfortunately, there is often no hyphenated identity for such women. As demonstrated for the Central and Eastern European region, prostitution actually has many grey zones (Demirdirek &Whitehead, 2004)

The historical emergence of the "Bush Lamp" and "Kaduna Come down" women represent an important component of female sex work in the Mamfe region. The slums of Mamfe town like the shanty towns of other Cameroonian cities today reveal a vivid picture of an ethnic red light district with women from this part of Cameroon being key stakeholders in the trade in flesh. In towns like Kumba and Douala, there are Bayangi quarters because of the alleged massive settlement of free women from this region in these quarters. In the latter location, it is equally called the "The Fence"- connoting an enclosed space used for certain kinds of illicit activities. In local Cameroonian parlance, the ethnic label Bayangi usually connotes a sex worker. In these ethnic red light districts, elderly women are usually the ones who place lanterns in front of their doorposts at night waiting on customers. Most often, young sex workers parade the streets while some elderly ones hang out in the shadow of street lights. Some merely sit in bars and beg for drinks at random as a covert mechanism of calling attention to themselves. This is because in most of Cameroon, for a man to offer a prostitute a drink is an implicit expression or symbol of the former's sexual intent towards the latter. Some other free women dance every piece of music played usually shaking their buttocks exaggeratingly with the aim of capturing the male gaze. The elderly women sex workers are usually believed to be selling at the lower edge of the commercial sex market because of their age. A male passerby is usually inundated with cat calls such as “cos come no” (meaning customer) or with unexpected greetings so as to attract attention to themselves such as “Good evening brother”. In these red light districts, age is not respected, so that to address an elderly woman as “Mami” is to disqualify her and to enlist her anger. Even among themselves, they call each other “sister”. This is not just because of a common regional origin but also to recreate a feeling of youthfulness in themselves. The elderly ones often get into conflict with the younger ones over sex customers. Sometimes, they openly fight over customers.

Their ethnic settlement pattern is partly informed by the need to serve as each other’s keeper in matters of security and to create a community away from home. In July 1997, I witnessed a nasty scene in one of the red light districts in Bonaberi, Douala. A customer, after having a quick fix with Bessem, refused to pay and was forced to drink from a bucket in which all the women present had washed their genitals. The story goes that he had lavishly spent all his money with Bessem drinking and feasting. After having sex, he is reported to have told her he was “flat”. Annoyed, the prostitute shouted for help in her dialect and within a short time span, her kinswomen came to recover her earnings and found nothing. They then took individual turns in washing their genitals in a bucket which they later forced upon the man and he drank from it. Such a practice in general but more specifically the throwing of this defiled water on someone is considered to be a sign of unending bad luck. It is also perceived to be a serious challenge to masculinity. When the police were summoned, they rounded up several sex workers. Some however bought their way either with money, sex or with both the same night and returned to the quarters. Women from this area have not only migrated to various Cameroonian towns, they are equally found in most other African countries such as Nigeria and Gabon. It is to one of the former group that I shall now turn my attention.

2.6.3 The Kaduna Come Down Women

In Nigeria during the 1980s, most free women from the Mamfe region of Cameroon settled mostly in Kaduna in the Muslim North. They equally settled in the then capital Lagos and in other strategic commercial towns like Calabar. The Ejaghams like their Bayang neighbours share a common culture and socio-cultural institutions. Despite some phonological variations, the Ejaghams further share a common language with some inhabitants of the Cross River region where Calabar is found. Those who remained at home settled in various Cameroonian towns like Mamfe, Kumba and Douala. In the wake of the SAP imposed on most African countries by the World Bank and the International Monetary Fund (IMF), Nigerian aliens were evicted from Ghana. The Nigerian government retaliated by passing a law obliging all aliens to leave the country. This was an economic strategy to nationalise the economy in favour of Nigerians. Cameroonians who had settled in Nigeria like all other nationals were forced to return home because of this "Nigeria for Nigerians" policy. Among them were Bayang and Ejagham women who had been living in Northern Nigeria and elsewhere. These returned migrant sex workers from the North earned the group label of "Kaduna Come Down".

Having lived a 'free' urban life in Nigeria, it seems that they no longer saw their place in rural society. This might perhaps have been an outcome of the stigma of sex work or because they wanted to continue with the same lifestyle in the urban environment out of the immediate purview of patriarchy. Most of them took up residence in Mamfe town. Given their familiarity with the Nigeria-Cameroon borders which they had crossed time and again visiting their families, some resorted to entrepreneurship as an alternative means of livelihood and accumulation. It further seems that the subsequent electrification of Mamfe town no longer favoured 'the bush lamp trade' as it might have led to a fall in the demand for "corner, corner love", although supply remained the same or even higher. This development would have scared off some (potential) customers since these encounters are fraught with discretion and 'secrecy'. Stated otherwise, some customers do not want to identify with sex workers in broad day light and only sneak into the red light district under the cover of darkness. Another prism could be that these returned sex-worker-entrepreneurs were eager to combine sex work with trading. In this regard, having monies of their own brought them status and they did not want to give the impression that they are depending on commercial sex. This seems to be a strategy to make the ugly look gentle and respectable. Taken in this light, their relatives believe that they are business women whereas they are combining this business with commercial sex. The Bush Lamp and Kaduna Come Down women have for a long time now dominated and monopolized the cross-border black marketeering business around the Cameroon-Nigeria border region.

Like other pre-capitalist African societies, the Cross River region is made up of kin-based societies in which case land is vested in males but women always have access for cultivation through their husbands or male relatives for unmarried women. In Southern and Central Africa, scholars have linked the development of sex work to colonial capitalism, particularly to the growth of migrant and sedentary labour and the freezing of legitimate cash earning opportunities for women (Van Onselem,1982, Cutrifelli, 1983:29-35). This has reminiscences to class-based explanations of sex work and exploitation. However, it is difficult to convincingly establish a relationship between sex work and exploitation rooted in capitalist social relations of production on account of the pre-capitalist nature of these societies, their kin-based social structures and access to land by women except under extreme circumstances where a woman is refused access to land as punishment. The 'freezing of cash' is an outcome of the articulation of modes of production and of women's dependence on men. Seeing societies as interconnected systems linked within wider ''social fields'' and modes of production permits us to capture intersystemic and intrasystemic relationships (Wolf, 1982:76). The capitalist and kin-based mode of production link and create contestation. Patriarchy implies monopoly over land and labour based on traditional relationships. It mobilizes the kin group and expropriates the labour of wives and daughters. As a social field of power, patriarchy is at the juncture of two modes of production because capitalism never destroyed but rather worked through the kinship mode of production, simultaneously stretched its field of operation into and over its mode of production. Some women asserted their agency by moving out of patriarchy for alternative ways of life such as trade mediated by sex work. Caught up between the capitalist and kinship modes of production, patriarchy works through but at the same time becomes contentious within the same framework.

The kin-based social structure of this society assured both individual and collective usufructuary right and equality to land. However, women's economic burden has been increased through the laws of property inheritance. Women are most often considered as "property" for inheritance. Forde (1937, 1950) has pointed out that almost all Upper Cross River groups shared a tradition of double descent. Patrilineal rights covered the use of both farmlands and dwelling sites to the provision of communal labour. Matrilineality on the other hand, took precedence over the inheritance of accumulated wealth (currency, livestock, and household goods), bridal wealth and its refund if the woman left her matrimonial home, redemption of debts owed by individuals among others. Wives and sons alike were excluded from inheritance, a man's mother's brother or sister's son succeeded him (Forde, 1950a:306).

This system of levirate meant the loss of social support network and labour by a man's wife and children upon his death. Although his successor was to take care of them in principle, this has most often, not been the case. Worst case scenarios occur when the widow refuses to remarry within her late husband's lineage. Despite her deprivation, a woman was further expected to bear a substantial amount of the funeral expenses. Against this backdrop, some women resorted to sex work so as to live up to these and other social and cultural expectations. Matrilineality further placed a man's children under the jural control of their mother's brothers. Men's lack of control over their daughters was partly responsible for women's proclivity to sex work. This is not to suggest that matrilineal descent definitely gives rise to commercial sex. This is an exception and not the rule. What is clear though is that patriarchy is the arrangement of authority within the articulation of modes of production, which necessarily results in contradiction and increasing conflict thereby expanding the opportunities for escape by daughters.

Patriarchy is just one among other factors that contributed to sex work in the Cross River region. It entails the social control of sex and procreation, the locking up of social labour in particular relations between people and its subsequent mobilization through access to people (Wolf, 1982:90-91). The men were against what they saw as the increasing independence of their womenfolk. A few elders pointed to short haircuts, which in the early United States was a symbol of women's freedom, as extremely threatening in those days. Even the carrying of traditional status objects like umbrellas, the putting of makeup, high heeled shoes and the smoking of cigarettes by women between the fifties and seventies was considered anathema to patriarchy. These restrictions instead pushed young women to migrate to urban areas where anonymity reigned, where they believed they were under the control of "government" and no longer "tradition" as represented by patriarchy in the rural environment. In this case, it might be stated that the colonial administration that preached women's liberty provided an alternative space for the public enactment of women's sexual liberation in the cosmopolitan environment.

Despite changing socio-economic circumstances, gendered divisions of labour in both production and exchange continued. Men were against women climbing palm trees to harvest palm nuts for the production of oil. This was based on the patriarchal and customary notion that palm tree climbing was a degradation of and an insult to womanhood and was therefore a male preserve. The ban against the planting of tree crops or even climbing trees to harvest fruits kept women away from competing with men in the economic sphere and maintained the *status quo* of women's dependence on men. But after World War II, things changed radically as women in the face of the post-war commodity boom became involved in all aspects of the production of palm oil, even exercising control over the full proceeds. Attempts to stem women's march towards economic empowerment and accumulation led to the prospects of even far greater economic freedom through sex work. In fact, the intensifying fight within traditional society about the labour and rewards of women actually led to women's escape to the city. ''Prostitution'' in the Mamfe area can be perceived as a form of protest against rural poverty, patriarchal exploitation and domination. However, it must be pointed out that it was not protest against male dominance and exploitation *per se* that led to sex work. It was rather the deliberate desire to make money caused by both internal and external forces, specifically shifts and contractions in the global and regional political economy of the region and the people's location within a "culture contact"(Bizzell,1997) zone: the transatlantic slave trade, colonialism and its linkage to the metropolitan economy, and the postcolonial Cameroonian state's marginal and peripheral position within the global economy in which it plays the role of mere primary producer.

In the next section, I will examine the dynamics of the traditional sexual organization of the Ejaghams while capturing the impact of patriarchy on women's bodies and their sexuality. I will make note of and account for changes in the specific institution of marriage such as in the category of match makers and in the pattern of female socialization over time. Secondly, I will look at various traditional mechanisms of patriarchal control over women's bodies and their sexuality and the local causes and representations of HIV/AIDS. This will provide a useful backdrop for understanding the debate between partisans and anti-FC advocates as well as the tension surrounding the Moninkim cult today. While doing all these, I will make note of instances of women's agency whenever they crop up in the course of the discussion.

2.7 Traditional political economy of sexuality

It is my contention that to better understand the institutional and social context within which FC takes place in Ejagham society and, by extension, the prospects for internal institutional change, we must necessarily look at the people's changing sexual political economy over time. To do this, we must pay specific attention to female socialization and changes in the institution of FC and marriage. Like in most African communities, female sexuality was (and is still) highly policed while males have always had the cultural license for freedom of sex with multiple partners. Whereas males can take sexual liberties, females are not permitted to exercise the same sexual liberty. In the past, sex was not meant for pleasure but rather for social and biological reproduction. This is the case because having children is considered as a source of prestige, a secured source of labour and a sort of safeguard/social insurance scheme against want at old age. As late as the 1980s, there was supposed to be no premarital intercourse for females. One of my key informants now in his early sixties, Pa Otang Martin recalls that:

> There was no premarital intercourse in those days (meaning for females) but today women are like gravel, they could be kicked and thrown anywhere. They start by dating and may not eventually get married although they might get pregnant. When you came across a girl in those days, she will escape, feeling that intercourse is painful. They used to run away from men. Maturity was determined through at least five menstrual cycles. Even my wife was running away from me for more than two years. I brought gifts, she will not take but the mother was taking. The elder sister informed me she is getting mature and might be tempted to sleep with somebody outside (Interview of 10/03/06, Eyumojock).

The ideal Ejagham woman was expected to be reserved and calm but today "girls are taking unwarranted liberties, they are always going to see 'unknown' friends". Informally, girls in particular and children in general, were taught self-respect, respect for parents and other adults in the community. They were taught critical thinking and critical judgment skills through the medium of riddles and jokes to brainstorm on, interpret and to imbibe the moral lessons behind these riddles and jokes. Formal education was gendered, it was not meant for girls but rather for boys only. Respondents pointed out that there were few educational institutions in those days and that the few available ones were located far away. This suggests that education was meant only "for the strong ones because they needed to trek for long hours and only boys could be up to the task" (Pa Etah, Educator, Interview of 05/07/06, Eyumojock).

Women were and are still considered to be weak. They were (and are) accordingly, supposed to be housekeepers. In this light, they were explicitly trained only for the home, marriage and domestic care. Institutions such as Njumepah and FC provided two avenues for the learning of social survival skills, matrimonial skills and conjugal roles such as respect for one's husband and his authority, talking to him in low tunes and without even looking into his eyes. In other words, women were supposed to be subordinates to men and to remain within the domestic sphere whereas only men were supposed to go out into the public sphere through the formal school system, which provided an avenue for social mobility. Community elders frequently pointed out to me that it was inconceivable in those days that women could be teachers, police officers, magistrates, nurses and even clerks. Any profession within the public sphere was considered to be a male preserve. A related conception in the past in this area was that schools were meant specifically for 'heady' children and children who were sent to school were therefore those who were hated by their parents. They were in the light of this idea, sent there to be beaten and shabbily maltreated by teachers because their parents did not like them. Those who were "liked"- (both boys and girls inclusive), were supposed to be kept at home and pampered and especially, first daughters were to be specially 'honoured' through the Mbogndem tradition and the Moninkim institution.

The formal education of the girl child was (and is) further stifled by the cultural conception that women are non-permanent members of the lineage group. They will eventually get married and therefore are members of their prospective husband's lineages. It follows from this cultural reasoning that educating girls, like allowing them to inherit family property, is a waste of resources because their husbands and their husband's lineage group will reap the benefits. Their bride prices and monies collected during their fattening periods and during the graduation ceremony proper for those who became Moninkims, as we shall see in the next chapter, provided school fees and bridal wealth for their male relatives. We should note here that today the Ejaghams export sisters and import wives, unlike in the past when it was a highly endogamous group in which as Talbot (1912:110) points out "there was nothing repugnant in the marriage of uncle and niece…". In other words, they largely practiced endogamy unlike today when they are practicing exogamy.

Despite this, most young women attribute their lack of marriage opportunities today to the fact that they are related to most of the eligible men and are therefore left at the mercy of 'outsiders' for marriage. It might be said that insiders' awareness of the sexual biographies of these young women is the main obstacle preventing their co-ethnics from soliciting them as wives as well as economic doldrums. One covert strategy of carving a path towards matrimony is to have children with these 'outsiders' who most often do not end up getting married to them. Most of the civil servants who come to the area and with whom they flirt are most often already married although they might not come along with their wives. Many, however, father children there out of wedlock before leaving the area and never continue to provide care for these children once they are gone. From my own observations, patterns of interaction among authochtonous people and the settler population, who are mostly from the Western Grassfield region, suggest that the stigma of 'slave' and free-born families of the colonial times still lingers on in the community. These settlers, some of whom are of former slave descent, are mostly having intimate relationships and inter-marrying only among themselves. Some actually continue to import wives from their home villages while or after going out with girls from the region. Talbot (1912:646) noted that free-born villagers were afraid of the presumed witchcraft powers of slaves who 'in the night banded together and ate out the hearts of the townspeople'. There was the widely held belief that since their own people had traded off the slaves, they were either criminals or witches and wizards and might therefore be a permanent danger. Marriage with people of slave descent was frowned upon and following Röschenthaler (2006:78) 'was considered a source of never-ending misfortune...'. This has reminiscences to getting married to an *osu* (an outcast) in Igbo society (Achebe, 1964). Slaves were socially erased from the realm of citizenship, marriage with free-born villagers, the ownership of important associations such as the Leopard society (Ekpe), barred from participating in prestigious social performances such as the staging of the Etokobiatu, (a warrior night dance which they could dance only on one leg). They were never permitted to take part in its night performances. Slaves were further used as sacrificial lambs for the burial rituals of outstanding men (Rösenchenthaler, 2006:83, 86).

In sum, there is rapid and unprecedented transformation in the sexual economy of the people as economic doldrums has eroded the authority of parents to provide for their children. Poverty has pushed many of the girls to commodify their bodies. Furthermore, male child preference in matters of education, because women are presumed to be passers-by in the family, and the subsequent confinement of women to the private sphere has left them to be economically vulnerable and dependent on men. Simultaneously, the distinction between freeborn and slave families and economic doldrums has left most women in the area with slim possibilities for marriage and political participation.

2.8 Marriage: continuity and change

In traditional Ejagham society, pre-arranged child marriage ('child wife') was one predominant culturally approved mechanism for match making. Upon the birth of a baby girl, a man might stop by the household with firewood and meat to announce his intentions as a prospective husband in his own right or for one of his sons or relatives. If it was approved, he went further and provided the necessary resources for the girl's upbringing from time to time and ended up paying the bride price as a way of culturally legalizing the marriage contract when she became a woman. But the girl, as Talbot (1912:111) points out, still had to decide whether to marry the man or not when she eventually came of age. In some cases, the man could marry her off to another man of his choice. Some women often jilted and rejected the men their parents had contracted them to at tender age when they became mature and native courts often granted them favourable hearings.

For a mature girl, the norm demanded that a man passes through the mother of his prospective wife by symbolically presenting to her a bundle of black plumbs harvested with their stalk intact. This is a symbolism of his marriage intentions. Immediately the mother of his prospective bride saw it, she knew that the man was asking for her daughter's hand in marriage. The mother is the key figure here because "she carried the child in her womb" and is considered to be the gate-keeper, guardian, and confidant of the girl. She will normally inform the suitor if her daughter is already engaged or not, should that be the case. If the mother gave her approval to the proposed union, she then informed her husband who was as of that moment socially mandated to take palm wine from the man and his kinsmen as the "knock door drink"(in pidgin English), called "Okparembi" in the Ejagham language.

Typically, a father will ask his daughter: "Do you accept that I should take something from this man?" If she answered in the affirmative, as was normally expected, he started receiving gifts from him and his kinsmen from then henceforth. Meanwhile before then, his wife would normally have been receiving gifts from both the individual and members of his kinship network since marriage is considered as a union of lineages, families and not as an exclusive affair between two individuals- the bride and the bride groom. If the marriage proposal is turned down because the groom is or members of his family are not considered to be morally upright, or are said to be witches and wizards, they still share the palm wine meant for the occasion together without any malice and disperse quietly.

The cultural expression of intent to marriage in those days did not entitle the man to appropriate the sexuality of his fiancée. This is "unlike today when girls have become like gravel". Several elders gave me to understand that a man could be fiancéed to a woman in those days for as much as three years without having sex with her. "She even slept with her mother on the same bed or behind her back" (Pa Otang, interview of 10/07/06). This implies that the society frowned on premarital sexual intercourse while privileging female chastity, an exotic reality today. Some of my ethnographic friends told me that in extreme cases, a girl even became an outcast if she got pregnant without having achieved the status of Moninkim in those days given the social significance attached to Moninkimhood. Things have however radically changed today.

In the past, mothers and other close relatives were key stakeholders in the matchmaking process. Today however, it is the prospective spouses who are the matchmakers themselves. This usually comes about after an intensive period of dating and even co-habitation during which both parties would have discovered each other in bed. Furthermore, teenage motherhood, usually resulting from unwanted pregnancies, leading to an unprecedented rate of female school drop out in the area, is the order of the day today. This undermines the cultural expectation of female discretion in matters of sexuality. Ironically, the boy who impregnates a girl, even if both are students is never forced to leave school. The national law is against the continuous schooling of a pregnant girl because she will serve as a bad role model to the rest. In other words, she will contaminate them and the school could eventually become a nursery for babies.

Formerly, despite the predominant role of parents in matchmaking, mature women however had some degree of latitude in the negotiation process. Talbot (1912:105-106) gives us to understand that the bride had to accept from the groom "... at least one wedding gift on the distinct understanding that it is received as such" and that this must of necessity be followed by a public announcement to the Chiefs and people after the ringing of the bell. He goes on to explain that "Ekoi women are too fond of inducing suitors to give them as wedding gifts, offerings which they afterwards declare they only regarded in the light of sweet heart presents (love bills) and therefore not binding them to marriage". Following him, women even used to bargain bridal wealth items with their prospective husbands and native courts often heard suits bordering on breach of marriage "contract". This instance like the need for a "child wife" to grow up and validate an earlier marriage contracted by her parents on her behalf, suggests that women at least had some agency in the matrimonial negotiation process and could manipulate it in ways favourable to them. Talbot (1912, 1965) further writes that:

> ...parents occasionally promise their daughters in marriage without the consent of the latter. Such an arrangement could never become binding, however, unless the girl herself agreed to it, when of marriageable age, and accepted the wedding gift (Talbot,1912, 1965)

This was particularly the case, (Talbot,1912, 1965) "when she received no marriage gifts from the man when she came of age". The divorce ritual was pretty simple. This ritual, as elders told me, consisted of a man rubbing white chalk on both hands of his wife. On the other hand, if a woman was eager to free herself from her husband's authority, she could either rake out the fire and pour water on the embers until they die out and simultaneously shave her hair and cover herself with white paint or enforce divorce by exchange. This implies that the woman could offer her husband a slave so as to gain her liberty. White paint carries the symbolism of irreconciliation and irrevocability of the separation of both parties. Talbot (1912:113) recorded the same a hundred years ago. But elders complain today that with the coming of the "White man", the process has rather become too long and demanding as divorce now implies lengthy court procedures and bargaining over the division of property even when women are not traditionally entitled to property ownership.

Furthermore, a woman could equally take advantage of her husband's inability to marry other women to unilaterally seek divorce. Talbot (1912:110) cites the specific case of Njabong of Oban who filed a suit against her husband praying the Native Court to grant her divorce "for his refusal to marry anyone else but herself". This is probably explained by the power and respect wielded by senior wives and the fact that extra wives in the immediate present and later on their children in future will help provide extra labour. In the same light, "An elderly woman has no cause to complain of neglect on the score of her advancing years, for what she loses in youthful attraction is made up by the reverence accorded to age" (Talbot,1912:110). A woman's only objection to her husband sweet hearting with other women as Talbot further points was that "if the latter received his attentions, they ought to do their own share of house and farm work for his family".

In addition to the above, the existence in the past of both pre- and postpartum sexual taboos was another mechanism of sapping the sexual energies and appetites of women and of simultaneously coordinating the sharing of sexual access between co-spouses within a polygynous family set up or of allowing monogamously married men to stray if they could not stay without sex while their wives were breastfeeding. Accordingly, pregnant and lactating women alike had to cede their places to their co-spouses who were not pregnant, menstruating or lactating. Policing women's sexuality further had to do with the transfer of property rights through succession. As a patrilineal group, property rights until quite recently used to be exclusively vested in male issues, although "malelessness" like childlessness is still considered as symbolic of the social and cultural death of an individual among these peoples. The traditional marriage contract is cemented with the payment of the culturally laid down bride price, which today is largely determined by the girl's level of education. Ironically, some parents still prefer to sponsor boys and not girls at school. In the past, it comprised of goods and services like working on the farm as well as the provision of some culturally defined articles in certain quantities.

Later on, bridal wealth changed to the payment of a symbolic quantity of cowries alongside some material goods to both the mother and the father of the bride by the groom and members of his kinship network. However, with the passage of time, urbanization and the subsequent monetization of the economy, bride wealth today largely depends on the level of the bride's level of educational attainment and has been largely monetized. Unlike in the past, it is most often, no longer used to import wives for male members of the kinship group. But rather for outright consumption by the father and the mother of the bride. At the same time, it is becoming more exorbitant, making co-habitation and single-hood more attractive choices for young men and ladies alike. This is the case because even enthusiastic poor young men who might want to get married cannot afford the amounts expected from them as 'marriage fee'. Cameroon is facing economic hardship following devaluation of the CFA franc and structural adjustment. In fact, the persistent ghost of the economic crisis is still hanging over Cameroon's economy and has affected all facets of national life with marriage inclusive. However, the monetary value of bride fees varies between families depending among other factors on the girl's educational level, the man's financial power, the size of the family and the decision of the girl's family. It ranges between 200 and 500USD.

After the settlement of the bridal wealth, the bride is usually rubbed with cam-wood dye and carried shoulder high by her age mates (*ekan*) and those of her husband to the groom's homestead for the culturally, official beginning of her matrimonial career. The payment of the bride price means that the groom is normally not supposed to have sexual intercourse with anyone else. In other words, the man and members of his kinship network have acquired exclusive rights over her sexuality and the children that will eventually be given birth to. Anyone who violates this right will be charged with committing adultery. The people practiced levirate, but today most widows are unwilling to transfer their love to another member of their latc husband's lineage. In retaliation, some are outrightly dispossessed of their husband's property by his kinsmen and even tossed out of the matrimonial home.

Although the institution of FC has remained the most explicit way of policing women's sexuality, other cultural mechanisms existed through which patriarchy policed women's bodies, their sexual and social reproductive labour. These included the existence of female fidelity oaths among the people. Two of such mechanisms which Talbot (1912:105) among others, points to are the swearing of a blood pact between a man and his wife before the juju Njomm Ekatt (The foot juju) which was supposed to keep wives faithful to their husbands. A woman's failure to comply was enforced by an induced illness whose only remedy was confession of her unfaithfulness so as to induce him to retract the curse. A second fidelity ritual also entailed a blood pact before Njomm Aiyung (The blood juju) whose contravention is thought to lead to the instant death of the woman "since her husband's blood will rebel at the first sign of unfaithfulness". If the woman abandons the man without a due refund of the bride price, any children given birth to belong to the man who paid the bride price because paternity is considered to be a social rather than a biological concept among the Ejaghams. She is further expected to be buried in his compound upon her death but in the case of the non-payment of bridal wealth, her corpse will however revert to her natal kin group when she dies.

Although there have been changes today in the people's value and sexual system as attested by rampant youth sexuality and the dominant role of prospective spouses in the matchmaking process, Ejagham women have always had some space within which to negotiate for some degree of agency over their lives. This implies that even within patriarchy there are always spaces for negotiation usefully suggesting that patriarchy does not imply closure, lack of dissent and contestation. A 'child wife' for instance, had to give her consent to a marriage contracted on her behalf by her parents when she eventually came of age. She could of course later on manipulate this clause to her own advantage by jilting and eventually rejecting the man selected for her by her parents in the final analysis. In the next section, I will attempt to account for these changes in the value and sexual organization of the Ejagham and then conclude.

2.9 Factors for change

Change has come about as a result of a complex interplay between endogenous and exogenous factors. These factors include Christianity, formal education and urbanization. This conglomerate of factors has led to the challenge of traditional wisdom. The situation is further compounded by lack of sexual privacy within most households, poverty, and lack of sexual education at home and in the national school system. These factors have heightened the debate between partisans and anti-FC advocates over female sexual morality in the wake of the HIV/AIDS pandemic.

Ejagham society like any other 'traditional society' has not remained static over time. Change, in the view of elders, has led to the collapse of the moral economy and fabric of their society, in which case the young generation are challenging both traditional wisdom and the authority of their elders as outdated. One evidence of this challenge is that the sexual knowledge which adults thought was limited to them-which they secretly guarded, mystified and were the custodians of- is now common knowledge. Madam Ayum Mary, 29 years old told me like many others that: "Children are becoming so arrogant because what you are doing, they too are doing it. They do not respect their elders." This means that children are having sexual intercourse and deriving pleasure from it like adults and therefore feel that they are on the same echelon with their elders. The past was characterized by blind obedience, subservience and subordination to the authority of adults no matter whether this authority was based on reason or not.

The coming of the "Whiteman" as epitomized by the so-called modern religion and the formal school system have all led to changes in the orientation of the present generation and they are increasingly questioning the wisdom of the past that was based on tradition. The 'Whiteman' here is used in a paradoxical sense among the old and the young generation. To the old, it represents anything believed to be both disruptive and repugnant: the contestation of traditional value systems such as FC, modern religion, the critical spirit acquired from formal education, claims over children and individual rights, television and pornographic films which display men and women kissing and making love, seductive dressing styles among females and in fact chaos and disorder, a contrast between traditional ideals and actual behavioural practices among the youths, etc. But to the youths, it is a short hand for modernity epitomized by freedom to question everything by the youths and the ability to make personal decisions and choices, to be free from the shackles of tradition as an aberrant past.

The acquisition of scientific knowledge has dealt a serious blow to traditional values and mechanisms of social control. Children are increasingly claiming their rights.

> "Children are trying to compete with their mothers. A child will tell you openly that you are not my God" (Nkoyo, Interview of 27/03.06, Eyumojock).

The main factor for change from the stand point of the elders who are the custodians of tradition is the presumed uncritical adoption of ''foreign values'' which children have copied and replicated through the watching of television, Western pornographic films, magazines and from the internet.

> Careless civilization is misleading children today as they watch foreign models on TV, copy and practice it and all houses have consequently become rotten. In the past, if papa was listening to a gramophone and saw you besides him, you were in for very serious trouble, but today, children watch men and women holding each other [kissing] on TV screens, copy and replicate it (Pa Otang, interview of 10/03/06).

To him, some aspects of modernity are incompatible with traditional values in matters of sexuality as children are increasingly taking sexual liberties, a thing they could not do in the past. Yelibi et al (nd) quoted by Nyamongo (1995:45) comment on the erosion of traditional patterns of sexual behaviour in Africa in these words:

> The rapid economic development of the sixties and seventies, as well as the continuous process of urbanization and modernization, have caused deep upheavals in the (socio)cultural life, and a major change has been the loss of traditional values. Their weakening, the presence of westernized patterns of life, the precarious conditions for women, and the men's attitude towards multiple sexual partners have exposed large social groups to sexually [transmitted] disease (Yelibi et al, nd, cf. Nyamongo, 1995:45).

A close reading of Talbot's (1912) seminal work on the Ejaghams against the grain offers some clues on the commodification of sexuality. It seems to suggest that the free fall in moral values epitomized by flirtation and prostitution among young people which adults condemn and point to it as one of the upshots of modernity ("The Whiteman") today is rather a reflection of the traditional norms of sweet heart presents in a mercantile capitalist society based on profit motive. Money, material goods and other favours are in exchange for sexual gratification. During my field stay, women in casual conversations often made mockery of men who had been tossed away by their paramours for failing to regularly pay their love bills, usually in favour of more financially capable and open-handed rivals. This state of things should therefore be seen as the very vestige of a past feminine culture in a new and more risky context with the ghost of the HIV hanging over everyone's head.

Another push factor for the presumed fall in moral standards and the subsequent disintegration of the traditional system of moral control is urbanization and the monetization of the economy. Whereas urbanization has led to the weakening of control and supervision over individuals by the members of their community, education, material wealth and no longer land ownership, membership of a secret society or merely being a free-born has become the main determinant factor for status. The elders who are usually poor because they lack marketable skills and have thus been relegated to the background and their authority is being constantly challenged by wealthy youths and mobile actors such as traders and drivers who are constantly passing in and out of the region. Apart from changing social relationships, it has led to a fall in moral standards as most parents have lost their authority partly because of their inability to provide their children with the basic necessities of life in the face of the unsparing economic doldrums that Cameroon and most African countries are going through. At the same time, competition among girls because of their presumed "madness with fashion", has heightened. And this presumed mad quest for the most fashionable things as a sign of modernity has its consequences for both sexual and reproductive health as the use of bodies amidst abject poverty has become the means to achieve this aim.

To live with the times like their peers elsewhere who are often their revered models, many young women have recruited a string of male sex partners in a bid to be able to capture the necessary material resources for their livelihoods from them. Most of the men and particularly the young men with whom I exchanged viewpoints often used two interesting idioms to describe women in general: "elephant meat" and "national cake". The former compares women to the flesh of an elephant which is so large that one individual cannot eat it all alone and there is often the need to share with other people as the people's tradition demand. The latter implies that state resources never get finished. Interpreted in terms of sexuality, these metaphors both imply among other things that, a woman cannot belong to one man alone. Every male who is capable needs to have sex with her and as many times as possible but she will remain the same. This is further buttressed by the fact that they see a woman's vagina as a 'silent object' which can be appropriated, without anyone knowing and which no one can effectively police. Having multiple partners among men here is one mechanism of constructing and at the same time, affirming one's masculinity, no matter the risk involved.

In the face of abject poverty, ways of selling sex by women have become the order of the day. Most single women have multiple sexual partners because of their anxiety to capture much needed livelihood resources. At the same time, they lack the power to negotiate safe sex. As a result of this, there is infrequent use of condoms, except to avoid pregnancy and venereal diseases. Infection with venereal diseases is reported to be partly responsible for abdominal pains, a widespread disease among most women in this community. This lack of knowledge about sexual and reproductive health issues is further accentuated by lack of communication between parents and children. This culture of silence in matters of sexual and reproductive health has led to lack of knowledge of both body care and body function among young girls, resulting in unwanted pregnancies, illegal abortions and an alarming rate of female school dropout.

The cumulative effect is single motherhood and one parent families. Evidence adduced from school heads in the area showed that in the 2005/2006 academic year, two primary school pupils and eight secondary school students from three of the existing educational institutions dropped out of school because of unwanted pregnancies. Most young men who are conscious of the sexual biographies of some of these young girls are unwilling to get married to them. In fact, most of the young girls here are teenage mothers abandoned to themselves by the men with whom they had babies. Only a minority of cases return back to school after 'maternity leave' as most parents in this community when confronted with the pregnancy of a daughter cease sponsoring her at school. They tend to perceive the education of a girl as a sheer waste of both valuable resources and time partly because women are considered as strangers within the family, "another person's property" and for fear that they might get pregnant along the way. This means that it is economically unwise to spend on the education of the girl child because she will eventually get married into another lineage. The same justification is given for why they are most often sidelined when it comes to property inheritance: they will take the lineage property and it will become their husband's own and in the eventuality of divorce, everything will be lost. This has partly contributed to the higher rate of illiteracy among women in this community.

Conclusion

In this chapter, I have examined the gendered political economy of the Ejagham region through the prism of the impact of various economic shifts and contractions on their social structure and value system, particularly the development of 'prostitution' as an adaptive system for women's personal accumulation. I have argued that the articulation of multiple modes of production- capitalism and kin-ordered modes have created contestation and that patriarchy as a social field of power is at the juncture of these two modes of production because capitalism never destroyed but rather worked through kinship mode of production. In protest, women have moved out of the patriarchal orbit for alternative ways of life such as 'prostitution' thereby creating conflicts between generations and sexes. Patriarchy works through both the kinship and capitalist modes of production but is at the same time, contentious. This analysis also shows that the people's historic contact with outside groups has led to the spread of new values and diseases with HIV/AIDS inclusive given the high mobility that characterizes the region. At the same time, the people's trans-border location and interaction with kinship groups in Nigeria allows for easy border crossings so as to circumvent a law against FC in either Cameroon or Nigeria. The dynamics of the Ejagham sexual political economy shows changes in the matchmaking process from close relatives usually parents to the prospective spouses to be and the increase in eroticized relationships. The advent of the HIV/AIDS pandemic reinvigorated debates over female sexuality and the need for control, a debate that led to increased tension over the institutions of Moninkim and FC and to conflict between generations. Pro-FC advocates pointed to the ritual cuttings as a useful 'native' antidote and solution to the pandemic while their opponents pointed out that FC could lead to the spread of the HIV.

In the next chapter, I turn my attention to the chasm between traditional and modern forms of rule given the conflicting landscape of institutions in which the Ejaghams find themselves today.

CHAPTER THREE

TRADITIONAL FORMS OF RULE AND CONFLICT WITH MODERN AUTHORITY

In the previous chapter, I have demonstrated that the Ejagham region has historically been connected to the outside world leading to constant changes in the people's values and practices, to conflicts between generations and sexes, and to the spread of both new ideas and diseases with HIV/AIDS inclusive. These changes are a reflection of the contradictions between the capitalist and kin-oriented modes of production. They are further reflected in the conflicting landscape and contradictions of the traditional and modern authority systems in place today, a situation in which tradition is sometimes simultaneously appropriated and contested. This is my preoccupation in this chapter.

I will capture changes and contestation in the Ejagham's gendered socio-cultural institutions over time. This is partly the result of intergenerational conflict, the clash between modern and traditional systems of authority and prestige, traditional religion and Christianity and shift from membership in various socio-cultural institutions of traditional society to urban jobs and education as arenas for the acquisition of status in contemporary society. These institutions include chieftaincy and a dense network of male secret societies such as Ekpe, Obhassi-Njom, Angbu, and Obhon, and female secret societies such as Moninkim and FC- the very instantiation of traditional womanhood and constitutive component of the patriarchal complex, Njumepah, Njumepah-atu and Mbogdem- another institution for first born daughters like Moninkim.

3.1 Traditional forms of rule and authority

In this section, I will in the light of my conflict-oriented notion of culture, examine some traditional forms of rule and authority systems among the Ejaghams that are most salient to my study. For an extensive study on the gamut of their institutions, cult agencies and dissemination histories, see Ruel (1969), Bonchuck (1997), Röschenthaler (2006, 2007) among others. Generally, these gendered institutions are responsible for socialization, social control, social hierarchy and the maintenance of social order. They include masculine institutions such as the institution of Chieftaincy, Ekpe (the Leopard society), Obhassi-Njom, Angbu, and Obhon and the female institutions of Ekpah also called Njumepah, Njumepah-atu, Mbogdem and the Moninkim cult. These institutions are interrelated as they all assure social and moral regulation despite the fluid gender divide, as I shall demonstrate later on. They provide a public arena for the enactment of social life and form the very hub of social activities. They therefore form the framework for understanding social mobility and social hierarchies between 'free-born' and slave lineages and simultaneously provide spaces for the construction and playing out of both masculinity and femininity among the Ejaghams. However, other social groups also exist in the community. While describing these institutions, I will simultaneously, take on issues of world sense and cosmology and highlight instances of conflict and contestation as they crop up along the lines. These institutions do not only assure harmony in the regulation of interpersonal relationships but equally reflect the people's world view, specifically, their relationship with the supernatural realm. This is probably the reason why they are usually categorized by scholars as 'secret societies' because they involve initiation rites.

3.2 Male Institutions

3.2. 1. Chieftaincy

Ejagham society during the pre-colonial and colonial period was a centralized kingdom but today various Ejagham communities are decentralized, segmentary polities (Bonchuck, 1997) under the leadership of a Chief. Chieftaincy is hereditary and only sons of the soil, not *nsung*, members of slave families, have the right to lay claim to this institution whenever it becomes vacant. Upon the death of an Ejagham Chief, members of the founding clans decide to choose someone among themselves to succeed him and to become the next *Ntuifam*. That individual following Ojong (2005:46) must be of good moral standing, show respect for everyone, especially the elders of the community, must be intelligent and demonstrate both tact and wisdom in solving problems in the community. He must also be literate as today's modern administration demands penmanship skills, specifically the ability to read speeches in public. It is these characteristics of changing times, particularly literacy, that led to a six year long succession conflict between various lineages in Otu village when the throne became vacant.

Following the death of the pioneer Chief of Otu village, His Royal Highness Chief Emmanuel Nyok in September 1992, two factions cropped up in the village and competed for the throne. Traditionalists wanted rotation of the throne in keeping with tradition. Modernists on the other hand, wanted that the new leadership should be educated. This is a clear instance of contestation, conflict between modernity and tradition. They invoked the qualities mentioned above. Unlike in the past, elections were conducted and Mr. Ayamba Ojong Ita was declared successful. The external elites did not deem him fit for the task since he is not literate. On the basis of this, they protested that the elections be repeated, not with the entire population as the electorate but rather among the ten elders and kingmakers of the village secret society, Mgbe. The Seniour Divisional and Divisional Officer oversaw the conduct of the elections and Chief Ojong Moses Ntui emerged victorious with six votes in May 2006. The loser camp boycotted various village functions such as participation in secret societies and cleansing rites and threats multiplied to outdo enemies using poison and or witchcraft. Ekpe was turned apart, the administration failed to reconcile both factions. Of late however, the Chief of Chiefs, Ntuifam Arrey of Ossing was able to broker an uneasy truce through a public reconciliation conference in May 2006 during which both camps pledged to collaborate with each other. The administration subsequently installed Ntuifam Ojong Moses Ntui, a retired civil servant as Chief of Otu bringing the conflict to "an end."

Before his initiation and subsequent enthronement, the prospective Chief is presented to the modern administration. The Divisional Officer or his representative usually installs him and he works in close collaboration with the modern administration as an auxiliary. The co-optation of the Chief into the postcolonial administrative set up has tremendously diminished his prestige and status. Chiefs often find themselves in landscapes of conflicting institutions as some individuals tend to invoke modern law in the resolution of conflicts of interest and no longer tradition, as was the case in the past. The prospective Chief is subsequently initiated into all the secret societies in the village since he holds the highest office in the traditional governing system.

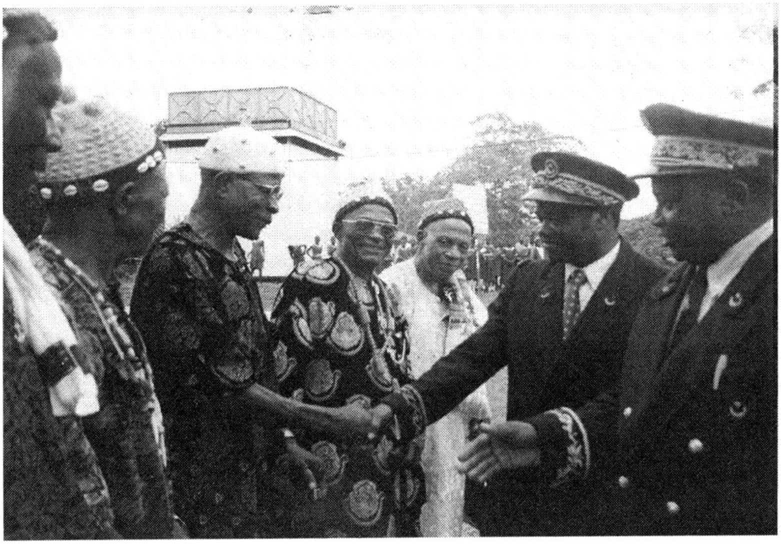

Fig. 3 Ejagham Chiefs with the Seniour Divisional and Divisional Officer

The Chief rules in collaboration with the village council (nju-Essere), the quarter heads (Abhonatui), the various family/lineage heads (Nne Nkwi Ndephenju) in the village and with the Ajom Etek (divinities). He is an intermediary between the living and the dead. He administers law and order through social institutions such as Ekpeh, Obhassi-Njom, and Njumepah and is directly answerable to the national modern administration. In the colonial and early pre-colonial days, they served as tax collectors for the administration. At times, he is assisted by the Regent Chief, especially when he is a civil servant. These Regent Chiefs are usually referred to as "administrative Chiefs", "Government Chiefs" and the Chief himself as the traditional Chief partly showing the erasure of their powers as well as the conflict between modern and traditional authority systems. The Chief, unlike in the Western Grassfield region of Cameroon where Chiefs still have exclusive right to marriage by capture as a mark of their distinctive status within society, is an equal among equals. He lacks power to enforce decisions and might not even be able to enforce a ban against FC as I shall argue later on in this work. In other words, he neither commands any special respect nor authority despite his high office. He can hardly "structure the possible field of action of others"(Foucault, 1984:428). He is however the custodian of the lores and customs of his people through the intermediary of a dense network of institutions to which I shall now turn my attention.

3.2.2 Ekpe

Ekpe popularly known as the Leopard society is designated differently among the different peoples of the border region including Southwest Cameroon. Among the Efiks, it is called Ekpe, Mgbe (Boki), Mgbe or Nyamkpe (Ejagham), the Mambila and Kaka people, call it SO but herein, I will mostly use the more popular name of Ekpe like most of my informants, except where necessary.

Membership into the Ekpe society entails, among others, several weeks of ritual initiation and sexual abstinence for as much as six months so as to instil the qualities of perseverance and stoicism in the initiate. However, today prospective initiates who reside out of the village can opt for a compressed syllabus into the society. This is the case with most top government functionaries who are appropriating these traditional institutions and status arena in this modern epoch by obtaining titles and ranks within these societies. The loosely woven costume of its members is decorated with large circles and other geometric forms that interpret the leopard's natural marks. There are conflicting accounts as to the origin of Ekpe. Informants told me that Ekpe was discovered by a woman while cultivating her farm and that upon her return home, she told her husband who later connived with other men and killed her to prevent her from revealing the secret to other women. The men then hijacked the association from them and obliged the women to create something similar for themselves called Njumepah. Through the slave trade, the Leopard society spread to Cuba among some Afro-Cuban groups and has been the object of cultural exhibitions in Europe and the United States of America.

To acquire membership, the prospective initiate has among other things to provide large quantities of food, limps of meat and money to the elders of the society before his initiation proper. It was (and is) therefore a type of social insurance scheme against want. It has a hierarchical structure with particular grades analogous to classes in the formal school system reflecting differential statuses, roles, rights but common duties and obligations. Descendants of slave origin could only gain membership within the lower ranks of Ekpe and the association's runners, executioners and other agents were deployed to discipline and maintain control over slaves (Röschenthaler, 2006 quoting G.I Jones). Some of the key roles and statuses within this hierarchical society among the Ejagham people of Southwest Cameroon in descending hierarchical order include: Iyumbah

(Seseko), Ekunimbeh, Ayumbeh, Ekumbi and the Obongo grade of neophytes.

The members of the Ekpe society use sign language, *nsibidi* for conducting their affairs partly as a mechanism to ensure that the secrets of the society remain among its members except during the Nkanda ("open door") session when non-initiates are present in their midst. The Nkanda juniour status group of Ekpe was responsible for the opening of the floor during the outdooring ceremony of a Moninkim. *Nsibidi*, the Ekpe society's secret communication code is the pictographic reduction into writing of sign language, where signs stand for ideas. Initially, it was considered sacred, known and closely guarded by the top echelon of Ekpe and was not to be divulged to junior members. It was further used to detect non-members and served as a secret code for transmitting love messages. White ethnographers considered it as part of decorative art (Sterk, 1998:116-117). This same pictographic writing usually connoting love between husband and wife was used to decorate the special calabash dish called *okpere* from which a Moninkim ate food as a mark of her distinctive status.

Ekpe was, and is still the secret police, the Supreme Court and the highest avenue for the adjudication of disputes in traditional Ejagham society. With the coming of modernity however, Ekpe's authority is at contest as some individuals often resort to modern institutions of law enforcement. At times, they are sent back to Ekpe. As the government of the people; it assured social control when there were no gendarmes and policemen, when modern institutions of governance were not in existence. It summons and tries defaulters, places injunctions on disputed pieces of land until the conflict of ownership is resolved. Furthermore, it assures social distribution and is like a social insurance scheme with resonances to FC and the Moninkim institution. Some people had no children and membership of Ekpe provided them with an opportunity to get shares during the sharing of items such as meat. It further ensures communal security as a killed bua snake is still brought to the Ekpe hall for everyone to ensure that its bile is removed and publicly disposed of in a pit toilet. This is because it is poisonous and can kill somebody instantaneously. In traditional Ejagham society, a killed leopard was abandoned on the spot in the forest and provided young men with an avenue for the enactment of masculinity as they had to carry it on their shoulders into the village and ensure that women do not lay ownership claim to it by touching it.

Members of Ekpe equally animate at the funerals of their dead members. They are supposed to be fed by the family of the bereaved each morning and evening for the seven days during which they are normally supposed to mourn their departed member. Feeding them ("cooking Mgbe") during a funeral is one way of paying back whatever the deceased consumed during his stay within the society. Ekpe is therefore reminiscent to a thrift and loan society. Even the progenies of a 'sleeping' Ekpe member are under obligation to reciprocate by repaying what their late father consumed as an absentee member of the society. This same rule is applied by members of the Njumepah female society, as we shall see in a moment. This traditional pattern of reciprocity is also displayed by the traditional obligation to circumcise, confine and publicly celebrate the graduation ceremony of a first daughter. As I shall demonstrate later on, this culture of obligatory reciprocity is still fuelling the continuation of FC among some segments of the local population, although it is gradually dying out in most villages. As the highest policy making organ, Ekpe supersedes any other institution in Ejagham land and symbolizes the group's power, authority and physical strength. As the 'backbone of the indigenous Ejagham political order'….. its judicial function approximates the European notion of law courts whereas its executive function could be compared to modern day governmental departments'(Bonchuk,1997:67). Ekpe's efficacy has however been undermined by the modern authority system in place. For instance, some cases are never referred to Ekpe today but rather to the modern court for abjudication. Apart from its political, legal, status symbol and recreational functions, it also performs a pre-eminent role during the celebration of the funeral of any of its members. Apart from guarding the Moninkim maiden during her confinement, as we shall see later on in this chapter, Ekpe formally certified the Moninkim graduate by offering her a staff of authority to connote her newly acquired status and role within her community. Ekpe also ensures gender equality by forbiding men from beating their wives.

3.2.3 Obhassi-njom

The Obhassi-njom association like other cult agencies and associations detects cases of witchcraft among the Ejaghams. In the worldview of the Ejagham people, witchcraft provides an alternative "native" explanatory model. It offers explanations for phenomena such as certain illnesses with infertility and excessive bleeding during the circumcision ceremony of an initiate inclusive. It is further used even to compel an initiate to circumcise or to oblige her parents to circumcise and organize a graduation feast for the people during the outdooring of his daughter. It is therefore deployed as one of several mechanisms "of tactical power" (Wolf, 2006) to ensure reciprocity.

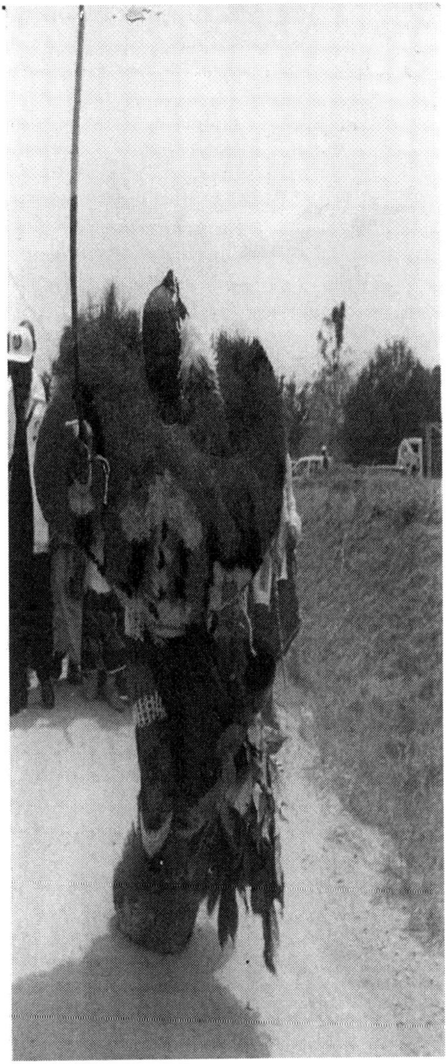

Fig. 4 The Ekpe masquerade in action

Etymologically, Obhassi-njom comes from two Ejagham words, "Obhassi" meaning "God is the creator of everything in the universe and anything created by God can be used for both negative and positive purposes". Obhassi-njom in the widest social sense is the god of protection against all kinds of imaginable dangers. Its function is to investigate, detect and expose witches and wizards, forecast and prevent malevolent acts that have already occurred or are still to occur. It has the power of clairvoyance. Individuals equally consult the institution for their own personal problems and to ensure their personal and family well-being because it is believed that the institution has mystical powers to cure and to protect using elements from the fauna and botanical universe of the people. These elements include herbs, barks of trees, roots for the preparation of various concoctions for therapy, for the fortification of members of the institution and for preparing the masquerade for their activities.

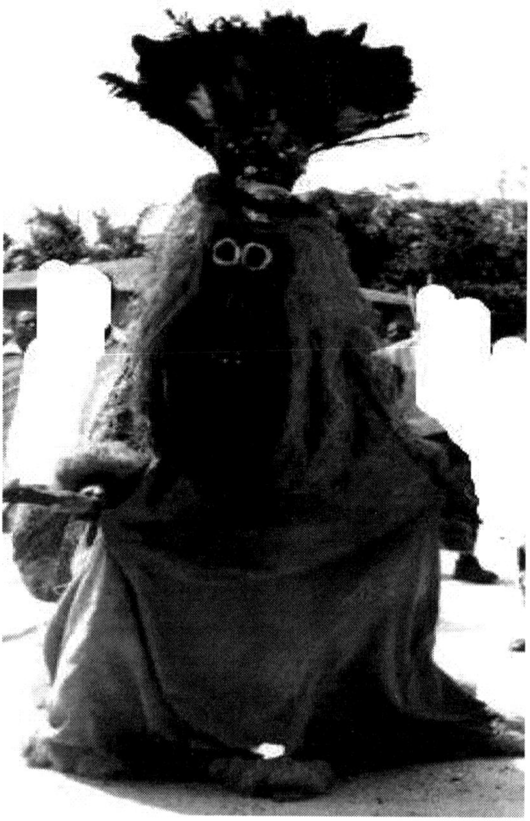

Fig. 5 An Obhasoin njom masquerade in action

The face of the Obhassi-njom masquerader (*Ebhu-Njom*) is decorated with varied objects of symbolism. Dressed in a black overflowing gown, only the eyes, hands and the legs of the masquerader can be seen. On the head are the feathers of the *nku ndap* bird, which is said to represent memory, wisdom, clairvoyance and intelligence. On the forehead are egg shells, mixed with the paste of a certain undisclosed concoction and the wooden statute of a baby. Both the egg shell and the pastry concoction serve as food for Obhassi-njom whereas the carved wooden statute of a baby symbolizes Obhassi-njom's love, care and protection of innocent babies, ignorance, purity of motive and neutrality, which marks the beginning of every investigation. The head is littered with fibres meant for decoration. It wears a tie made of leopard skin, denoting power and authority.

Membership is open to all mature males who are judged to have respect for the elders and the customs and traditions of the people and who are capable of paying the initiation fee. This entails the ability to provide large quantities of food, four legs of bush meat, a goat, plantains and palm wine to the members. Although I was constantly told that membership is open to every male who is considered to be morally upright, Ojong (2005:49), expunges this view by maintaining that the trumpeter, the soldier and the interpreter are co-opted by the Chief of the institution whereas all other members are selected. Initiation partly entails participation in a blood pact during which prospective initiates are scarified and they mix and consume each other's blood vowing in the process to keep the secrecy of the inner workings of the institution from non-members. The bloodletting and exchange that this initiation entails can facilitate the transmission of HIV. Initiation, which used to take as much as two weeks, ends with a ritual dance in the course of which the neophytes dance around the knife of Obhassi-njom which is placed at the centre of the hall. The egg of a locally bred chicken is attached to the handle of the knife and a pasty concoction smeared on the handle. The individual who picks the knife goes straight into the sacred forest and upon his return after cutting the Obhassi-njom tree *Eti njom*, he becomes the masquerader.

During its performances, Obhassi-njom holds a knife (*Essome-njom*) in the right hand and a woven basket in the left hand. The knife is believed to be a telephone for the transmission of information from the spiritual realm through telepathy whereas the basket serves as the telephone receiver. The transmitted information is made public through the interpreter, *Ossame-njom*. The masquerade lingers around the village and from time to time, goes into a trance once it has received information about what is under investigation or about something that is going to happen in the future. Although members claim equality in terms of role and status within the society, it is hierarchically organized. Following Ojong (2005:50-53), there are five interrelated statuses and roles within Obhassi-njom. At the top of the hierarchy is the Chief, *Ebhangne-Ne-njom*, the masquerader, the soldier, *Agune-njom*, and the trumpeter called *Eru-njom.*

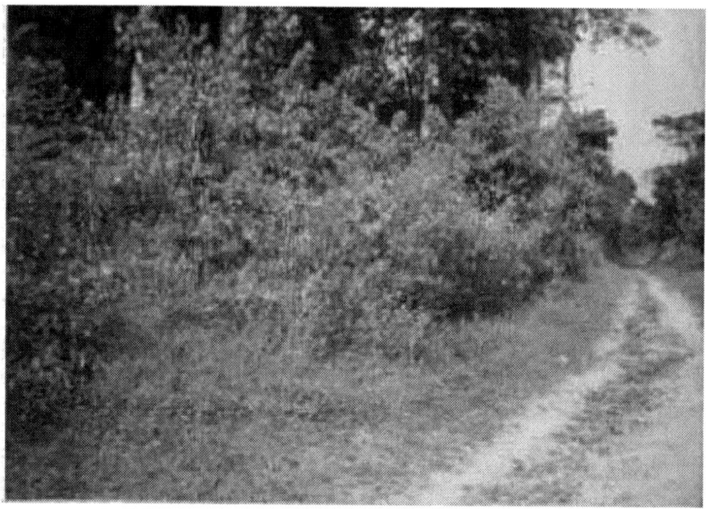

Fig. 6 Obhassi-njom sacred forest

Although an entirely male institution, a girl child, usually the daughter of one of its members however plays a symbolic role within the society during public performances. The Ma-njom, as she is called, plays the symbolic role of "wife" to Obhassi-njom. She can be seen clapping and singing to impress him whenever he is dancing in the course of his public performances. Her role ends whenever she starts menstruating. Menstrual blood is considered as symbolizing pollution and seems to suggest why she vacates her symbolic office at this point in time. It is said to be incompatible with the ritual purity of the Obhassi-Njom masquerade secret society.When she eventually starts menstruating, she goes out and shouts at the top of her voice: "Nti Egbe oh, Nti Egbe oh". This is considered to be a tacit invitation to prospective suitors to come forward and ask for her hand in marriage.

The institution further serves as an intermediary between the people and their ancestors since the sacred forest is believed to be the abode of the gods. It ensures the protection of people and property against contagious magic and regulates the use of the forest by conserving the sacred forest for future generations.

3.2.4 Angbu

Angbu is another masculine, security organization and an agent of moral restitution and social order. Initiation into this mystical society was compulsory for all Ejagham males. Upon attending maturity, the members of Angbu might pay a surprise visit to an individual whom they deem courageous enough and morally upright. The initiation proper entails a very long and elaborate process because the individual is entering the cycle of manhood. Before bringing the individual(s) to the ceremonial hall, he/they would have been seriously tortured. According to one of my key informants, Nkom, (35), "they take you there through torture and you are treated as a criminal. After this torture, the initiation proper starts piecemeal during which the novice is shown a few things at a time". This torture undertaken by the Priest is meant to imbibe in the novices, stoicism. On the next day, they are taken to the bush for the second phase of the initiation ceremony. They are secluded during the two-week time span as nobody apart from those carrying out the initiation see the neophytes. The masquerade will constantly be dancing around the hall during the entire procedure while outside, men will be dancing and feasting all through the two weeks. On the final day when the initiates are exposed to the public, they would have gone through the initiation and accordingly acquired the status of full-fledged members of Angbu.

This mysterious society is used to chase away evil spirits and ghosts from disturbing the peace and serenity of the community. It exhumes the corpses of troublesome individuals and burns them up publicly using herbs so as to prevent them from coming out as spirits and disturbing others. In the recent past among the Ejagham, tradition demanded that every corpse be buried with protective herbs either placed on the chest of the individual or the liquid from the herbs squeezed into the eye of the dead to prevent the individual from coming out as a ghost. This is in consonant with the Ejagham world view of reincarnation. Those who refused were warned and a predetermined punishment laid down in advance for the family in question in case the ghost of their dead kinsman is seen lingering around. There was controversy in Ekok in August 2006 when the son of a reputed witch refused her dead mother from being smeared with the herbs to prevent her from coming out. The adoption of Christianity is undermining the role of institutions such as Angbhu.

The people believe in reincarnation and to forestall this most corpses are smeared with medicines to prevent the individual from coming back to life as a ghost. While the adoption of Christianity has led to the waning of this practice, some individuals are still continuing with it. My ethnographic friends constantly made mention to me of one particularly wealthy individual in Eyumojock who knew he was going to die and accordingly, dug a hole in his cocoa plantation where he reserved 10 million Cfa (approximately 200.000 USD), so that when he eventually dies, he will come out as a ghost, collect that money and begin a new life elsewhere. A soothsayer unveiled the secret to his family, who decided to place medicines on his corpse before burial so as to prevent him from resuscitating and they then went to his cocoa farm and collected the money. Members of Angbu also recover debts or ensure that fines are paid.

The members of Angbu therefore act as traditional bailiffs, soldiers, the executive branch of Ejagham traditional government, cleansing the society of ghosts and evil spirits as well as collecting unpaid debts when the indebted party has refused to pay off.

3.2.5 Obhon

This is a wrestling group which is usually made up of age mates, *ekan*. It is therefore one alternative arena for the achievement of status and for the simultaneous enactment of masculinity. The test for membership comprised of the demonstration of maturity in terms of strength and stoicism. Before a group of initiates enter the hall where everybody is assembled, other peer groups that are already full-fledged members are already present, waiting to challenge them to a wrestling match and once they show evidence of manhood and strength by putting up a brave fight with them, they definitely gain admission into Obhon. And once a group of individuals are conferred membership, everything remains social. They henceforth come out on ceremonial occasions, demonstrate strength, dance and perform some traditional rites. They usually eat together and make merry. One of their aims is to entertain people during various ceremonies. In traditional Ejagham society, wrestling was a fashionable artistic undertaking and provided one avenue to the achievement of masculinity.

Through Obhon, the Ejagham construct masculinity in terms of physical strength which is partly displayed through wrestling. Obhon equally provides entertainment and offers social support as members commune together to celebrate the dead ceremony of their members or on invitation.

This far, I have described and shown instances of conflict, contestation and change within various male institutions. Membership into these groups and one's rank marked out a freeborn Ejagham man from those of slave ancestry. I have further shown that they provided a traditional avenue for social mobility and for the construction and subsequent playing out of masculinity. Membership in various secret societies was the badge of ethnicity, maturity and masculinity- gendered masculine knowledge which distinguished adults from children within the tribal social structure. But today, modern jobs and education are undermining these traditional status criteria that depended on membership in various associations. Despite change, there is the selective appropriation of tradition and modernity by village elites showing the co-existence of both tradition and modernity at the same time. The coming of modernity has led to a new form of social stratification as shown by the supposed falling moral standards among the youths and their lack of respect for elders. However, given the complementary role played by both male and female institutions in Ejagham society in the maintenance of social order and harmony such as the provision of an avenue for the adjudication of conflicts, I will turn my attention onto the female institutions in the next section. One general characteristic of these institutions, be they exclusively male or female, is their use of masquerades as a symbol of their mystical powers and presence.

3.3 Female Institutions

Females have various groups within which they stage out their lives such as mutual help groups through which they share their troubles or pull their resources or labour together on a rotatory basis, working from one individual's farm to the other or have their collective labour hired by somebody in need. However, the main cultural group in charge of female socialization is called Ekpah or Njumepah. In what follows, I will deal with the Moninkim association, the very instantiation of commercialized patriarchy and its entanglement with wider patriarchal social fields, Njumepah or Ekpah, Ekpah-atu and the Mbogdem association of first daughters.

3.3.1 The custom of 'fixing women' and the Monikim Cult

Until the 1980s before FC became a rather contentious issue, both males and females were traditionally circumcised among the Ejaghams. But unlike FC, male circumcision was and has remained a banal process locally without any socio-cultural ceremonies. This culture therefore seems to 'honour' only womanhood. This is perhaps explained by the high premium paid to women's fertility which ensures the continuity of the society through biological and social reproduction.

One other bodily modification practice which is still common among the people is the existence of facial marks for both sexes. These facial marks are said to serve as lineage, tribal and family identity, as beauty marks, and for magico-religious purposes: severing an individual's link with the spiritual world and protection against malevolent forces. Some of the ways of 'honouring' females included the institution of the Moninkim cult which preceded FC and the Ngbogha-ndem association which like Moninkim consisted of being a first-born daughter, circumcision, strict seclusion and an elaborate graduation ceremony.

The circumcision of both sexes has traditionally been the norm among the Ejagham of Southwest Cameroon and of Southeastern Nigeria until now that FC is done in secrecy and without the usual pomp and pageantry of the 1960s and 1970s. A complex and intertwined set of beliefs about the human body, its anatomy and functioning has sustained both institutions over time. Both male and female circumcisions are considered to be functional to the social structure of Ejagham society although only the latter is marked by elaborate celebration. Most women with whom I spoke categorically stated that they will feel uneasy having intercourse with a man with an uncircumcised penis. On their part too, the men still see male circumcision as normal. It seems that from the very beginning, FC was an imitation of male circumcision but eventually came to carry far more importance as demonstrated by the ceremonies and rituals surrounding it unlike male circumcision, which has remained something banal over time.

My ethnographic friends reported that male circumcision took place for reasons of aesthetics, gender identity so that a child should resemble his father and above all, suggesting that it has always been done because an uncircumcised penis is inconceivable. Are these same reasons valid and to the same extent as they apply to FC? The complex body of beliefs and practices sustaining FC include: tradition, aesthetics, moral considerations and ethnomedical health concepts. I shall now examine these reasons one at a time to demonstrate how they cohere and make sense within the cultural prism of the Ejaghams before describing the bodily mutilation ritual and its significance. I highlight changes and contestation of the ritual along the lines.

The maintenance of tradition and, by extension, a specific cultural identity is the strongest reason proffered by partisans of FC. They often point to their ancestors and presume to be respecting what the latter had laid down and had been doing on females for centuries. This group of adherents see tradition as cast in stone, as unchanging despite changing circumstances. This is contrary to the views of progressives among them who ridicule this 'blind' adherence to tradition and point to modernity while casting FC as the very vestige of a primeval past. Most elderly men and women with whom I spoke on the subject constantly invoked tradition to justify the ritual cuttings. However, this tradition should rather be understood as part of a much larger complex cultural and continuum. They want to look like their ancestors, perhaps explaining why uncut women who died were cut in the past before their burial probably so that their ancestors should be able to recognize them in the spiritual world.

We should note the people's belief in reincarnation and the transitory nature of death as I pointed out earlier. Simply stated, to get to the world of the ancestors, an individual should, among other things, have to look like the ancestors and to look like them means being circumcised. One aged woman justified FC to her daughter, who was circumcised in 2002 despite the ongoing anti-FC debates within the HIV/AIDS context in these words: "My own mother did not leave me like that, so I cannot leave you like that"(meaning with your clitoris intact). Status anxiety is at play here. Her mother is worried of her not conforming to the laid down standards of femininity, success and therefore fears that she will lose the respect and consideration of the others. According to Anjezza (2005) quoting Albanny (2004:2) status anxiety is the longing to be somebody, to be within the mainstream, for respect, attention and visibility for fear of social erasure and invisibility as failure will lead to a negative self-image and uncertainty.

Another reason informing the ritual cutting of FC is the need to preserve gender identity and feminine personhood. A cardinal assumption of Ejagham theosophy is the belief that human beings are bisexual animals. Following this, it is assumed that males have a feminine organ, the shield on the tip of the penis, whereas females have the clitoris, a male organ. Curiously enough, this society either defines individuals as masculine or feminine with no group willing to identify with the other. In other words, there is no third gender in the Ejagham worldview. For women, they will face "social public sanctions" and eventually erasure which therefore prompts them to "have a body feel feminine" (Barkty, 1990:38). Stated otherwise, to maintain their ethnic and gender identity and to avoid de-sexualisation, to avoid being "annihilated" in Barkty's term, the internalization of beauty standard (here meaning circumcision), provided women with a secured sense of mastery and identity as females. The refusal to be circumcised was negatively rewarded. It was like "to diskill embodying the feminine" (Barkty, Ibid). To look 'good' and to come out of this physiological ambiguity, it was deemed necessary to circumcise both sexes so as to do away with the organ that represents the opposite sex as a mechanism of sexual identification with others of one's sex. Taken as such, male circumcision was meant to "masculinise" a man whereas FC was aimed at feminizing a woman.

Respondents frequently said that the standard Ejagham woman was the one without a clitoris and keeping one's clitoris intact was considered as belonging to a "third gender" that did not even exist in the Ejagham imagination. In other words, this traditional beauty standard pressured the uncircumcised to suffer from status anxiety. Circumcision is therefore a form of body construction, a form of repair from an abnormality since they are supposed to get transformed "to meet the other woman" (Wolf, 1991:287) (those who have already conformed by getting circumcised in this case). They are in other words, made to get disciplined by undergoing practices that meet the beauty standards set by patriarchy with the 'complicity' of matriarchy. Since women are under persistent surveillance by patriarchy/the opposite sex, they are socially conditioned and made to stick to patriarchally induced and internalized requests through various practices with regards to their body image (Wolf, 1991:287) which FC is one.

As most circumcisers put it, ''the individual should look nice". They frequently invoked the expression ''to fix'' with reference to FC. This means that 'bodies, then, are not born: they are made. The body becomes a conglomerate of practices, or 'body techniques' which represent and regulate bodies in time and space (Turner, 1992). Since women who had been "fixed' were the models of womanhood, paragons of beauty, or the equivalents of local Helens of Troy, they stood the most prominent chances in the matrimonial market thereby forcing all others to follow suit. For one thing, they were believed to be fertile, well behaved and therefore, to be embodiments of womanhood.

> To us, we have reasoned that the clitoris is not nice. When a woman goes to the stream to take a bath, her private does not look nice. When not cut, you are both a woman and a man at the same time (Bassey Erica, 28, interview of 10/05/06, Ndebaya).

> Yes, to me, I feel there is a difference. The difference is that when you are having sex, look at the genitals of a circumcised woman, you cannot find dirts there unlike that of an uncircumcised woman. Some people like me, when I see it, I can even run away from you. It seems she is a man and I am also a man. A cut woman is nice, she is clean (Ndom Jonathan, 40, interview of 23/05/06).

> The clitoris of a woman who is not circumcised grows and becomes long. It will disturb both the man and the woman when they are having sexual intercourse. At a certain age, the woman's clitoris grows as she is growing and this is done (circumcision takes place) to stop it from growing by trimming it (Robert Mbi, interview of 28/06/06, Ndebaya).

> ...It was like an abuse if you were not circumcised. Whenever you go out with friends, they will be abusing you "Go away, you are not circumcised". They had a name. When you died, before you were buried,[if not already circumcised], you were circumcised using an okarang before your burial in those days. But this is no longer happening today (Anonymous woman, Ndebaya market, informal chat 23/06/06).

The above interview excerpts lay bare the aesthetic belief associated with being circumcised as well as the presumed contrast between the circumcised and the uncircumcised. The clitoris is presented as being an unfeminine organ, as being unsightly and as posing an impediment to the consummation of sexual relationships between couples. The interview excerpts further demonstrate that the aim of FC was partly the conferment of gendered ethnic identity, personhood, and that it provided an aesthetic appeal to patriarchy. The failure to conform was reminiscent of social death as it was punished with mockery by significant social others. Social exclusion further extended to a woman's inability to get married because of her presumed lack of the moral virtues and values that circumcision inscribes and imbibes such as reservation within the matrimonial home through "dislike" for sex. A heavier workload was further imposed on the uncircumcised during community activities such as keeping public places clean, all with the aim of forcing conformity. When seen from this perspective, FC becomes a psychological mechanism aimed at transmitting the basic personality traits of a "real standard" woman, a moral check and a mechanism for keeping women in matrimonial service.

FC is presumed to be one way of maintaining restraint over women in particular and girl children in general. The Ejaghams often believe that women have revolting sexual energy inside their bodies as represented by the presence of the clitoris on the female body. This finding corroborates Foucault's (1979) representation of the body as the ultimate site of political and ideological control, surveillance and regulation- a focal point for the exercise of disciplinary power. Through the body and its behaviour from a Foucauldian perspective, state apparatuses such as medicine, the educational system, psychiatry and the law define the limits of behaviour and record activities, punishing those bodies which violate the established normative boundaries, and thus, rendering bodies both productive and economically useful. The widespread cutting of the clitoris was one mechanism of exercising power over women by maintaining exclusive sexual rights to culturally recognized individuals through the institution of marriage to the exclusion of all others at the same time. This is based on the belief that circumcision reduces sexual desire and prevents women from being wayward and is therefore a "native" mechanism for upholding their dignity. Within the context of the AIDS scourge, partisans invoke this function of FC as a "native" therapeutic model with which to fight against the pandemic. This should rather be seen against the backdrop of the patriline on which Ejagham society is based. Fatherhood unlike motherhood is a social concept and the society believes that "it is only the mother of a child who knows the real father of that child". The society defines fatherhood in terms of the individual who pays the culturally prescribed bride price. In this light, when the marriage breaks down and the dowry is not refunded, the children given birth to by the woman remain those of her 'former' husband both in principle and in practice. In the case of a spinster, they are her father's children. Hodson and Mcurdy (2001:159) have rightly noted that:

> There are competing definitions of fatherhood: a jural definition anchored in rights established through marriage and bridewealth, and a more "social" definition, based on the duties and responsibilities of a "father". Therefore, separation without refund of bridewealth still entitles a man to children given birth to by his wife. Any children conceived, whoever their genitor or biological father, will therefore be recognized legally as the children of the bridewealth payer. Bridewealth exchange is one way of contributing and expressing patriarchal authority (Hodson and Mcurdy, 2001:159)

Unwarranted sexual activities by women are therefore seen as a form of pollution for "it can bring bad blood into the family" through the birth of (a) child/ren out of wedlock. One of these children might eventually come to succeed the man and might wreck havoc and disaster on the entire lineage group because it is presumed that he does not feel as belonging to or secured among them. This is a clear instance in which both biological and social characteristics are fused together and it is assumed that the child might grow up and have a different, usually bad character, reflecting that of his biological father in that case. To forestall this and to maintain 'family blood', women had to be circumcised. Another reason related to this is the sustenance of polygyny, in which case co-spouses had to individually wait for their sexual turns. The following interview excerpts are in order here:

> According to oral tradition handed down to us, when a girl used to bath with friends, her clitoris used to show outside, there was the need to trim it so that the body becomes normal and to reduce excitement. Women too are erotic just like men. And a man who had several wives was in danger of lossing control, if these women were not circumcised. The aim was partly to avoid women within a polygynous home from prostitution because the clitoris makes women curious to have sex. The rate of sex today has increased but you became an outcast if you got pregnant without having achieved the status of Moninkim in those days. There is a period, according to our grandmothers when the clitoris of a woman gets up like the penis of a man and a woman will want to have sex (Regent Chief, interview of 14/03/06, Eyumojock).

> Our people say it is nasty (clitoris) when women grow with their clitoris intact, uncut. It is dirty, may be when you meet with a man it looks very dirty and it spurs a woman more into sexual activities which is clearly a danger in a polygamous home. By cutting it, it limits you more on your sexual life and you can do many other things….You can now go to a place like a bar, or where you can mix up with boys, you will not be easily excited into having sex….You will always maintain yourself, your dignity. (George, 38, interview of 25/04/06, Eyumojock)

> They (our ancestors) believed that if a girl child is not circumcised, the child will always feel like making love whenever she is in the company of men. She will always be yearning to have sex with a man. I feel that with the removal of the clitoris, the child's curiosity for sex will be reduced…It was believed that a woman, who has not been circumcised, will always indulge in high rate of sex…'therefore cannot contain her marital home [Bernadette]. The aim was therefore to confine women's sexuality within the matrimonial home (Nkoyo, 33, FGD session of 27/03/06, Eyumojock)

It is this contention that women are guided by their sensuality or could revolt at any time by engaging in uncontrollable sexual activities that undergirds the arguments of most pro-FC advocates. They hold that the non-circumcision of girls has given rise to a free fall in moral values as epitomized by multiple sexual encounters. Against the backdrop of the HIV/AIDS pandemic, hard-liners therefore see FC as a useful, "native" response to the ravages of the pandemic. This brings to light the argument against the mind/body dualism in which the female body is turned into a metaphor for the corporeal pole representing nature, emotionality, irrationality and sensuality. Put differently, the female body is always the 'other': mysterious, unruly, threatening to erupt and challenge the patriarchal order, symbolizing all what needs to be tamed and controlled by (dis)embodied masculine rationality (Lupton, 1986:3-4). The social gaze is accordingly always on women and not on men here because male sexual escapades are socially sanctioned and even licensed unlike female sexuality. This stance is even more clearly articulated by the following interview excerpt in which the respondent contrasts the behaviour of girls in the past with those of today which suggests that FC instils the virtues of sexual reservation in the initiate:

> The circumcision that was given to girls cooled down their anxiety for sex (men). The high numbers of uncircumcised girls today are the ones prostituting all over. It should still take place so that anxiety and immorality will reduce (Ayum Mary, 29, interview of 20/03/06, Boki, Eyumojock).

Although this informant does not subscribe to FC, in the face of the sexual immorality and sexual, moral panic engendered by prostitution, she feels that uncircumcised girls are at the core. She would therefore recommend FC as a necessary moral check against the spread of the pandemic. She does not subscribe to circumcision for her own daughters. She however maintains a ‘double discourse’ when confronted with the perceived ills of FC and the AIDS pandemic. She told me she escaped from the ritual cutting because of the pains it entails. Her husband is equally against it because the circumcision of one of his daughter (given birth to, with another woman, out of wedlock) almost led to disaster as she bled profusely. The category of uncircumcised girls includes the daughters of some educated individuals in this community and those whose parents did not circumcise them because their relatives had suffered from excessive bleeding.

Another reason informing the practice of FC is ethnomedical health assumptions. Every society has its health system which pulls together illness causing beliefs and practices and their solutions. These beliefs and practices may not cohere in the view of individuals from other cultures. This brings to the fore the chasm between local and scientific knowledge, suggesting many varieties of truths, many rationalities.

Among the Ejagham, the failure to circumcise a woman might partly account for her inability to conceive. In the same light, if a woman has not given birth to other children for a long time, and she had not been originally circumcised, they deem it necessary to circumcise her with the belief that thereafter she will give birth. Coincidentally as most respondents pointed out, it usually came to happen. FC is being presented here as one of various “native” therapies against any degree of infertility. We should keep in mind however that even the concept of infertility is gendered. It is always women who are considered to be infertile, not men.

Because of the enthusiasm to give birth to children partly as a certification of, and to earn the status of motherhood, females were under pressure from society to circumcise or face the dire consequences of infertility. To reinforce this cultural expectation, infertile women are abusively referred to as unproductive plantains. Bearing children implies having security at old age because an individual normally expects to receive care and support from his/her progeny at old age or curse them. Having many children is symbolic of wealth, it is not considered to be a burden: "When you have the scabies, you will also have the nails. When you have many children/many wives, God will provide you with the means for you to take care of them" (Pa Otang, interview of 10/03/06).The inability to have children of one's own is considered to be a type of social death for both genders. The contention is that only one's child can treat that individual well and not those of one's relatives, although every child belongs to the lineage group and to the society at large for his or her upbringing.

The body is a text on which specific cultural impressions and behavioural traits are written, an 'instrument of order and control', 'an anatomical atlas' (Foucault, 1979) and conformity through circumcision is the internalization of the gaze of society, of the opposite sex, as the "surveying gaze", transforming women into the agent of the panopticon-"the self-policing subject, self-committed to relentless self-surveillance" (Barkty, 1990:43). Psychologically, women are kept in negative feelings of self-hatred and low self-confidence about their bodies- the obsession becomes that of acquiring the status of being circumcised. Turner's (1992) concept of somatic society- in which the body is a metaphor for social organization and social anxieties, the main field of cultural and political activities is appropriate here since the somatic society regulates, surveys and monitors bodies and the spaces between them.

Certain implicit and explicit cultural contrasts were and are still being made to reinforce FC. Through social conditioning, the circumcised are still believed to be the equivalent of 'local modernity', paragons of beauty, perfect bodies, fertile, normal without the zeal for inordinate sexuality, assumed to have higher statuses and higher self-esteem. On the other hand, the uncircumcised are considered as 'primitive', ugly, imperfect bodies requiring perfection, infertile, as socially abnormal because of their presumed wanton sexuality, having lower statuses and paradoxically as suffering from complete loss of self-confidence. I will take up this critical issue in the next chapter in greater detail as the contrast between this laid down cultural ideal ("tradition") and counter-ideal ("modernity") partly explains the state of both contestation and acceptance of FC and articulates the need to fight against stigma in anti-FC advocacy. Mary Douglas's argument is therefore still appropriate here, that bodily rituals 'enact a form of social relations' and by conferring on 'these relations visible expression, they enable people to know their own society'. '. Ritual works on the body politic through the symbolic medium of the physical body' (1980/1966:128).

3.3.2 The female circumcision process

At the turn of the twentieth century, FC was universal as every female Ejagham was under strong social pressure from significant social others such as parents to either circumcise or be ostracized from her community. The failure to comply by circumcising meant the loss of community support networks since resistance was interpreted as constituting the highest act of deviance. Parents in general and grandmothers in particular were consequently bent and determined to ensure that their granddaughters be 'fixed' as part of their socialization process because failure to circumcise was interpreted as a clear evidence of parental negligence, in this case motherly negligence. Both the individual and her family alike were ridiculed without any pity. To become a circumciser like to become a Moninkim entails initiation as well as a sacrifice.

The circumcision process usually begins with a sacrifice and an early morning bath. This pre-circumcision sacrifice comprises of cooked beef, mixed with palm oil alongside fried corn mixed with palm oil and salt, and some palm wine. Once everybody is assembled, the ancestors are invoked to guide the circumciser in the performance of her duty, to forestall bleeding and to be witnesses to the ceremony which they had laid down in the dim past. Then these ritual food items are shared out and consumed. My ethnographic friends and acquaintances told me that the aim of the sacrifice was to prevent those with evil eyes from causing the initiate(s) to bleed and that after this, the circumciser will then circumcise the initiate(s) without any fear of cutting too much, leading to bleeding. Consuming these food items implies that an individual can neither bewitch any of the initiatees nor mystically block the circumcision process by making her or them to bleed. In other words, taking part in this ceremony is believed to weaken the evil powers of any malevolent individual because it is held that the ancestors are now in total control and will not allow any interference with the ritual procedure. This pre-circumcision ritual no longer takes place today.

I was told by a circumciser in Ogurang, one of several Ejagham villages close to the Nigerian border that she normally receives two bottles of palm oil placed in a basket at the centre of the floor and a negotiable amount of money (at least 2,000 frs CFA, 4 USD) for her services for each circumcision session per initiate. She further takes part in the meal and drinking that usually follows the ritual cutting ceremony. The people assisting at the ceremony are expected to individually drop whatever thing they have as a mark of gratitude to the circumciser into the basket. Another circumciser said she receives at least 5,000 FRS, CFA (10 USD) for each clitoris that she cuts. This really depends on her relationship with the family of the initiate, although her mother who initiated her into the art had set down a specified, undisclosed amount. What is clear is that the amount of money received for circumcision services varies from one circumciser to the other.

Talbot's (1912) observation made at the beginning of the twentieth century gives us a clue as to the age and various categories of initiates, although a seemingly inconclusive one for that matter. He observed in passing that:

> Usually before leaving the fattening-house, the girl undergoes clitoridectomy, but this operation is sometimes performed in infancy and sometimes not until after the birth of the first babe (Talbot, 1912).

He states in the excerpt quoted above that there was fattening before confinement and circumcision after confinement. Until recently, several categories of initiates existed among the Ejaghams, two of which Talbot has hinted at above but my fieldwork shows that in reality, there were actually four different categories of initiates and functions of the ritual cuttings.

The first category of initiates was to be specially 'honoured'. They were cut after the birth of their first children. This was the normal cultural timing and expectation. They were expected to become Moninkims after their confinement and subsequent graduation. Most of the women in this category with whom I spoke painted glamorous and glaring pictures of their having enjoyed their confinement periods and some even expressed the wish to go back into confinement if given the opportunity so as to continue enjoying.

The second group underwent the ritual process in childhood. This suggests that this group of initiates did not go through the fattening house period. This is understandable as the general rule was that circumcision was mandatory for all females. Those who were to be specially 'honoured' were however entitled to later confinement if they were to become Moninkims depending on whether they were first daughters. There is a return to this pattern of initiation today in the face of criticisms of the ritual procedures from within and from without the Ejagham community. Although respondents reported that it is because "children are still young and will not feel the pains too much", the actual reason is that they should not grow up and start contesting the ritual procedures under the influence of the "Whiteman".

A third group was made up of those who were initiated at maturity when they had not yet given birth. Initiates in this category were later confined when they eventually gave birth particularly if they were to become Moninkim, a form of "symbolic circumcision". It seems that their parents lacked the necessary resources for taking care of them to complete the initiation process at the time of their circumcisions. It could equally be that some individuals were mature whereas others were still young. Their parents therefore wanted to cut down on cost by circumcising all of them at the same time.

The fourth group comprised of those who had "stayed for too long without procreating and it was suspected that it was because of their non-circumcision status" (Ma Sophie Otang, interview of 10/04/06). This seems to have been those who initially resisted the ritual cuttings but were eager to have issues or were constantly under provocation for their non-circumcision status as well as those who, although fertile, were still being provoked for not having been circumcised. For instance, a woman was circumcised in 2002 following social pressure from her mother after she had already given birth to her fifth child and despite the ongoing anti-FC campaign within the new institutional context and dynamics triggered off by the HIV/AIDS pandemic.

The various categories outlined above suggest that some of the initiates were virgins whereas, others were not and perhaps differences in the socio-economic status of parents either led to earlier or later circumcision ceremonies and confinement as the case might have been. It is not quite clear from my field research which clans practiced strictly earlier or later circumcisions. It is however clear that FC was a general practice in the whole region. Their Bayangi neighbours are said to have totally abandoned FC as far back as the 1950s. I got faint echoes from a few informants that among the Ossing, FC too was fashionable but was unrelated to membership of the Moninkim society. This reflects the general pattern in the Central Ejagham area as a whole unlike in the Lower Ejagham region where most circumcised women especially if they were first daughters were 'honoured' through initiation into the Moninkim cult (see also., Nkongho, 1999). Coincidentally, this region is the most resistant to change and is very enclaved lacking even access roads. The people here forward their resistance to part with the ritual cuttings by invoking the fact that government has marginalized them. In other words, they are only symbolic citizens in their own country since they lack everything that makes human life colourful: a road network, potable water, electricity, a health care facility. Some said that the day that a road network will reach them, they will abandon FC. They are the most enclaved and very few NGOs reach them unlike the Upper Ekwes who are urbanized and in the centre. This poses problems for the spatial geography of intervention against FC in the area, an issue that I take up in the next chapter.

Usually within a week after the birth of a woman's first child and in some cases, barely a few days later, she is instructed by members of the women's secret society to take an early morning bath and not to oil herself in preparation for her circumcision. She will normally have to be rubbed with white kaolin locally called calabar chalk after the circumcision ceremony to make her beautiful. It is believed that the morning bath numbs the body and that too much blood will not flow. Thereafter, she is either made to sit on a stone or lie on a mat. Other women will hold her down on both legs and hands and on the chest. The circumciser, usually an elderly woman, will then take her clitoris using her hand and cut it implying her break away with and from the vestiges of childhood and gender ambiguity. This is usually amidst shouting and crying from the initiate. A local anaesthesia made out of a plant and called *Okimi* like the plant itself, will be squeezed and applied to the wounded genital to stop blood from oozing out. In the past, the ritual cutting was done with the help of a small pen knife called *okarang* but today with razor blades.

Up to the 1980s a group of girls were circumcised using the same *okarang* but now probably as a result of anti-ritual FC campaigns and HIV/AIDS, the people report that it is one individual per razor blade ("one individual is equal to one blade"). Pro-FC advocates pointed out that the change has equally affected bodily scarification for therapeutic reasons. The cut genital is then buried behind the house so as to inform the ancestors. The great significance attached to a successful circumcision session makes it obvious that this ceremony is symbolic of status appropriation- a process of appropriating and expropriating, that which is desirable and undesirable at the same time. In other words, the yoke and ignorance of childhood has been thrown off and adult gendered but secret knowledge symbolically inscribed and acquired.

In the midst of singing and dancing, the group alongside the age mates of the initiate will lead the initiate into the house. The initiate's mother is then usually instructed to warm water three times a day-morning, afternoon and evening and massage the initiates' genitals with it so as to kill the pains and to facilitate the healing process.

Gloria, now in her thirties and mother of four kids was circumcised while she was nine years old. She was however, later secluded and went through the fattening period when she gave birth to her first baby. She vividly recalls her own circumcision process and the immediate and subsequent trauma she went through in these words:

> In the morning of your circumcision, as early as five o'clock, you are taken for a cold bath, forced onto a mat behind the house. Six people held me on my legs, hands, chest, they pressed me down. It is not all that very easy to cut part of the body of a human being. I shouted. If it was now I am not sure I can do such a thing. It is a vein that is cut. I bled for three days. On every occasion, whenever I attempted to ease myself, I bled. They said that was not the way. They used to insert the medicine into the vagina and pad you. You are supposed to join your legs before easing yourself. Once the urine mixes with the medicine, you feel more pains. You are padded with gloves.
>
> If this child were circumcised now [pointing to her two weeks old baby which she was carrying in hand], I will wear her a napkin. Each time that she urinates, the medicine will mix with the urine and enter the wound. The aim is to make it to heal easily. It is painful; I cannot tell you a lie. I think that might be why they are refusing circumcision. But if they are saying that circumcised women do not give birth, that is a big lie. That is a big lie. Even I myself as I am here in Eyumojock, I have been giving birth to my children safely, nothing disturbs me. How does circumcision disturb? It has no effects [on fertility] (Gloria ,interview of 10/05/06)

Some initiates reported that after their circumcisions, water was boiled and put in a bucket and they were instructed to sit on top of it so that the vapour should help in healing their circumcised genitals. This needs a lot of courage because if the initiate is not courageous enough, she can collapse due to the heat generated and the pains she is feeling at the same time. Yet this pain is viewed as a mechanism to tame and regulate the female body. That is to instil bodily discipline. Every female was entitled to circumcision but only first born daughters were specially 'honoured' through the institution of Moninkim, which entailed further initiation. It is to this that I turn my attention in the next section.

3.3.3 Becoming a Moninkim

The word "Moninkim" in the Ejagham language is a title conferred on a woman who has been duly circumcised, confined and ceremonially presented at a public ceremony in front of the Ekpe hall. Thereafter, she is culturally certified and permitted to dance the "Nkim" dance. The title of Moninkim is added to her name for life as a mark of her circumcision status and dancing ability. In fact, they are revered as local popstars. For "Social /Modern Moninkims", some were confined and fattened without circumcision. Others have merely been integrated into the group with no ritual largely due to their dancing ability and social status. Until the late 1980s circumcision, "NKIM" was traditionally the precondition for dancing the Moninkim dance as other members of the band played only minor roles- holding the Moninkim's mirror, beating the drum, gong and singing for her or for the "awuounokims" (plural for a group of circumcised and confined first daughters).

Historically, Moninkim began among the Ejagham upper class and later on diffused to the entire society as even the so-called slave families (*nsung*) later came to adopt it as a way of identification with the mainstream society. The people distinguished between 'free born' Ejaghams and those of slave descendants. Upper class here refers to the former group who among other things, owned the land, and could easily acquire membership in most secret societies. They could purchase cult agencies and could rise to the highest rank within these secret societies unlike the latter who had only limited rights of participation and at times, had to dance on one leg (See Rősenchaller, 2007, Limunga, 1999). Talbot (1912, 1965) observed that:

> "before their wedding, all free-born Ekoi girls, of well-to-do parents spent time in the "fattening- house" and during this period, they may not wash their faces" (Talbot, 1912, 1965)

Becoming a Moninkim as a mark of 'honour' was the exclusive prerogative of first daughters although all females like males were circumcised. Being a first daughter among the people is considered to be a sign of good luck. However, today, the uncircumcised are dancing the ritual dance unlike in the past. This is partly explained by the ageing of the initial initiates and the need to replace them, the debate set in motion by the HIV/AIDS scourge, formal education and intercultural contact, as I will demonstrate below.

After the circumcision process, they were taken into seclusion and confinement during which time they received red carpet treatment. A Moninkim aspirant took part in no household chores, and in virtually no activities within both the private and public spheres. She only slept, was bathed and was fed with highly nutritive food items. She became healthy, smooth and fat. This is the prototype of ideal feminine beauty among the

Ejaghams as I was made to understand. Moninkim received the very best of everything. For instance, she received the blackest plums from the forest, the best and largest fishes from the streams and the largest *yamagoros* (snails). Chief Ojong Moses Ntui, in his 60s, of Otu village vividly captures the special treatment received by a Moninkim thus:

> The woman (meaning Moninkim) who was confined remained indoors and was fed like a small chicken; she could not even go out (laughing). They made her look beautiful. There were women whose sole role was to decorate her with white chalk every morning and so as to make the place look animated, they taught her songs and dance. During the dancing, people were admiring her, looking at her buttocks, her body. Then tomorrow, you see a young man like you, say "I will go and try". And if that young man is accepted, he becomes a jackass to the family. He will kill and bring all the animals he is capable of killing and bring to the bride's parents for the feeding of the Moninkim. He digs palm trees, and brings all the palm wine taped for the same purpose (Chief Ojong Moses Ntui, Otu village, interview of 23/07/06).

The length of the confinement period varied from a few months to years depending on the socio-economic status of the initiate's parents, her suitor/ husband or both. The basis of socio-economic status here included ownership of farmland, cult agencies and slaves. The owner commanded the labour of slaves while some owned and traded in the transfer of cult agencies. It should be recalled that the Ejaghams were middlemen in the transatlantic slave trade between the Western Grassfields and Old Calabar, in Nigeria. During her seclusion, she was under the protectorateship of Ngbe, the men's Leopard Society and her father gave its members palm wine at the beginning and at the end of seclusion announcing both her entry and exit from the fattening house (Röschenthaler, 1998:40). This fact seems to suggest the ambiguity, danger and uncertainty surrounding this period of confinement.

Moninkim was never seen free of charge, something had to be offered in advance. Any visitor who wanted to catch a glimpse of the initiate during her confinement period had to offer something for her upkeep to the elderly Moninkim women who were teaching her the skills and secret knowledge commensurate with her new status. She remained inside the room, could not even sit in the sitting room and was taken care of by some elderly women who themselves had been initiated into the Moninkim cult. This seclusion period was meant for intensive indoctrination and tutoring by these elderly women, an endurance test to inculcate control, adherence and submission to authority as well as a mark of rupture with the initiate's past life. A favorite pastime for the initiatee during this period was learning dancing and making artistic marks on the walls using chalk. To catch a glimpse of Moninkim during the confinement period, an individual literally "had to break the door to see Moninkim" with gifts and money no matter the value. In some cases, bells were even placed on the door post and any visitor had to ring the bell to announce his/her presence and then get ready "to break the door" and see Moninkim.

In the presence of a visitor, the elderly women taking care of her will intone a song, sing, and clap their hands while Moninkim will dance in the room with them to the admiration of the visitor(s). The old mothers kept an eye on the way the initiate placed her legs, her body movements and gestures. The dance entails a lot of body movements partly explaining why as the old members are ageing; they need young and energetic women to keep up with the tradition. In other words, she does not just dance anyhow. They will in turn give you food and drink if available. If it was absolutely necessary to go out, she had to pass behind houses, through footpaths to avoid the gaze of others. Even for the husband to share food with her, he had to 'bribe' his way through by providing drinks to her family before they will permit him to serve himself from Moninkim's dish. Moninkim ate in a specially decorated calabash dish carrying love messages using nsibiri signs.

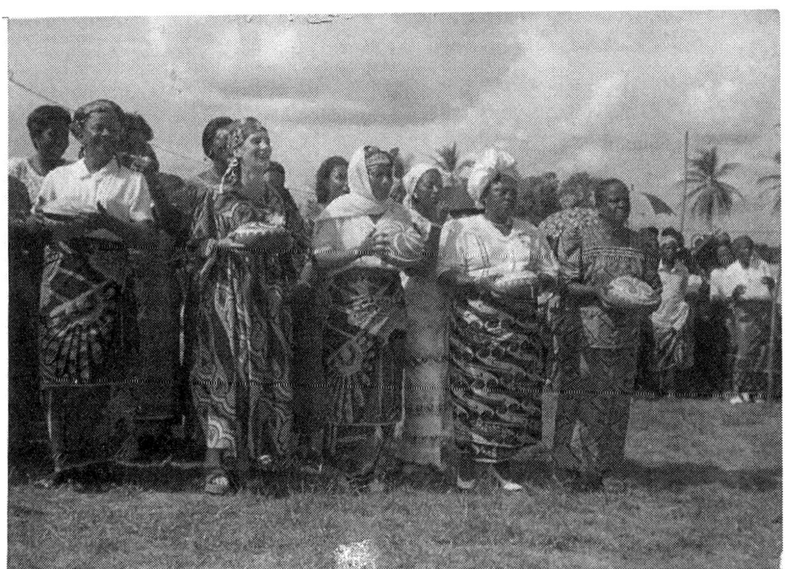

Fig. 7 Typical dish from which Moninkim ate. Copyright, the author.

People had to pay to embrace her even when she was on the dancing floor like with a striptease dancer in European cities. One old man said in a focus group discussion session that:

> Even if you were Paul Biya (President of Cameroon), and came around, Moninkim could not greet you with her hands or you could not just go forward and embrace her. You could only embrace her when she was dancing on the floor and you had already given some money. If she liked you, she embraced you. (Sub Chief, community interview of June 03/06/06, Inukon)

After the healing of the circumcised genitals, the women taking care of Moninkim had to start rubbing her with cam-wood dye and later on, white kaolin, popularly called calabar chalk. These ointments are symbols of beauty and fertility in the Ejagham cultural universe. They further have an aesthetic effect on the body of the initiate. Then they will put waistline cowries and beads on the waist called "ajij ta bangles". The father and mother of the Moninkim took their individual turns to put bangles around her legs if they were rich enough because very few families could afford it. The father will put on the right leg, the mother will do the left leg. Until the 1990s, some initiates slept with the Moninkim regalia while some others even carried theirs to school. During her confinement, the fiancée/husband kept a symbolic grinding stone and snuff for visitors to collect and sniff. The snuff ritual appears to carry the symbolism of an engagement ring and to represent the physical presence of the prospective husband at all times besides his wife. It was therefore meant to scare away his love rivals.

3.3.4 The outdooring ceremony

After spending some time in confinement, a ceremony had to be organized to mark the initiate's re-entry into society. This ritual ceremony had reminiscences to a fashion parade and was a unique occasion for parents to showcase the beauty and care they had given their daughter during her confinement and consequently to become popular. The father, husband of the maiden and their close relatives will normally invite their friends; from within and beyond their village. The age mates of the initiate, her husband's and father's age mates given their roles as we shall see below as well as members of the Ekpe society were all invited. A special day was then set aside for the graduation ceremony of the initiate from childhood into adolescence and her subsequent re-entry into society with her new status.

Her perception has now been shifted towards her rightful place, status and role in her community and a new perception of her community has been re-engineered in her alongside more demands and obligations. Of primordial importance, however, initiation is about the creation, maintenance and longevity of the community- a sort of insurance scheme for the continuity of the community (Crow, 1994). She has been well schooled in the traditions of her tribe and the secrets, behavioural codes, survival tactics that have ensured the continuous survival and power base of her community. She has to suppress her own individual needs for the well-being of her kinship group and community. Malidoma Some (1986) has rightly observed that "a true community begins in the hearts of the people involved. It is not a place of distraction but a place of being. It is not a place where you reform, but [rather] a place where you go home to". She is now conversant with the mysteries of the female secret society and armed with gendered knowledge. She can now be said to have moved from social insignificance into signification as a full woman.

In preparation for the ceremony, palm trees had to be felled to prepare good quality palm wine because if the wine was not nice, she was sent back into 'the house'. Assorted food stuff and meat were equally prepared in large quantities.

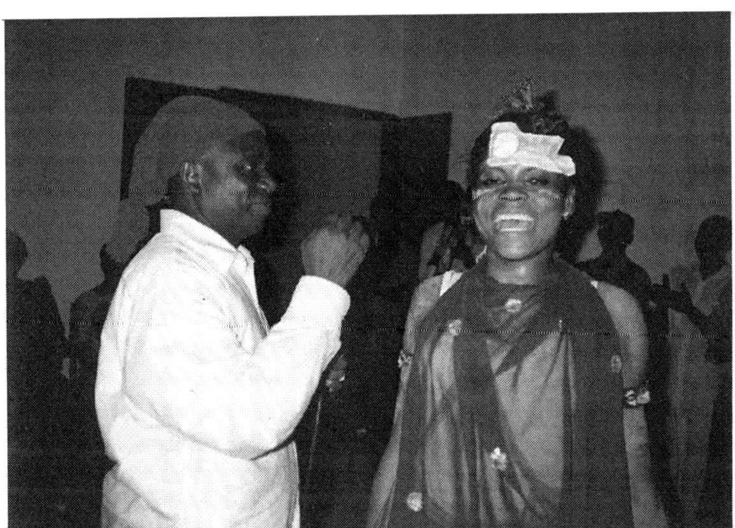

Fig. 8 Moninkim Dancer being rewarded. Copyright, the author.

On some occasions the feasting and dancing went on for days and Moninkim, and indirectly her family, was showered with gifts and monies. She was "spread with bank notes" (ABEMO, 2002). These gifts and monies were meant to provide her with capital with which she could start her own life and to permit her to continue to dress well when she came back into the public sphere as a mark of her new status, knowledge, skills, and change in both her self esteem and role. In other situations, the monies were used to sponsor her brothers in school, pay the bride price of close relatives (brothers, uncles etc) or her parents consumed it as profit accruing from this investment enterprise. Taking part in an outdooring ceremony was in itself implicitly signing a social contract that one will one day refund what one had eaten by sponsoring such a feast in the near future.

> Everybody wanted to do it, let it not be as if you have eaten and do not want to refund. If you ate and did not celebrate a feast in turn, people will be annoyed with you. Everybody was obliged to do it, it was like pride and once you did it, you are free. People hear about you (informal chat with Madam Martha Nkongho, 50, 20/05/06, Ndebaya market).

It should be pointed out here that people often expressed their 'annoyance' with an individual for failing to circumcise and host a feast for his daughter through witchcraft practices. Some informants probably in this light reported that failure to circumcise one's daughter could lead to subsequent infertility or to her mysterious death because of the expectation to feast during the outdooring ceremony.

As a likely demonstration of the family's status, Moninkim was well clothed for the ceremony. She literally wore her Sunday best. Bonchucks (1997:66) has noted that "on graduation day, the girls [or Awuonokims] were decorated with beads, assorted colours, manila coins and various sound producing objects, flowery patterns, and styles, smeared with camwood-dye, chalk and indigo with well plaited hairs, etc" before appearing at the ceremonial grounds. Röschenthaler (1998:41) notes that her choreography includes "a skirt of bells, a decorated fan and a flywhisk, and white ornaments on her body and face" and black juiced nsibiri signs on her checks and forehead at the turn of the century. On his part, Talbot recorded that:

> When a girl leaves the fatting-house, it is an occasion of much rejoicing. A great feast is made and dances are given. The girl herself is smeared from the waist downward with a red dye made from the cam-wood tree. Fattening-house ornaments, consisting of tassels and chains made of dried palm-leaf fibre also dyed red, are hung round her neck, while a cross-piece

> of the same is usually passed beneath the breasts. Her girdle of beads, cowries and palm, is also rubbed over with the same dye. Her face is painted in various patterns and colours, and her hair dressed in a very elaborate way and decorated with combs, and large " pompoms " of white feathers, while over all nods a plume of the dark green and creamish feathers of the Nkundak (Greater Plantain-eater) (Talbot,1965: 191).

The ceremony usually took place in front of the Ekpeh hall. This cultural museum is always located at the centre of the village and serves both as the town hall and as a public cultural arena. Members of the Nkanda, a junior grade of the Leopard society, performed the opening of the dancing floor while Ngbe roared in the Ekpe hall. Röschenthaler (1998:41) vividly captures the scene in these words:

> Then the Monenkim performs a Ngbe dance dedicated to the large slitdrum of the village, using Ngbe mimes learned during her seclusion. She next entertains the relatives, villagers, and guests with the repertoire of songs and dances she rehearsed during that time. The girl imitates the Nkanda dancers, miming the content of her songs, the women in the audience answer as a choir. The spectators comment avidly on the monekim's performance, if they appreciate it, they will give her many presents and urge her to continue for several hours. At the turn of the century the monenkim would dance around with a large calabash, beautifully decorated with nsibiri signs, to collect gifts for her parents (Röschenthaler, 1998:41).

When respondents were constantly pressed as to why in the past women had to be circumcised before they could gain membership of the Moninkim cult, they constantly said that the aim is "to make girls light to dance". The underlying but un-echoed cultural meaning seems to be that cutting as a precondition to dancing the Moninkim dance had to do with ritual purity. Taken as such, it will logically follow that Moninkimhood as an institution in itself had to do with ritual purity.

However, from my own observations, the dance requires a lot of energy, flexibility and body movements particularly the incessant shaking of the buttocks probably meant to capture the gaze and attention of the opposite sex. The pitch of this highly dramatic and erotically intensive scene is usually enacted in front of the largely male audience at the grand stand during public performances on various occasions: during the visit of a top politician, administrator or during national holidays. Two or three Awounokims constantly stage together. They dance on their toes, turning spontaneously in all directions, wriggling their back muscles down to their waists usually in tandem with the drummers. Meanwhile the jigta adds beauty to their attire and erotic effect to the dance as they mesmerize everyone present, attracting money gifts in the process. In fact, I never observed a situation in which only one Moninkim was staging during my nine month's field stay in the area. Given the similarities between the Moninkim and the Efik Abang dance which is a modified version of the latter (Onyile, 2000:4), several Awounonkims staging together seems to be a dramatization of polygyny in traditional Ejagham matrimonial arrangements like among the Efiks. This is more likely the case because both the Ejaghams and the Efiks have a common family and kinship structure partly characterized by polygynous unions. Taken as such, dancing becomes a love contest among co-spouses fighting over their collective husbands' love, with each one of them trying to outplay the other(s) so as to win him over. This is more likely to be the case because the dance is the public re-enactment of a fertility ritual. It is therefore a celebration of both life and the feminine virtues of all women although it is overtly a medium of entertainment during ceremonies marking various facets of individual, local, national, regional and international life. It is enacted on occasions such as the visit of an important personality and during ceremonies commemorating various national and international days. This in itself is a modernization of the ritual showing that it has been transformed from a ritual to a spectacle, from chastity to commercialization.

It was usually at the end of this ceremony that both parents of the maiden had to remove the bells from her ankles- the father undoing those on the right whereas the mother, those on the left leg in the vicinity of the Ekpe hall. Right and left in the cultural universe of the Ejagham are simultaneously complementary and contraries but both are nevertheless, symbolisms of gender, power, authority and strength. The 'left' is seen as "the woman hand", which, when compared to the right is believed to be weaker. Women are accordingly represented as the weaker sex. Acquiring the status of Moninkim means acquiring power as depicted by the Ekpe symbolic staff that formally certified initiation. The father and his age mates as well as the mother and hers took turns to dance with Moninkim and showered her with gifts at the very end of the ceremony. The maiden was then presented with the traditional walking staff reserved for members of Ekpe as a symbol of her newly acquired power and strength amidst shouting and clapping. Röschenthaler (1998:41) notes that 'late in life, she may take part in Ngbe as an honorary member'.

This implies that we can partly understand the persistence of the Moninkim tradition only within the larger context of the complex social, economic, power and authority structure of Ejagham society. As Röschentaller (1998:41) has pointed out, old Moninkims were co-opted into Ngbe as honorary members. Gender in African societies is a social construct rather than a biological category, which constantly enacts and re-enacts a complex web of social relations within a dynamic historical context. It regulates various patterns of daily social interaction between the sexes and between culturally defined norms of masculinity and femininity. Secondly, age mediates gender making relationships more dynamic and fluid over time say between an aged woman and male members of her community. This is because in most African communities, aged women are considered to be 'men' and like aged men, are also said to be closer to the ancestors (see also Amaduime, 1997). They are unlike young girls because they can keep secrets.

If a graduated initiate is not given the symbolic Ekpe staff of authority, it means that the Moninkim is a fake because she and her family had been unable to muster the necessary resources to host Ekpe and members of the community at large. In fact, not to award this staff of authority was considered a protest of dissatisfaction meaning that the outdooring ceremony had been poorly organized and had to be reorganized altogether with all the huge expenses that this implies. Only rich families could perform the Moninkim tradition on their daughter accompanied by bangles as part of her choreography showing status differences among families. In the case of an appropriately married woman, she left the ceremonial grounds and was carried shoulder high by her age mates and those of the husband to his homestead for the official beginning of her matrimonial career. This seems to be a dramatization and re-enactment of marriage by capture.

3.3.5 The social significance of Moninkimhood

Circumcision and later confinement as a badge of 'honour' and a prelude to becoming a Moninkim had certain cultural undertones. These cultural significations are both explicit and implicit. It provided a period of cultural respite for a woman and served as a forewarning to her prospective husband. It was also an educational and matrimonial workshop thereby offering an opportunity for transmitting and subsequently imbibing gendered personality traits. At the same time, it is linked to the politics of marriage and the conservation of lineage, community identity, and provided spaces for simultaneous protest and resistance. It also offered an avenue for the assertion of women's individual and collective agency. I elaborate on these covert and overt cultural logics below.

Most women were nursing their babies while confined. They had been traditionally circumcised after the birth of their first children. The fattening house session therefore provided a period of respite to both the mother and child. She was excluded from the normal routines of everyday life with all its associated psychological stresses since everything was being done for her. She only took care of her baby, slept and rested. This seems to be functional for reproductive health as her reproductive system and entire body rested during this period especially as there were prohibitions in place backed by negative sanctions against violation of the postpartum sexual taboo. Among other things, the child will be attacked by kwashiorkor if she violated the postpartum taboo because it is "feeding on the food of another child" (Pa Otang, interview of 20/05/06). The people reason that sperms will weaken and destroy the child's immunity and lead to changes in the body chemistry of a lactating woman. This is one traditional mechanism of family planning. Some women stayed in the confinement room for years and their children and others were conceived and given birth to and these children even began walking while they were still there.

Furthermore the fattening period served as a pragmatic lesson to the future husband and his family to take good care of their wife. In other words, the woman was supposed to be looking fresh and healthy at all times as if she was just coming out of the "Njumkim". I am in line here with Bonchuks (1997:66) who quotes Monday E.Noah as saying that the significance of the fattening house system has been misconstrued:

> One motive of the fattening house system was to afford the girl's father an opportunity to demonstrate that he was capable of maintaining his daughter even without his in-law, and that the prospective husband was warned before hand to follow the footsteps of the father in-law in maintaining the daughter after marriage.(Quoted from Bonchuks, 1997:66)

This point of view is further given impetus by Talbot's (1912, 1965) observation that if the parents of the maiden are unable to provide for her during the fattening room period, their daughter will be "looked down upon by her companions before marriage" and also by members of her husband's family when she (eventually) joined them. Elders further brought it to my attention that the inability of a prospective husband or of a socially recognized husband to provide "good care" during the fattening period could lead to instant breakup of the (prospective) union. It was therefore equally an avenue of protest within which a woman could change her mind independently or with the influence of her mother. If the latter did not like the former's spousal choice, she could engineer her by complaining that had she a different man, she might likely have received far better red carpet treatment during her confinement. This was usually the case if a mother had preferred for her daughter somebody else. This is understandable given the pivotal role of mothers in the match-making process. This is a clear instance of both individual and collective female agency.

Confinement as part of becoming a Moninkim was "like a father sending his daughter to school", "Confinement was the school as most people in those days were not sending their female children to school" (Nkoyo Otang, interview of 27/03/06). Formal education was and is still gendered. Females are mostly trained for marriage unlike males. During this "fattening room" ("Njumkim") period, Moninkim took lessons in cookery and housekeeping, childcare, personal hygiene, matrimonial counseling on the secrets and intricacies of the man-woman relationship and proper mannerisms among others. She was taught moral values through stories, riddles and jokes. Röschenthaler (1998:40) adds to the above that the maiden equally received instructions on the preparation of ritual food and on Ejagham art traditions. It was in fact, simultaneously an educational as well as a matrimonial workshop meant to prepare the maiden for marriage and for social life.

Seclusion in my view further has a deeper layer of meaning. It carries the idiom of reservation and interiority, key personality traits expected of women, since there were mechanisms in place to ensure feminine fidelity such as the pro- and post-partum sexual abstinence taboo, blood pacts as we saw in the preceding chapter and ritual circumcision as I pointed out above. This seems to resonate with Boddy's (1982) concept of the womb as a symbol of interiority in the Northern Sudan.

The ideal Ejagham woman was culturally expected to be sexually reserved. This is probably because of a sexual political economy that extolled feminine reservation as a mechanism of keeping the family intact and sharing sex among co-spouses in a polygynous set up. Although polygyny has waned here (and is being gradually replaced by serial monogamy) partly because of economic forces at the global, regional and national scales, there was the need for the sexual restraint of women because the inability of a polygynist to sexually satisfy all his wives could spell disaster for him as extramarital sexual escapades could have become the rule. Secondly, to associate women with interiority means freedom from danger for them and the possibility to remain within the household and to take good care of children. Circumcision is therefore a mechanism to transmit the virtues of reservation into women and girl children and in relation to the Moninkim cult "when a girl is circumcised, it is assumed that as the wind is blowing, the way the leaves of plantains are shaking, that is how she will be dancing"(Otang Effa Nicoline, 22, Interview, May 10/06). In other words, she will be smart and pro-active within the household as a way of outsmarting her co-spouses within a polygynous set up.

Getting married to a Moninkim was the dream of every young man in those days because Moninkim was an incarnation of the standard Ejagham woman. This is probably the case because initiation was certification of fertility and sexual reservation. She was considered to be the prototype of Helen of Troy. Initiation into this cult clearly marked one out as being of a particular social status. It was really a pride to be associated with a Moninkim through marriage.

The graduation ceremony proper further provided disenchanted women with a public space within which to sanction their "wicked husbands". This is a blanket expression for all 'non-conformist' women who resist patriarchy as used by Hodgson &McCurdy, (2001). Many people told me that the Moninkim could tacitly reject her husband and his age mates' snuff and this will spell danger for the man and members of his entourage who just have to quietly sneak away with their snuff in humiliation. The ritual therefore seems to provide a space for women's empowerment. Talbot (1912, 1965) points out that if a woman was disenchanted with a man with whom she was sweet hearting or who had amorous intentions towards her, she could symbolically declare his love suit hopeless by calling for water and washing her hands in front of him. Before undertaking such an action on an outdooring occasion, the woman would normally have stricken a love deal with someone else who will now come forward with members of his family and age mates to perform the snuff ritual and at the end of the occasion the lady will be taken to his homestead. It therefore provided for 'positive deviance' as maltreated women sanctioned their men and members of their entourage by bringing them shame in public. In other words, it offered a space to democratize love relationships and for husbands to constantly 'negotiate' with their wives at any one point in time given the high status of these women. Not to provide one's wife with "a good fattening-house" could equally be used as a pretext by an unwilling mother-in-law to induce her daughter to give up the man contrary to a situation in which she had chosen her mother's favoured suitor (Talbot, 1912, 1965). Such an act was like consciously sending your fiancée into your love rival's arms, a type of social suicide indeed. This again is another space for agency, and through which women could manipulate situations to their own favour and for their own interest. The ritual celebration might therefore be said to provide women with power for agency.

The ritual celebration proper therefore provided a political avenue at which some women demonstrated their agency and will. At these matrimonial trade fairs, suitors came to admire prospective wives and it came to have the coloration of ball room dances during the medieval ages in England where matchmaking was one of the central concerns for attendance. On the one hand, parents were eager to get to know and may be become acquainted with those admiring their daughters. On the other, other young men and women alike observed each other within this public but simultaneously enclosed space offered by confinement and subsequently outdooring. One of my key informants, Nkoyo, summarized the Moninkim cult as "a mechanism through which parents garnered resources and at the same time, showcased their daughters for marriage through public exhibition provided by the graduation ceremony since bachelors usually fought over the possession of the Moninkim's heart". Some people are even reported to have resorted to the use of magic to outplay their love rivals in either winning Moninkim's heart or in deterring their rivals from winning her over.

Moninkim is today seen merely as a dancing association. As I have argued above, it is in fact, the core of local pride and gives anyone a sense of recognition, even men. It is now only perceived as a dancing outfit, both within and beyond its own locales. It is famous for its dances by the FC women. Although the methods for the ritual procedures are being modernized, it is not the practice that is being modernized *per se*. The Ejaghams are increasingly using a single razor blade for every individual. There has also been a drastic reduction in the confinement period over time dictated by the need for girls to go to school unlike in the past. The ceremonial celebration is also waning but the commercial aspects such as payment for the services of a circumciser, and dancing for money have remained. At the same time, the youths are increasingly seeking a much more fulfilling sexual life and tend to see FC as an impediment to romantic relationships particularly as they go beyond the village nexus. Most first daughters who were born in the 1940s are today out of service because of old age and the on-going anti-FC campaigns have led to intense debates and contestation. There are now non-circumcised girls dancing the NKIM dance. The Otang family has nine daughters and one son. Although Mr. Otang's wife was circumcised, his daughters were never. For one thing, apart from living in town and being an educated man, he was opposed to FC. He complained that when his wife was confined, she became too fat and bulky and he literally begged his in-laws to end the fattening house period. In villages such as Ebinsi, Ajah and Ayukaba, this commercialized dancing is largely undertaken by 'Social Moninkims' as a profession. In these three villages I came across 12 individuals who are acclaimed uncircumcised dancers.

One bone of contention between partisans and opponents of ritual FC is over the issue of 'Social Moninkim'- that is women who have been co-opted to dance the NKIM dance strictly on the basis of their dancing ability. While they serve as evidence that change is underway and needs to be embraced, it is widely held that they have been circumcised. This is the case because at least up to the 1980s, it was unimaginable to dance the NKIM dance without being circumcised. These women have not gone through the ritual process which entails among others seclusion and a public graduation ceremony. Five of the 10 circumcised Moninkims with whom I spoke felt that they had been slighted by their parents through circumcision and that their uncircumcised colleagues were cheating on them by staging the dance without ritual initiation and accreditation. However, the other five saw the new generation of Moninkims as growing up at a time when change has come, when FC is being decried because of its harmful effects. This conflict between maintaining the *status quo* and change in the procedures of the dance is exacerbated among the old and young generations.

To some people, uncircumcised Moninkims are fakes. One of my respondents, Etchi Moses, 36 years old when asked why there are uncircumcised Moninkims dancing the NKIM dance had this to say:

> Yes, there are people dancing the dance who have not been circumcised. But that is an act of imitation. It is just like when a musician is dancing and you are watching him on the screen. You can imitate the action and do the same thing even without necessarily being a musician. As far as you have the dancing talent, you can dance Moninkim whether you are circumcised or not. But the origin of Moninkim is through circumcision. It is the same thing like the Ekpe tradition. Whether you are a member of Ekpe or not, you can still sing, you can still beat the drums, dance even better than somebody who is initiated. But it is the signs that you will not know. And even if you know the signs, you will not know the meaning associated with those signs. But when we talk in signs and you are initiated, you will know the meaning, what happened before the sign was put in place. But with Moninkim whether you are circumcised or not, you can still dance. But the recognized one is the one who has been circumcised although both of you can dance (Etchi Moses, 36, interview of 26/05/06).

I will argue that social Moninkimhood is part of a larger process of modernization brought about by the criticisms levied against ritual FC, the advent of formal education and Christianity. Within the context of the HIV/AIDS pandemic, procedural reforms such as the use of a single blade for every initiate so as to avoid transmitting and fuelling the spread of the virus among participants through the bloodletting that the ritual cutting entails. The coming of formal education has led to the waning of the confinement period from years to a few months. Parents too are beginning to realise that girl children cannot only be trained to become housewives as in the past but that they can enter professions in the public sphere, a domain that used to be the sole preserve of men. Some people even find it foolish to continue to groom women through the institution of Moninkim. 'School has come and there is no need to put women at home so as to make them Moninkims'(Agbor, interview of 23/05/06). Some Christians, particularly those of the Pentecostal denomination, apart from arguing that the Bible does not condone FC, pointed out that the institution of Moninkim is not just about commercialized dancing but also about spirit possession and interaction with the supernatural world. Mary stated for instance that:

> I am against Moninkim. People say that it is a traditional dance, something like that. It has been modified; it is a spiritual type of a thing. To me, it has something that has to do with spirit possession. Women dancing Moninkim are possessed. If you go to the river, you will see them there. They are pythons. As they manifest in the physical world, that is how they manifest in the spiritual world. There is a sickness called arem, before it starts, people start dancing the Moninkim dance (Mary, interview of 26/05/06, Eyumojock).

I have argued above that the waiving of the criterion of circumcision for some members of the Moninkim cult, a clear evidence of an emerging change that needs to be consolidated has engendered conflicts between the old and the young generation of Moninkim dancers. The former like some segments of the community are increasingly feeling that they were cheated and violated through ritual circumcision and continue to see the new uncircumcised members as fakes in the profession. For one thing, they maintain that new counterparts did not complete the laid down syllabus for membership since some were merely confined without appropriate indoctrination or co-opted by virtue of their ability and agility to dance the NKIM dance.

Moninkimin in fact, represents 'traditional womanhood'. It is the cultural apogee of the institutionalization of Ejagham femininity and personhood. It is in fact, the instantiation of local patriarchy and its entanglement with ritual FC and other wider patriarchal social fields such as marriage and kinship, labour and revenue, male monopoly over property, makes it the bone of contention for contestation and resistance between modernity and tradition on the one hand and scientific and local knowledge on the other.

3.4 Njumepah

Njumepah, one of the traditional arenas for female socialization, is equally called Ekpah. It is the female equivalent of Ekpeh and membership is strictly restricted to old and elderly women because "young girls do not keep secrets". This seems to be a reformulation of the statement that women are excluded from Ekpeh "because women do not keep secrets". To seek membership, an elderly woman has to accompany them when they are dancing in public with their walking sticks and once they are holding their public sessions; the prospective candidate can come around with food, palm wine and tell the members that she wants to join them. They will examine the prospective candidate's behaviour and if she is of good moral standing, they will ask her to pay the admission fee of 200 CFA (approximately less than 50 cents). This association has no clear hierarchical structure but for the presence of a female Chief called "Atukah" who is considered as one among equals.

Traditionally, Ekpah was one avenue for the socialization of female children, monitoring their behaviour and reporting back to their parents for improvement. But today unlike in the past, social and economic transformations have dealt a serious blow on this specific function of the institution. These changes have led to an individualistic ethos among women. Children are accordingly, no longer seen and treated as the collective property of the community but rather, mostly, in individual and sometimes lineage terms. It equally adjudicates in issues concerning women, settling differences as a result of gossips, intrusion into privacy, fighting among women, acts of public indecency such as getting drunk and being rowdy. It is a taboo for anybody to insult an Ejagham woman's genitals. Even to declare for instance that a woman smells, attracts a huge fine comprised of crates of beer, jugs of palm wine, money and large quantities of soap to be used in cleaning that particular woman. Men can equally take their personal matrimonial problems with their wives such as a woman's failure to take instructions from her husband and extra-marital entanglements to Njumepah for arbitration. In some cases, the man with whom a married woman is having an affair is fined and the fine reverted to the husband of the woman in question as payment for damages.

As a secret society, they cleanse Ejagham society against epidemics, illnesses through their nude night dances. They equally curse people who have disobeyed them through this nude dance variously called *etatuh, ma-wu*. It is this particular aspect of their activity that many non-members with whom I spoke were reluctant to seek membership partly because of its presumed incompatibility with modern religious beliefs. They term it as a satanic society but its members hold there is nothing secret in their activities although the inner workings is shrouded in secrecy. Bonchuk (1997: 63) has observed that:

> Ekpah [is] for women and it operate(s) at night with the women going around nude. Men [are] not supposed to view the women. The assumption [is] that a male observer could be paralyzed (Bonchuk, 1997:63)

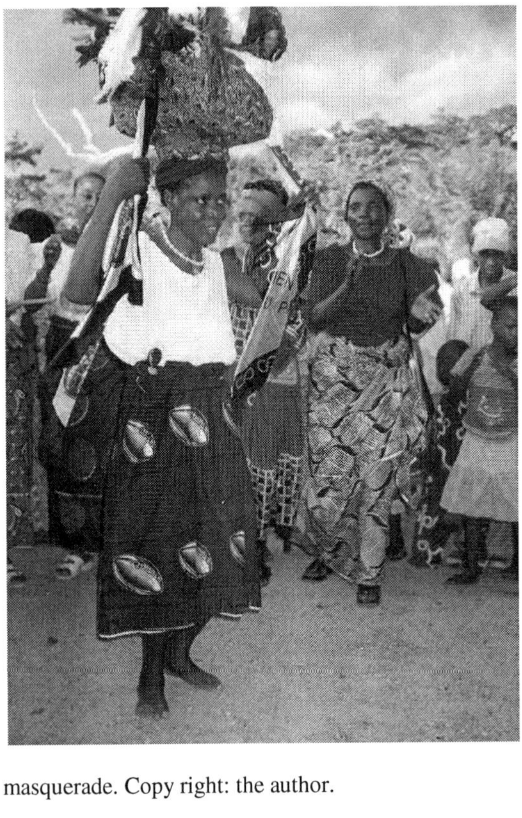

Fig. 9 Ekpah masquerade. Copy right: the author.

They provide animation at the funeral of their members and keep the place lively. They are expected to be entertained with food and wine at least twice daily by the offspring and family members of the bereaved. They have "to cook Ekpah". Like the members of Ekpeh, all what they receive during funerals ("dead taxes") is said to be what their late member ate while holding membership of the group. Membership is not hereditary as the daughters of bereaved members can either choose to join the society or not but must "cook Ekpah" all through the funeral of their kinswoman. Like in Ekpeh, the members are out to recuperate what their deceased member had consumed all through her membership and probably to lure any of the deceased's daughters to join them in the process. Though a secret society, Ekpah equally has a public culture: animation during public ceremonies like during the graduation ceremony of a Moninkim, usually on invitation when they dance alongside their masquerade.

In a nutshell, Ekpah settles conflicts among the womenfolk and with their men, purifies society, wards off epidemics and through the intermediary of the ancestors pray for blessings towards communal progress in Ejagham society. Christianity too has affected membership into this female socialization institution as most women are no longer enthusiastic joining the group because of its presumed association with the devil and thus, its incompatibility with their faith.

3.5 Ekpah-atu

The Ekpah –atu is a women's night ritual dance which like Ekpah, the women's society is totally out of the reach of men. My informant friends told me that traditionally only free-born Ejagham women and not descendants of slave families gained membership into this group. It is composed of married women from the age bracket of 17-60 years. Its members are entitled to dance the mid-night dance with the exclusion of lactating women with male children. Before the Ekpah-atu demonstrates in the village, the men are forewarned by the sound of a gong not to go out of their houses between 9 pm and 1 am. Any man who ventures outside within this time frame and is seen pays a fine of one cow but if not seen, it is assumed that he will have an everlasting curse throughout his life because he has seen his mother's nakedness, except he is ritually purified. To see one's mother's nakedness is reminiscent to some sort of symbolic incest. The purification ceremony for a man who violates the above rule entails washing the individual using a concoction of water which the women have used in washing their genitals alongside some undisclosed herbs. During this cleansing ceremony kind words are recited to the ancestors to forgive him. During the cleansing rite of an individual or of the village from malevolent spirits, the women dance naked with their dresses on their heads, with water in which they have individually washed their privates within their homes. This water is then poured into a basin at the Chief priestess' house.

They equally use this same water to cleanse the village with from evil spirits, to destroy powerful charms that have been buried by malevolent individuals so as to thwart the progress of their enemies in the village. It is also believed that this dance is performed at the beginning of every planting season to call for good harvest even when the rains delay or there is a drought. One strong believe here is that there are witches and wizards with powers of transferring through mystical theft an individual's yields on to their farms. It is equally enacted to wade off epidemics such as rampant sickness among children or women not conceiving and giving birth to children. All these functions were performed in the past until the coming of Christianity. Some of its members have joined various denominations and now brand the society as an incarnation of the devil.

In sum, Ekpah-atu is a female institution that safeguards the interests of the Ejagham community through purification, killing powerful charms, performing fertility rituals and exiling undesirable elements from the community.

3.6 Mbogndem

The word 'ndem' in the Ejagham language refers to a fairy spirit. Fairy spirits in the people's cultural universe are equally designated as "arem". This fairy spirit can either be an already born or a yet to be born child. According to the people's theosophy, all new born babies have fairy spirits in them. This is because when a child is sleeping; it sometimes laughs, smiles, or cries without any apparent reason. These fairy spirits are believed to be of two types-bad and good. The bad ones are called *obanje*. The good ones are said to be frequently sick, and are often suspected of being Mbogndem. If a lot of medical care is given to such a child, yet there is no improvement, the parents are usually advised to take the child to an *arem* shrine and to perform a sacrifice so as to unveil the real personality of this child. At times once this sacrifice is performed, the illness stops abruptly, implying that the child is a Mbogndem. The child might then grow up to maturity without any signs of illness again. Such a child is then considered to be a natural gift and a blessing to the family. This child might one day want to proof to the world that he is a mbog. The spirit commands it on certain days not to exchange words with anyone, and on other days not to cry. At times, nobody passes around such a person and nobody is even supposed to wear anything black and come near the child. People are not even supposed to enter a house where he is there with their shoes on.

Contrary to Rösenchenthaler (1998) who recorded fainting memories of an association of Mbogndems and maintains that they were only females, male mbogndems equally exist. In fact, for a first daughter to become a Mbogndem, she had to be circumcised, confined and 'honoured' through the organization of an elaborate feast like for the Moninkim female institution, which is at the centre of the present enquiry. From my own research, it is clear that Mbogndems are both men and women. This is my impression from what my respondents told me although most of those I observed doing fortune telling in various Cameroonian towns were all women. Whatever the case, it seems that this culture paid a high premium to 'honouring' only women and not men. This is the case if we look at the fact that only circumcised women had ceremonies, whereas, male circumcision remained something banal with virtually no ceremonies.

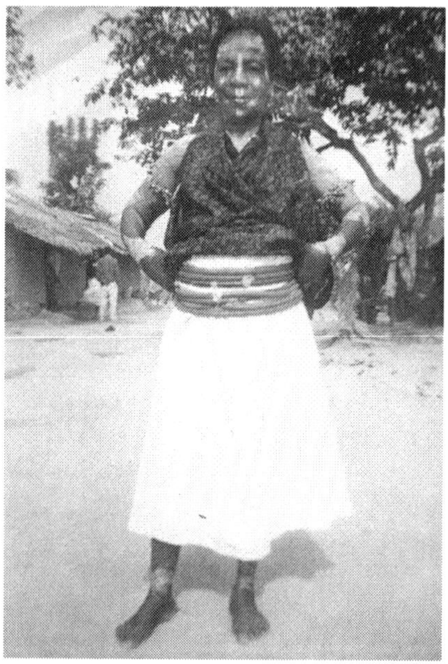

Fig. 10 A Mbog-ndem. Copy right, the author.

What is worthy of note at this point is that membership into these female like for the male institutions was initially the sole preserve of 'free-born' Ejaghams and created a system of indigenous stratification reinforcing the people's specific group identity in the process. Both male and female institutions have elements of reciprocity. In the new context of a dual authority system and Christianity, they have witnessed transformations. Although Moninkim is strictly not about rule, it is about commercialized dancing within and beyond the village nexus.

In summary, Mbogndems are spiritual beings from the fairy world who usually come into the world with a specific mission to accomplish. They however do not just start until they go through torture and several tests and tribulations. It should be recalled here that apart from the Mbogndem association, first born females were also 'honoured' through the institution of Moninkim, the very hub of contestation and debates among proponents and opponents of FC within the institutional context of the HIV/AIDS pandemic.

Conclusion

In this chapter I have argued that the Ejaghams are caught up between the contradictory logics of the modern state and the capitalist economy on the one hand concentrated in the cities and traditional, village-based self-rule on the other. A traditionally stable society is now marked by contestation over shared values. For instance, the institution of Chieftaincy has been weakened by the advent of and subsequent co-optation by the modern administration of the Chiefs. At the same time, there is contest over the authority of Ekpe and other traditional institutions as some individuals prefer the modern court for the adjudication of conflicts. Despite this conflict between tradition and modernity, elites are still appropriating tradition by taking titles within institutions such as Ekpe. I have further demonstrated that the institutions of Moninkim and FC, components of the patriarchal complex have been subjected to changes over time. Contestation by the youths who are increasingly opting for self-fulfilling sexual and romantic relationships has instead led to earlier circumcision on neonates so as to circumvent resistance. Although the methods are being modernized, the procedures remain violent. The ritual is intertwined with the political economy and politics of marriage, kinship, property and the appropriation of labour. Even the change to 'Social Moninkimhood' due partly to the ageing of the initial initiates and sensitization undertaken by NGOs among other factors has been a bone of contention among ardent traditionalists in some Ejagham villages. The 'Social Moninkims' are often branded as 'fakes.

CHAPTER FOUR

HIV/AIDS AND ANTI-FC CAMPAIGNS COME TO EJAGHAM LAND

In this chapter, I will demonstrate how the moral panic generated by the advent of the HIV/AIDS pandemic became an ambivalent framework for support, resistance and contestation of the institution of the Moninkim cult and FC. This contest pits western rational science represented by NGOs and the state against local culture and knowledge system represented by various loose actors in Ejagham community. Both knowledge systems, I argue, can be harnessed and the outcome will be both democratic and progressive. In line with my power-oriented vision of culture as contestation, I will therefore examine state and NGO initiatives geared towards change in the practice of FC and the position of local stakeholders such as Traditional Birth Attendants (TBAs), the medical corps, local community leaders and members of the Moninkim cult- the very source of all the conflicts going on among generations and sexes in the Ejagham community.

4.1 HIV/AIDS pandemic and its relationship with FC

Following the results of Cameroon's third demographic and health survey (CTDHS), the total national HIV/AIDS prevalence rate stands at 5. 5% (CTDHS, 2005). The total national gender ratio is 6. 8% among women and 4.1% among men, showing that more women than men are affected by the pandemic. Ajaga (1999:41) proffers the relative dependence of women and cultural biases towards them in the Cameroonian society to explain this gender disparity in the rate of HIV/AIDS infection. According to him, women are less likely to be gainfully employed than men. They have a higher propensity to depend on men for both financial and material support and many of them still need the go ahead from their husbands or other male authority within the household to engage in activities that demand substantial financial burdens such as health. Lastly, he maintains that they have a higher aversion to health risk than men with particular reference to STDs and pregnancy-related infections.

By age and sex structure, between the age bracket of 15 and 19 years, 2 girls versus 1 boy per 100 are said to be HIV positive. Between the age category of 20-24 years, 8 girls and 3 boys per hundred are reported to be HIV positive. In the 25-29 years age bracket, 10 girls per 100 are reportedly HIV positive as compared to 5 boys (CTDHS, 2005). The above age brackets are composed of people with great economic and social potentials. This is in consonant with the findings of other scholars (eg Nyamongo,1995:45) who rightly observed that "…..AIDS predominantly affects young and middle aged people, those in their prime productive years". The World Bank (1989) observed that "among the African adult population the largest amount of infected people are between 16 and 29 years".

The Southwest province has 5.1% male and 11% female HIV infection rate. The other two provinces where FC is also practiced are the East and Far North Provinces. The former has 7. 6% male and 9.4% female rate of HIV cases whereas the latter has 1.7% male and 2.2% female rate of HIV infection respectively. These figures seem to undermine the view that associates FC with high prevalence rates of HIV/AIDS infection. Nevertheless, these statistics clearly show that women are more at risk than men.

The same trend is reflected by the data for Cameroon's main cities of Douala and Yaoundé where the male to female percentage ratios are higher for the former than for the latter category. Douala has 3.7% male and 5. 5% female rate of infection whereas for Yaoundé it is 6% male and 10.7% female rate of infection. The findings here like for the whole of Cameroon reflect the worldwide infection rate in terms of age and gender structure. In other words, all over the world, young and able men and women are affected but more women than men, probably owing to women's vulnerability and lack of power in negotiating safer sex. The table that follows captures this information for Cameroon displaying the percentages in terms of gender by province and the average. The same pattern is shown for the main cities of Douala and Yaoundé.

Fig. 11 Distribution of HIV/AIDS by age and sex for Cameroon

PROVINCE	Male	Female	Average
Adamaoua	4.1%	9.8 %	6.9 %
Centre	2.2 %	6.8 %	4.7 %
Douala	3.7%	5.5 %	4.6 %
East	7.6%	9.4 %	8.6 %
Far North	1.7%	2.2 %	2 %
Littoral	4.4%	6.5 %	5.5 %
North	1.7%	1.7 %	1.7 %
Northwest	5.2%	11.9 %	8.7 %
West	5.2%	4.3 %	4.7 %
South	4.5%	8.4 %	6.5 %
Southwest	5.1%	11 %	8 %
Yaounde	6%	10.7 %	8.3 %

Source: CTDHS, 2005

Social mobilization against HIV/AIDS in Cameroon is hierarchically organized. At the top of the organizational structure is the Ministry of Public Health which makes and ensures the implementation of HIV/AIDS policies in the country. The ministry works in close collaboration with the Provincial AIDS Control Committees who oversee social mobilization at the provincial levels. They are assisted at the Divisional levels by Health Area Committees, who are further assisted by local AIDS Control Committees in various villages. Each Health Area Committee is financed at a meagre total of 500, 000frs CFA (USD 1000). This amount is portioned out as follows: 120.000 frs CFA, (USD 240), 24% of the total amount is designated to the activities of community leaders. After organizing a trimester of activities, each community leader is entitled to 2500 frs CFA (USD 5). A further 180,000 frs CFA, (USD 360) amounting to 36% of the global total amount is allocated to peer group educators.

The fight against HIV/AIDS like many other aspects of development and especially rural development in particular and national life in general, is bedecked by inaccessibility to rural areas, lack of logistics, opaque management and inordinate corruption. Most often, the money ends up in private pockets at the top and never trickles down to the grass roots. This has led to the acute lack of logistics such as sensitization materials, means of transportation and lack of motivation on the part of community educators. And to compound matters, there is still underaction to and negation of the existence of AIDS probably due to ignorance among some segments of the population.

Local reactions to the HIV/AIDS pandemic in these communities varies between recognition that AIDS exists and is a global threat with no biomedical answer in sight, to a culture of silence that revolves around negation, resignation and subsequently the outright denial of the existence of the pandemic. In other words, although most people are conscious that AIDS exist and that it is caused by unprotected heterosexual activities usually with multiple partners and the sharing of sharp instruments such as needles, syringes, razor blades and pins with an infected individual, there is still under-reaction to the HIV/AIDS scourge. Some individuals attribute it to the activities of personalistic agents such as witches and wizards.

The Ejaghams are located at the Cameroon-Nigeria border region, an area marked by intense mobility. Their borderline location has been a trade outpost since colonial times with people passing in and out of the region spreading both new ideas, lifestyles, fashions and diseases in the process. This passage of people, ideas, goods and services has led to the people's interaction with others and a high number of temporal partners is maintained by some traders, long distance truck drivers and uniformed officers in the area.

Given women's vulnerability, the overall consequence has been the spread of venereal diseases, including HIV which causes AIDS. This has further resulted in the visibly large number of fatherless children and single mothers in the area. Orphaned children are clearly seen as a burden to social networks as grandparents and other close relatives of AIDS victims are at times saddled with the responsibility of taking care of them. I could observe teenage school girls dating mostly elderly men at the hotel where I usually stayed each time I went to Mamfe town. These school girls carrying books, who had probably left their homes under the pretext of going to read and sleep in school, could be observed leaving the hotel as early as 4-5 am each morning. In the internet cafes, online dating is a fashionable pastime for many youths in Mamfe town. Their target is usually wealthy whites who would get married to them and eventually take them abroad.

Probably lured by some traders and long distance drivers in the early 1980s, and pushed by economic doldrums, most single women in the area, like their neighbouring Bayangs-who are stereotypically presumed to be famous for urban prostitution in Cameroon, migrated out of the villages into various towns of Cameroon and even across the border as far as Gabon and Nigeria to work as commercial sex workers. Most of them often send remittances back home, thereby luring others to see the overt advantages of sex work in the process. At times, they come home and recruit young women for their "secuire businesses". They often return home when they are ageing and therefore selling at the lower end of the commercial love market. Alternatively, some return home to die due to infection from AIDS so as to spare relatives of the burden of transporting their corpses across long distances.

Some people, despite the general awareness that AIDS is an existing disease with no therapeutic solution in sight, however, attribute the cause of the disease to 'slow poison' and witchcraft. In other words, they see patients as those who, because of hatred and animosity with others, have been mystically bewitched. They have been mystically injected with the virus and they will get slim and eventually die. It seems that witches and wizards are now using AIDS symptoms as one way of doing away with their victims while at the same time covering their tracks. Being attacked by 'witchcraft' has become an alibi to suffering from AIDS. This rejectionist attitude to AIDS is partly fuelled by the fact that it is still a terminal disease. Some individuals have accordingly resigned to fate, holding that if it was preordained that they will die by contracting AIDS, then, there is virtually nothing they can do about it. This is reflexive and reminiscent of the initial attitude of the Cameroonian authorities when the pandemic was first reported in 1987. For fear of lossing much cherished touristic revenue by frightening tourists away, the authorities in Yaoundé downplayed and even falsified HIV/AIDS statistics, under-reporting initial cases at the very beginning of the pandemic (Ajaga,1999). This government ambivalence actually brought traditional medicine to prominence as a last resort since it has a holistic vision of patients. In fact, traditional healers and vendors of medicinal plants alike took advantage of the government's ambivalence and invaded urban centres with billboards carrying among others, pictures of pale and wasting, scarry-looking, infected individuals. Variously nicknamed euphemistically as "slow poison", "maladie d'amour" and associated to malevolent spirits, they put up billboards explaining that they had a ready cure for the "slim disease", "seven plus one", "nine minus one". One of several billboards carried the epithet "Pharmacie qui "traitent" les maladies depassant la medecine moderne"(Pharmacy which treates diseases that are above modern medicine) referring among others, to HIV/AIDS (See Pemunta, 2001). Given their track record in the treatment of venereal diseases, biomedicine's lack of an immediate response to the scourge and the collapse of the health care system in the wake of the structural adjustment programme imposed by the Brettonwoods institutions on Cameroon and other African countries, they enjoyed a boom.The government's public acceptance that 'only prostitutes were carriers' (the most easily identified and stigmatized risk group) would have scared away tourists from the country (Ajaga, 1999).

It is against this backdrop of contestation, denial and resignation to AIDS that pro-female ritual circumcision advocates maintain that it instils calmness and sexual reservation in women and is therefore a moral check against the presumed ravages of non-circumcision. They argue that the sexual immorality, which has today become the order of the day is because females are no longer circumcised and are freely exercising their sexuality. Although there is a likelihood of a relationship between FC and HIV/AIDS (though scientifically still unestablished but hypothesized about), this group of "hardliners" continue to claim that FC has nothing to do with HIV/AIDS.

Although heterosexual intercourse is the main mode of transmission of HIV in this region, FC can fuel transmission and has psychological and psychosexual impact reminiscent of suffering from AIDS. For a detailed account of the stigma of HIV/AIDS, see for instance Campbell et al. (2005). First and foremost, it has been hypothesized that HIV infected sharp objects such as a blade, if used on several individuals, one after the other, can lead to the transmission of diseases with HIV/AIDS inclusive. Further, a circumciser will also be at the risk of infection with the virus if she wounds herself while cutting the clitoris of an infected initiate. Depending on the type undergone, FC can further leave scars on the vagina that can render the woman more vulnerable to a man infected with HIV during intercourse.

In some cases, sexual difficulties caused by circumcision can even cause separation between couples and social insecurity for the woman.

Psychologically, the shame and stigma resulting from non-circumcision through social ostracization by significant social others has reminiscences to suffering from AIDS. Apart from being a likely threat to health security, it threatens women's social security networks. Despite the possible associations between FC and HIV/AIDS, 'hardliners' advance various defensive arguments. Among these is the fact that circumcision like scarification of the body for therapeutic purposes is now being done with one razor blade for every individual and with modern anesthesia to stop bleeding. This is simultaneously a reaction to the presumed violence and risk of the ritual bodily procedures and an appropriation of the concept of health security. On the one hand, some people among the population even claim that AIDS is a fiction. On the other, some attribute its cause and spread only to heterosexual intercourse. Both groups therefore point to the need to tighten control over women and their sexuality as a 'native' response to the scourge of the pandemic.

This group of "hardliners" further attribute the presumed falling moral standards to the impact of the sexual revolution from the West. Accordingly, they accuse the West of trying to balkanize and see to the eventual collapse of their cultural system and its eventual disintegration by preaching non-circumcision for females. Some even conceive AIDS "to be a Whiteman's way of fooling people not to enjoy themselves" because they say that they do not achieve sexual fulfilment when they have protected sex. "How can I eat sweets in a wrappen paper?"(meaning to have sex while wearing a condom, 'with socks on').The following interview excerpt is in order here:

> People are being infected every day. There are some areas where people still believe there is no AIDS. It may be that the few learned people there, especially the men, still tell these young girls they want to have sex with them, that there is no AIDS. It is the Whiteman's way of fooling people not to enjoy themselves. Because they say they don't enjoy protected sex. "How can I eat sweets in a wrappen [polythene]", they say. That is what they feel. That is the problem. They don't believe that there is AIDS. And then mothers too, when their daughters are in town schooling say in the university, in secondary schools, staying out of the village where there are no such schools- the children come [meaning come back infected], they say it is slow poison. That people have poisoned their daughters. They find it difficult to accept that it is AIDS, even when tests have been conducted. They refuse to admit it because when they admit it, you see, it will be very effective. The next mother or family will know and then, will say no, it has happened to my friend here, just next door. Let me look at how I can talk to my daughter just to prevent it. So, there is a culture of silence and denial. But I think that there is hardly a family here in the Division, that you could say, which has not been touched [by the scourge of HIV/AID] .If I say Division I just want to be cautious but if not, I could say in the whole Province, which is not touched. (Madam Nyenty Henriette, Divisional Delegate For Women's Empowerment, Mamfe, Interview of 18/05/06).

Despite the scientifically documented existence of HIV/AIDS, the interview excerpt cited above like many others, emphasizes that some people still say it is 'slow poison'. In other words, witches and wizards have mystically infected their loved ones with poison so as to eliminate them. Some people equally conceptualize condoms as a capitalist weapon meant to drain people's money and to cut down on the population. One young lady, Anni, questioned the economic logic behind the existence of several categories of condoms with different prices and concluded that AIDS is a disease for the poor since the poor cannot afford to procure expensive condoms, which are believed to be safer and effective in the prevention of HIV. They are therefore discriminated against because they are poor. She reasoned that they are accordingly allowed to die. She further said that some men are against condom use because it seems as if the woman is determining or keeping count of the number of sexual episodes that a man is having with her. But in reality, it seems that poverty is part of the real issue at stake here since most men are unable even to afford condoms constantly. This has partly led to the inconsistent use of condoms, usually only with suspected disease carriers, "easy going ladies", but not with others and for the womenfolk, usually to forestall the eventuality of pregnancy. This 'discrimination' in the use of condoms and inconsistency has implications for the spread of venereal diseases with HIV inclusive.

> They look at condoms as a foreign thing [body] that has been brought into society to reduce their sexual taste, the pleasure of sex. They prefer going them live, flesh to flesh. Very few use condoms. Some women even become pregnant before they know that they have taken in because, some are embarrassed. You see a woman giving birth to 5-8 children, not because she likes it, she fails to know that she can protect herself and they hardly come out to ask for medical advice. Most of them don't even understand their system, how they operate, which is the safe or unsafe period. When they become pregnant, they only struggle to abort and when they do not succeed, they decide grudgingly to give birth. But to prevent or go for family planning with their husbands, most do not. The lack of medical facilities and illiteracy are the main factors behind this. If a woman gives birth and stays for long, say, eight years, without giving birth again, it is looked upon as being abnormal as being the handiwork of witchcraft. She is normally supposed to be giving birth, year in and year out, without resting (Ofuka Jacob, interview of 18/07/2006,Otu village).

In the above interview excerpt, the respondent Ofuka, a Parent Teacher Association employee and drug vendor in Otu village points to lack of knowledge about family planning and the failure by the population to use condoms because it is a foreign object meant to interfere with sexual pleasure. Most people prefer "to go live, flesh to flesh". The end result of this ignorance is multiple unwanted pregnancies, abortions and naturally, the risk of infection from venereal diseases with HIV inclusive which is even compounded by the lack of medical facilities within reach. The people love children so much so that infertility is a cause for concern, usually associated to witchcraft. It might be said that because of this penchant for children, the woman's reproductive and sexual health is always at stake.

In the face of the HIV/AIDS pandemic, most protestant religious denominations in the study area present the disease and the lack of a medical breakthrough as a form of divine retribution for sins presumed to have been committed by the people. This reflects the presence of all the ingredients of HIV in the community. The churches are using this discursive repertoire to uphold morality in matters of sexuality but the hardliners within the local population are calling for a return or reinforcement of FC to achieve the same aim. The AIDS discourse therefore seems to be working both ways here whereas a third discourse presents the ritual cutting as being capable of facilitating the transmission of HIV/AIDS.

I have thus far described the people's attitude towards the moral and sexual panic generated by the advent of the HIV/AIDS pandemic. I have further established the likely link between HIV/AIDS and circumcision, the causes and representations of the pandemic among the people as well as their underaction to the pandemic.

In the next section, I will examine local state and NGO-delegated initiatives and their entanglement in international activities and institutions aimed at curbing FC among the Ejaghams. This leads me on to an evaluation of the anti-FC campaign messages as well as the people's perception of various intervening NGOs. I begin with state initiatives before examining the activities of local NGOS. I argue that the issue of FC is subject to various knowledge practices whereby it is understood as a particular type of social, political or economic activity. The issue of FC juxtaposes Western science, rational knowledge and medicine against tradition and local knowledge. I argue that there can be points of convergence and dialogue among these centrifugal forces. The state and NGOs like some segments of the local population are in alliance with the former as represented by the harmful health effect model of NGO activism. I begin with state initiatives before examining those of a selected number of NGOs.

4.2 State and NGO initiatives

Cameroon has signed an avalanche of both regional and international treaties aimed at protecting the rights of women and children. Among these treaties are : the Convention on the Rights of the Child (1989), the Convention on the Elimination of All Forms of Discrimination Against Women (CEDAW), 1981, the African Charter on Human and People's Rights (1986) and the Programme of Action Adopted by the United Nations International Conference on Population and Development (ICPD) in Cairo (1994) among others. While the signing and ratification of these and many other treaties shows the state's commitment to the welfare of women and children, it further provides evidence for the government's subscription to international norms aimed at protecting women and children.

Furthermore, Cameroon is one of the several beneficiaries of the Regional Action Plan co-sponsored by the World Health Organisation (WHO), the United Nation's Children's Emergency Fund (UNICEF) and the United Nations Population Fund (UNPF) with the aim of accelerating the eradication of FC. It was launched in Yaounde, Cameroon, in 1997 within the framework of a seminar to strategize on culturally appropriate strategies to fight against F C. This action plan is based on three interrelated approaches: to educate the public and legislators on the necessity to abandon FC, to fight against this practice as a violation of the human rights of the woman as well as her right to health and to encourage the conceptualisation and the eventual putting in place of a National Action Plan Against FC which is specifically adapted to various local cultural contexts.

The support programme to initiatives for the abandonment of FC is executed by the German Technical Co-operation (GTZ) on behalf of the German Federal Ministry for Economic Co-operation and Development. This project encourages innovative activities in diverse countries of West and Central Africa, reinforces the putting in place of networks and evaluates approaches adopted for the fight against FC. In Cameroon, it has supported various activities elected by the national branch of IAC in the development of information, education and communication tools for the mobilisation and sensitisation of change agents at the community level and for the organisation of sensitisation seminars in regions where FC is practised. Change agents could be members of a given community, capable of playing a pivotal role in decision-making processes in relation to the practice of FC such as parents, health workers, and teachers, religious and political authorities or the youths. The project equally brings together governmental and non-governmental institutions so as to reinforce the efforts of the public administration and of judicial institutions in a bid to bring an end to FC.

The Cameroon Ministry of Social Affairs and Women's Empowerment (MINASCOF), in collaboration with NGOs launched an anti-FC campaign and adopted a National Action Plan in 1999. The national Chapter of the Inter-African Committee For the Fight Against Harmful Traditional Practices (IAC), a network of national associations found in FC practising countries in Africa and Europe, played a primordial role in drafting it.

However, the scope and funding of this ambitious programme is in contest and curiously enough, the state party has never implemented it.

In June 2004, a Private Member Bill against FC tabled by the opposition Social Democratic Front was defeated in parliament and the ritual procedures have continued unabated. At the Dakar Parliamentary Conference of 4-5 December, 2005, Cameroon and eighteen other African countries observed by Switzerland and the United Kingdom pledged to develop and enforce legislation for the abandonment of FC, develop and implement national strategies and to adopt adequate national budgets as well as to fully collaborate through international and regional co-operation in the fight against FC. Despite these rather positive strides, there is still no law against FC in Cameroon. Suffice it to state here that the Cameronian state only frames the issue of FC and allows NGOs to conduct sensitization at the grass root level.I will attempt to explain the legal vacuum within which FC is practiced in Cameroon below.

I have argued in the preceding section that the government of Cameroon currently has no law against the practice of FC. However, general assault laws can be readily invoked and applied if a circumciser in the process of circumcising an initiate causes harm. My analysis shows that some frantic but abortive efforts have been made over the years in an attempt to criminalize FC (see above). The Cameroonian state seems to be aligning with those who support the *status quo* for political gains probably because outrightly condemning the culture of various practising communities could lead to alienation and the loss of electoral votes to the opposition. The validity of such a strategic explanation however seems doubtful (but is plausible like the situation in Sierra Leone seems to suggest). The Cameroonian State's refusal to criminalize FC has reminiscences to the Sierra Leonian situation. Although the latter has signed treaties to protect women and children's rights, politicians still appropriate the Bondo secret society for their own aims. In Sierra Leone where there is an approximately 80-90 percent prevalence rate of FC (Skaine, 2005:235), there is simultaneous open state alignment with and co-optation of the Bondo secret society whose membership procedure includes FC. Many politicians prefer to court and cajole members of the Bondo by building them initiation centres or "bushes" in their constituencies, providing money to meet up with the initiation of large groups of girls into the society rather than enlist their wrath by condemning them.

Although the Cameroon People's Democratic Movement (CPDM) party has always 'won' a landslide majority in the various FC practising communities all over the country, the conduct of the various elections is never fair and transparent. A more convincing argument to explain the legal vacuum with regards to FC in Cameroon is an institutional explanation. The supporters of the procedures who are predominantly the community leaders and traditional birth attendants have elaborated and successfully used various discursive repertoires based on self-autonomy, the preservation of tradition and the upholding of moral values particularly in the face of the HIV/AID pandemic. The pandemic has become an ambivalent framework for both support and contestation of FC with "traditionalists" arguing that FC provides a "moral native antidote" against the ravages of the pandemic while anti-FC activists point to the prospects of the ritual cuttings to fuel the spread of HIV. A third group wants medicalization so as to do away with the harmful effects of the procedures.

Another possible reason for Cameroon's failure to enact a law against FC is the fear of violating minority and individual rights. This is ably illustrated by the following interview abstract:

> When I just came here and was staying down there, a woman gave birth to a baby. Her child was circumcised and the very next morning, the child died. They did not report to the police. It is their culture and it was their child. How will they tell the police?(Mami Celina,interview of 07/03/06, Eyumojock).

The respondent cited above points to a conspiracy between family members in not bringing cases of death occasioned by circumcision to the attention of the forces of law and order, and invokes both individual and cultural rights as justification for such acts of complicity. The latter view is best illustrated by the interview abstract below, in which the respondent opts for continuity through medicalization while highlighting the issue of individual rights and choice. He further points out that anti-social behaviour (like FC because of the various health risks it entails), is decried but people still submit their daughters to the ritual practice.

> If instruments are clean and safe, circumcision can still be good to those who still wish. Some time a canoe capsizes in a river, people still go by it. You see a train can derail, people will still continue to travel by train. A plane can crash but people will continue to travel by air. We refuse stealing but people still steal (Tambe Robert, interview of 03/04/06, Eyumojock).

Cameroon's 1996 Constitution states for instance that "the state shall ensure the protection of all minorities and shall protect the rights of indigenous populations in accordance with the law[1]". The various

[1] At the same time, this Constitution is curiously silent on the use of native law although it could be argued that the protection of indigenous rights as they exist

communities where FC is practised in Cameroon are in the minority when compared to other ethnic groups. This is the case because in the national constitution, the government has expressed its commitment to respect the culture and customs of every ethnic group as well as the freedom of any ethnic entity to pursue its culture. This constitutional provision certainly places the government in a dilemma with regards to outlawing FC.

Moreover, in the wake of the present economic crises that most African countries including Cameroon are going through, the tendency is to enact legislation as a means to capture much needed international resources which are thereafter diverted to solve other pressing problems if ever, since corruption and inordinate embezzlement of state resources are key issues in the management of public finances in Cameroon. We should recall here that the American State Department in the 1990s packaged and tied human rights and, especially the rights of women and children to its financial and developmental aid packages to African countries with FC practicing communities ("donor democracy"). For most countries, instituting legislation will imply setting aside resources for the implementation of such laws. This is partly given impetus by the fact that the lack of resources with which to implement such laws by countries like Tanzania, Togo and Burkina Faso which adopted anti-FC laws has led to failure.

Lastly, seemingly in keeping with but contrary to Mcknight's (1986:415) axiom for critical health action that "to convert a medical problem into a political issue is central to health improvement", the Cameroon government's reduction of the complexity of the issue of FC into a health issue alone, the same narrow basis of NGO activism, has frustrated intersectorial collaboration. Medical doctors as administrators in the health ministry of various countries with Cameroon inclusive generally wield a lot of power in the ranking of government health priorities. Officials at the Women and Family Empowerment Ministry and its Provincial and Divisional delegations constantly hinted at this issue in discussions bordering on FC in particular and the status of women in general with me. Although they claimed at the same time that the government was following the provisions of the CEDAW convention to stem the tide of FC and to improve upon women's status in Cameroon. The fight against FC ought to be part of a holistic plan to fight poverty. The practice has to do with differential power between men and women as well as with the economic and social livelihoods of both the women who

---

under customary law is provided for in the light of this principle. As Njoko (2006) points out, the protection of indigenous rights under customary law has not yet been put to contest in the courts.

undergo the ritual practice and the perpetrators who have vested interest in the ritual procedures and will not want an end to it.

To compound matters, corruption is a key issue in the award of contracts in every facet of national life. NGO representatives are always sidelined when it comes to discussions on women's issue or only called in if they have powerful networks within the upper echelon of the administration. Social education campaign funds from government sources are mostly doled out to political clients of the regime. This has left most NGOs without the right network at the mercy of international and multilateral donors, which partly presents them as agents of the "whiteman" in the eyes of the local population since he who sponsors a dance definitely determines the tune of the music. To give more vent to this perception, they hardly domestic the health concepts used in the anti-FC advocacy campaigns, a situation that creates both resistance and contestation.

4.3 Local NGO initiatives

A dense network of local NGOs including the Inter-African Committee for the Fight Against Harmful Traditional Practices (IAC), ABEMO, the Youth Development Centre and the Association for the Fight Against Female Genital Mutilation (ACAFEG) are intervening in the fight against AIDS, FC practices and other harmful traditional practices. Alongside the state, they have adopted the modernist health paradigm which sees FC as a harmful traditional practice, calling for the need to eradicate it.

The IAC is a regional and international organization with affiliates in 24 countries and branches in immigrant receiving countries such as Britain, Switzerland, France and a liaison office in Geneva. The Cameroon national chapter sensitises opinion, religious leaders and the general public against the harmful effects of FC, undertakes the retraining of health personel and TBAs. This organisation like all others is the point of connection between locally based and international organisations.

Another local NGO fighting against FC in Ejagham land is ABEMO. They focus on issues of rural development with a specific focus on women through legal awareness. The underlying philosophy of this organisation is ''Knowledge is the first step towards a better life'' and 'Keep women intact, women need to be themselves''. They are out to train women so that they can become their own change agents by knowing their rights through economic empowerment and the acquisition of both survival and marketable skills. The activists use two interrelated strategies in the fight against FC. First, they undertake community sensitization on the harmful effects of FC at all ages.Secondly, they are attempting to build a general consensus among opinion, political leaders, parents, men and women alike usually by casting the traditional motivations supporting FC against a counter modernist health belief paradigm. Knowing fully well that circumcision was the main criterion for dancing the 'NKIM' dance, they point out that the agility to dance has nothing to do with cutting and that an uncircumcised girl can perform just as a circumcised one, if not, better. This is the case in villages such as Ebinsi, Ajah and Ayukaba. They also cite women with established sexual biographies to show that sexual desire is a mental process and not in the genitals and that prostitution is explicitly meant to garner resources rather than just to offer sexual pleasure to many partners.

This signboard in Otu village, also implanted in other Ejagham villages by ABEMO carries the religious ethos that "FC is Against Christian beliefs", is dangerous and against human rights. This is of course, the donor's ideological stamp and label. It further enumerates some of the long and short term consequences of FC and shows the organization's affiliation with the First Presbyterian Church Ithaca-New York, USA, the sponsors. Critics of FC and the organization are quick to point out that it is an idle sign post as most villagers are "illiterates" and that it has no meaning to them.

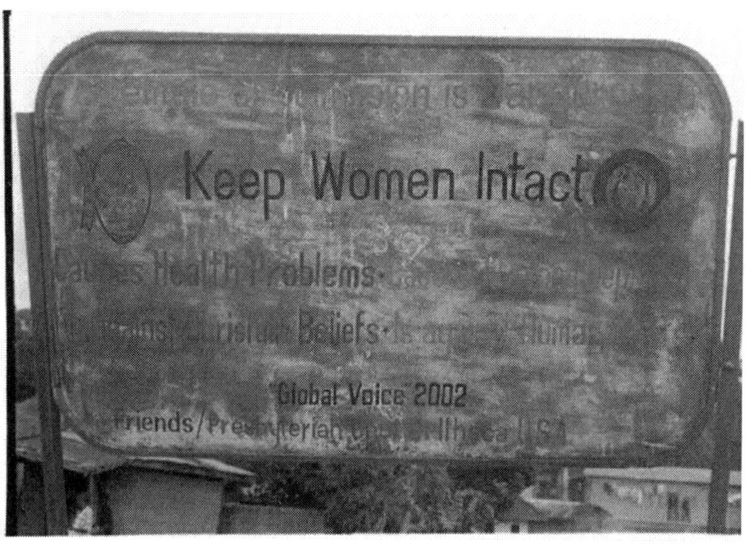

Fig. 12 ABEMO anti-FC advocacy bill board at Otu Village. Copy right, the author.

The Youth Development Centre also uses empowerment approaches against economic hardship, rising youth unemployment, juvenile deliquency, illiteracy, ignorance and the scourge of the HIV/AIDS pandemic. They have held seminars in the Ejagham area on the various likely associations between HIV/AIDS and FC. Their main philosophy is to use a gradual but integrated approach to talk the people out of the ritual practice of FC through young men and women who represent a counter version of modernity. Like other intervening NGOs, their main goal however is total eradication and not modification as a first step.

The Association for the Fight Against Female Genital Mutilation (ACAFEG) focus on the political, economic, social and cultural education of rural women. They are engaged in identifying cut and uncut girls and women within practicing communities in the Upper Ekwe region where their activities are concentrated. They equally operate an adult literacy programme and have so far graduated 13 people among whom are three TBAs. Graduants are expected to be role models and to ensure that uncut women are not ostracised from their communities. They provide formal education to children at risk of mutilation as a pre-emptic major against forced child marriage which is very rampant in the area.

The underlying politics and philosophy behind these NGOs is to act as agents of governmentality through the modern health concepts that they use in their anti-FC campaigns. They are accordingly perceived and represented as agencies of the Whiteman, a perception that has reinforced both resistance and contestation among certain segments of the local community. Furthermore, transnational mobilization against FC through regional bodies like the IAC might be interpreted as a mechanism to limit immigration and asylum claims based on the effects of apparently negative cultural practices such as FC. It might be stated here that FC is connected to a far broader world and field in which the local intrudes into the global in a way: modern medicine and western scientific rationality confronts local cultural practices and knowledge systems. This has implications in the way that FC is conceived, be it as violence, a threat to human security, human rights, the rights of women and children, and it becomes an object of knowledge and power practices through the activities of NGOs and then get relayed in other fields such as medicine, law, gender, migration and development.

It might be argued that my 'multiplex identities' as an insider/outsider (male, black man, Cameroonian and African affiliated to the 'Whiteman' by virtue of my western education and therefore an agent of neo-colonialism), and therefore presumed positionality in the anti-FC advocacy camp as well as the people's diverse and often shifting reactions reflect the larger global context of power in which the contentious cultural practice of FC is enmeshed and how, this power nucleus may be shaping the practices on the ground as evidenced by the ambiguous and often shifting positions of internal stakeholders especially when faced with the global network of local, national and international NGOs calling for eradication of the ritual procedures and the increasing privatization of FC on younger girls. The increasing internationalization of the world through processes such as trade finance, technology, threats to human security, communications, research, education and culture has led among other consequences to the mutual penetration of economic, political and social forces among the nations of the world (Smelser, 1992:371). As Smelser points out, it might also be the case that the governments of nation-states are progressively lossing degrees of direct control that affect them and this implies rethinking the fundamental social science assumption that the primary unit of analysis is the nation, the society or the culture. Social change should therefore be seen as the outcome of a complex fusion between external and internal, endogenous and exogenous forces. These external forces include the presence and influence of other societies in a given society's environment (international, intersocial, and intercultural forces) while internal factors are comprised of the mutual interrelations of values, social structure, and classes as they are institutionalized in a given society. Both forces fuse to either generate or block social change.

Given that the underdevelopment of the Third World does not rest only on internal factors but on the fact that they are an integral part of the world economy, it might be argued that given their dependency on the First World, a dependency that gives the latter power and leverage, increased dependency in the face of global economic downturn has led to a surge in national and international concerns about the practice of FC. In the light of world systems theory, different patterns of relations largely determine the internal economic fates of nations in each category. The state becomes the agency charged with executing and implementing or resisting the strictures imposed by other national governments, international banking agencies and transnational organizations. In the internationalization of the FC debates, it is clear that states with practising ethnicities have less control over their economies and therefore their political fates. They are told by the international community to eradicate FC practices or lose development aid. Faced with this situation, different states have adopted different positions. On the one hand, some have criminalized the procedures, at times without implementing the ban because of a conspiracy of obstacles embedded in both state structures such as weak legal systems, lack of funds and in the socio-legal structures of the local communities, particularly their kin-based social structures and a conspiracy of silence among family members.

The state plays a delicate balancing role: reconciling local sentiments and institutions on the one hand and resisting the imposition of supposedly external norms and on the other, adopting international normative standards of human rights. In the case of anti-FC campaigns, national interests and international norms calling for eradication clash and there is the need to reconcile local, national and international ideals. Despite the increasing internationalization of the national economy, 'national politics remains national' (Smelser, 1992:391). States are increasingly finding themselves arbitrating economic contradictions and political conflicts that are fuelled by them. They must therefore respond to forces that are neither of their own making nor of their own society's making. These forces are played out in different ways. In the first instance, external political and financial agencies join the domestic political arena as they attempt to influence economic policy. They also enter domestic politics as they are singled out as politically responsible agents. The linking of development aid to the eradication of FC can be read and understood in this light. Secondly, there is the presence of international political movements, human rights, peace and others (NGOs and their allies at various scales) which often constitute political pressures on domestic governments. Thirdly, the development of systems of international politics in the UN and various regional federations and coalitions such as the IAC involves interplay among national political interest and international processes. Fourthly, cultural diffusion through the mass media is out of the control of national governments as they tend to influence popular attitudes, values, political understandings and sentiments. This has exposed but at the same time dramatized the effects of FC cutting practices and created resistance among certain segments of the population in practising societies. Simultaneously, countries that resist presumed alien cultural influences such as the call for the eradication of FC have difficulties in doing so because once the door is opened to international exposure through mass media; it is difficult to shut it again. Cultural influences are shaped by domestic traditions, values and interest illustrating the interplay between external and internal processes.

Governmental and NGO-informed interventions and concerns against FC merge over the issue of human security. They are independent but interrelated power fields and vehicles of domination. In their own right, NGOs are agents of power, at the same time, they represent state power and both the state and NGOs are preoccupied with security, an issue over which they converge and which has kept the flames of anti-Fc activism alive.

4.4 NGOs as agents of state power and the issue of security

Countries in which some ethnic groups practice FC are called upon by national and international NGOs to eradicate the ritual procedure of FC. This is to happen through the enactment and subsequent enforcement of legislation based on the health security discourse. This discourse is framed in terms of the protection of women and children's human rights and health through the '*challenge of the growing shared risk of disaster, disease and disruptions*' (Missiroli 2007). This is evident from the health concepts used in the anti-FC campaigns and materials. Low income countries are mostly influenced through the linking of development aid with democratization, good governance and the respect for human rights ('donor democracy'). One of the implicit aims of such policies is to decrease the influx of refugees into wealthy donor countries. Some potential victims have been granted asylum on the basis of their risk of undergoing FC should they return to their home countries (See for instance, Boyles and Preves 2000).

Transnational stakeholders have invoked the notion of health risk and, by extension, the comprehensive concept of human security to justify their presence and dominance in FC practicing communities and countries because of two main reasons. First of all, they aim to protect the human security of individuals, in this case women and children, enables transnational stakeholders to legitimately influence the authority of the state. Secondly, human security and state sovereignty are not incompatible when a '*cautious approach to human security is used…[while] a broader understanding of the concept challenges state sovereignty more fundamentally*'' (Oberleitner 2005:193). However, most states, Cameroon and Egypt for example, while publicly endorsing the international commitment to end FC, at the same time distance themselves from that goal at home and assert their sovereignty. While intense emotions and power underpin the interest and concern of transnational stakeholders and their local allies who seek to end FC, the issue must, I argue, be contextualised in the historical responses and relationships of colonizing powers when they first encountered the procedures. Styled as 'irrational, immoral, and uncivilized' by the horrified British colonial administration in Sudan (Abusharaf, 2006:209), historical responses can and must be placed within larger questions of gender, power and colonial governmentality' whose aim was to 'police women directly and indirectly through kinsmen, chiefs and clerics.....[a process that came] to occupy centre stage in colonial legislative agendas' (Ibid). Following the colonial perspective, women's power needed to be circumscribed and their bodies governed, in order to inscribe colonial rule. There is a clear need here for the abandonment of the West's 'positional superiority' (Said, 1978) and the need to advocate a single standard in ethical and legal evaluations of the practices.

I suggest that NGOs and other transnational actors appropriate the concept of health risk and security also to reinforce their status and to promote their own self-interests. Such interests include the promotion of neo-liberal ideology and 'third way' welfare development (Kemshell 2002:133). The preoccupation with health security in low income countries is a reaction to 'tradition' where 'modernity' is supposed to confront the high level of risk created by the neo-liberal paradigm. Kemshall (2002), for instance states that '*risk is replacing need as the central principle of social policy formation and welfare delivery*'. On her part, Joyce (2001) makes the claim that the management of health risk has become the most essential form of governance within the neo-liberal health discourse. Following her advice, citizens are supposed to act cautiously as consumers of health care. In his application of the notion of risk and secure development, Duffield (2001) points out that '*development is a new, largely privatized form of security,... aimed at changing the conduct of populations*'. Taken as such, this indicates that the risk-conscious society perpetuates neo-liberal ideology and that transnational actors who oblige states to adopt it help construct that social model.

NGOs become vectors for the dissemination of information about risk among the population. It is assumed that since they work at the grass roots, they are able to effectively transmit issues of health security because of their presumed rapport with local communities. As professionals with roles of medics and other kinds of caregivers, they '*are trusted and highly regarded*' (Coutler 2003:235) by some segments of the local population as vectors of modernity. However, even those NGOs have both the power to do good and bad. In terms of governmentality, the closer NGOs as transnational agents '*become associated with the delivery of welfare (such as the provision of human security), the more well defined and institutionalized professional autonomy becomes and individuals become passive consumers of collective health care provision* (Joyce 2001:296-297) and information. Local NGOs who might be regarded as the 'professionals' in the anti-FC campaigns are highly dependent on the financial and logistic resources of powerful transnational stakeholders and have virtually become transmission belts for information from the latter. I argue that this hierarchical relationship impacts negatively on anti-FC campaigns as they are regarded as agents of neocolonialism, thereby fuelling resistance and contestation in the process.

Local NGOs as grass root development agencies assist the state and transnational actors. There is an overlap in the roles of these three stakeholders. The former, for instance, help to establish health security in cooperation with the latter two stakeholders. While local NGOs may be said to be playing the role of the state at the grass roots, the state uses them to reinforce its authority especially where they tend to execute state and transnational projects and agenda. Gibbens and Reimer (1999:120) draw our attention to the fact that states create structures and construct 'defense spaces' as a mechanism of retaining power and to subvert the decision-making processes of other superior actors. Relying here on two notions, Foucault's 'disciplinary power' and governmentality and the Gramscian theory of hegemony, I will argue that FC practicing countries use risk discourse as a tool to garner scarce resources from multinational organizations and Western governments. Local NGOs function as facilitators for this purpose. The state allows them to conduct sensitization campaigns. The notions of development and health thus become one 'operating unit of power' (Adams 1966, 1975 in Wolf 2001) for maintaining their authority. They simultaneously permit the state to 'resist' imposition from transnational stakeholders with their financial and ideological clout while both are appropriating those same resources for other ends. Risk should be conceived in the light of the governmentality paradigm as a way of constituting society and as a functional governmental rationality (Strydom 2002:45). Since the population becomes subjugated to surveillance and self-regulation, the notion of risk by extension should rather be viewed as a state mechanism for controlling and tightening security over its population and borders.

The state articulates and preserves its power by appropriating the notion of security in a bid to transform the people into 'docile bodies', a population that is increasingly focused on non-local norms. Here the state determines what it takes to be human - care for children and the protection of the nation become effective tools of influence over individuals. On the other hand, the people rely on the state for their health security. The official discourse emphasizes the responsibility of the individual which is at the same time not centered on the individual *per se* but rather on the preservation of a greater social collectivity. The ideologically defined good of the people isolates individuals temporally but at the same time draws them into a social collectivity. State and individual interest interpenetrate each other and create a moral link between the individual and the state. The state guarantees an individual's security to conduct a particular form of life, a version of a protection racket that is designed to preserve state power.

The state uses this security panopticon in a complex and covert manner through which it is able to effectively influence and control the population. Government, Foucault maintains, does not exist for its own sake but rather for the presumed improvement and welfare of the population. Government deploys a range of capillaries and mechanisms of power (Foucault 1994:95) through which it exerts its influence on the population, a conglomerate that is collectively called 'the art of government' (Foucault 1994: 98). This is a particular set of mechanisms used by the state for the imposition of its power on its citizens. The state constantly reinforces its position face to face with various transnational actors through subscription to, and construction of, the notion of health security allegedly to protect its citizens from risk and danger. The more the power of transnational stakeholders threatens state authority, the more the state asserts its dominance over the population by prioritizing human security issues such as FC. The interests of both the state and NGOs therefore overlap over the issue of security.

As they facilitate sensitization on behalf of the state, NGO staff become 'agents of state power' (Castell 1994: 293). As stakeholders of medical knowledge, parts of 'a biopolitical strategy' of the state (Foucault 1994:137), they are presumed on the basis of their knowledge to have access to the individual's body, 'biopolitical reality' (Foucault 1984: 137) and private sphere for the manifestation of state power. In the face of the bird flu virus for instance, health professionals received information from the state and passed it down to the people through the media. State authorities in some countries like Hungary were paraded on television devouring roast chicken to demonstrate that the epidemic was not yet in the country and that the state was doing something to safeguard the population's health. This was partly a mechanism of 'injecting' confidence into the body and minds of individuals that their health security was guaranteed. Confronted with the state as an omnipotent actor, individuals are virtually helpless. This explains why in the absence of laws prohibiting FC and despite contestations of the harmful and traumatic effects of the violent ritual operations by segments of the population in Cameroon, people still talk of a 'government ban'. This shows their awareness of the states' 'monopoly of symbolic violence' (Bourdieu 1992). In this way HIV bears a relationship to FC which highlights the need for health security but paradoxically strengthens the position of advocates of FC.

4.5 Evaluation of the anti-FC campaigns and perception of intervening NGOs

The multitude of NGOs intervening in the Ejagham area against FC in particular and gender and reproductive health issues in general may be said alongside the state to be in an uneasy alliance marked by lack of collaboration as the latter has abdicated its responsibilities to the former. Although they represent modernity through the various facets of the empowerment approaches that they use, there is lack of collaboration between these NGOs and the state on the one hand and on the other, between the various NGOs themselves. Most of the change agents do not even know about the other activists working in the same area as themselves. They can even be said as Sogge and associates (1996) point out to be more secretive (and even suspicious of each other) than the American Central Intelligence Agency (CIA), a situation that has partly frustrated collaboration. The anti-FC campaigns may thus be said to be fragmented, lacking collaboration and giving even contested meanings in the assessment of success. The spatial variation in their pattern of intervention reflects underlying processes of immanent development (Bebbington, 2004).

The modernity paradigm that these NGOs use however seems to clash with tradition as perpetrators of the practice of FC persistently see them as conniving with the "Whiteman" to bring down the moral fabric of their community and female identity and personhood which FC represents to hardliners. This call for change is seen as donor driven, "donor democracy" in the words of Kereta (2005). Local change agents who are mostly indigenes of the area are in league with international actors to bring about change in the state of contestation to the practice of FC and all other practices deemed to be anathema to the health of women and children. They are in fact embedded in global networks and transnational aid chains since the very notion of NGO implies multiple flows (Bebbington, 2004). They have however been able over the years to raise public awareness about the harmful effects of FC and the issue is now being openly talked about. They advocate with the Chiefs, opinion and political leaders in the region in particular and in the nation in general. They further use information, education and communication tools which are sometimes usually designed in collaboration with the local masses although the message of the campaign always carries the dominant health concept norm stamp of donor agencies. There is in fact insufficient domestication of the information, education and communication tools. These tools usually target pharoanic circumcision, though the aim might rightly be to shock and frighten the people to abandon FC but the people also forward counter arguments to the presumed health effects they are usually presented with, thereby producing both contestation and resistance in the process.

The anti-FC advocacy campaign is further seriously affected by the enclaved nature of the most interior regions where there are still strong sentiments in favour of FC, the seasonal access roads and by the bare bone budgets on which most of these NGOs operate. Given that most often they rely on foreign funds, the campaigns are usually sporadic partly due to the bad condition of the roads and the paucity of these funds. This is further compounded by the geographical location of the stakeholders. As Bebbington (2004) rightly points out, an NGO intervention constitutes a new form of connectivity for the area of intervention. 'If places are articulated moments in networks of social relations and understandings' (Massey, 1993:66) and 'are constituted by economic, social, cultural, and political relations and flows of commodities, information and people that extend far beyond a given locality' (Mohan, 2002:134), then the presence of NGOs becomes part of a place-making project. They are all urban based with no outreach offices in the area and although mostly insiders in the culture, they are more of 'insider-outsiders' given their connections with foreign funding agencies to whom they act as a transmission belt for information. At times, the government organizes conferences and seminars usually meant to coincide with important transnational events such as the International Day of the Woman, of the Family and Children's day among others. This might be forwarded as part of the government's strategy of appropriating the new international modernity discourse while simultaneously maintaining silence over the issue of FC.

The people further see the various intervening NGOs merely as agents of neocolonialism. Development in this sense, is equated to the reproduction of various forms of Western hegemonic power over the Third World (Kapoor, 2004). After all, we are positioned within a 'development discourse' (Escobar, 1984, 1994, Sachs, 1992) where there is the dominance of the north over the south because of its assumed superiority. The anti-FC campaign seminars have reminiscences to the seasonal visits of urban-based local politicians to the area who come only during political campaigns at the verge of every electoral contest. Most of the people usually come out for these seminars like during political campaigns only to take advantage of the opportunity to have a free dish and beer. One circumciser told me in April, 2001, during a workshop sponsored by the IAC Cameroon that if they stop FC, they will not have the opportunity to be invited to Yaounde annually, drink coffee, be lodged in hotels and make some monies for themselves. At the end of the workshop however, they all pledged to stop the cutting, a pledge that ended there at the conference centre because when I went back to Ejagham land in 2006 for my fieldwork, she was still in active service circumcising young girls. This suggests that the persistence of FC really depends on demand.

However, all the stakeholders recognize the fact that gendered poverty is at the very heart of the FC dilemma and other social problems blighting the life of women and children in the region. In recognition of this, most have consequently resorted to various facets of empowerment approaches- be it political, economic or social empowerment with the hope that once women recognize their rights and have the requisite means and skills, they will eventually be in disavowal of FC. This is probably the case because in the hinterland villages of Araru, Babong, Mbofung, the people constantly attribute their resistance to stop FC as a protest against government's neglect. They lack pipe borne water, a road network, a hospital and have been virtually forgotten about and left to themselves except at the verge of every election when elites come to solicit their votes. Although they allege that they never even vote, results showing that they voted 100% in favour of the ruling CPDM party are always cooked up on their behalf by and for the elites to continue to secure their places in the various rank and file of the national administration. This calls for the need for an integrated rural development model that reflects the rather truncated and multifaceted nature of the FC problem.

4.5.1 Perception of intervening NGOs

In this section, I argue that intervening NGOs who form and are the connecting point between the local and global nexus in the debate on FC are perceived as agents, outposts of neocolonialism, agents of the "Whiteman". This neocolonialism perception has partly fuelled resistance to FC among some segments of the population. This is the case because the concepts, programmatic approaches disseminated through educative and sensitization materials are supplied by international NGOs. This is despite the steady decline in the funding of these NGOs (Igoe and Kelsall, 2005). While they maintain that they are out to 'ameliorate the disordered faults of progress' they are not static entities and must be seen as an ongoing and emergent process because of differential power relationships (Lerio et al, 2004:281). Since most of the pathological concepts they use do not often reflect local realities and are not sufficiently domesticated, some members of practicing communities see them as part of a neo-colonial conspiratorial system and a transmission belt for hegemonic concepts from above meant to silence practicing communities. This perception really has to be seen through the lens of the hierarchical locational "mechanics of power within networks" through which even values are reconstructed (Lerio et al, 2004: 853). We should further note that 'collaboration' between northern and southern NGOs is usually based on what Silk (2004:229) calls the Resource Transfer Model. This is marked by donor domination and low level of reciprocity despite the rhetoric of partnership and participation due to "asymmetry of power" (Elliot, 1987:65) which simultaneously controls and limits recipients.

NGO activists are the ones conducting anti-FC advocacy at the grass roots. Partly through their own concerted efforts, they have been able to bring the issue of FC to world attention. However, in the eyes of the local population, they are and remain outposts of neocolonialism given their strategic location in a complex, network of powerful agents, be they state or non-state actors. This view is given impetus by the fact that as the point of intersection between the local and the global scale, they are mostly funded by international finance capital and the concepts they use in the campaigns are donor stamped and dictated by their financiers. In return, as 'donor darling NGOs', appearances and correct status have replaced action: an office over membership, projects rather than geo-physical locus of action. An emerging norm has been the overemphasis on artistic representation of images of action rather than on actual development. In this light, a language of development emerged that put more focus and premium on projects and their 'sympathetic' projections to external audiences with the concomitant graphic imaging of local poverty and need (Fisher, 1997).

Their structures, ideological frames, principles and terminologies, practices and technologies are pregnant with ambiguities and debates partly as to whether they are mere buffer zones and transaction vehicles between exploitative local and global regimes and popular struggles and resistances (Petras and Veltemeyer, 2001:131) have intensified. With particular reference to FC among the Ejaghams, their overemphasize on harmful effects, on health, usually based on findings from the drastic cuttings in the Sudan, Ethiopia, Egypt and elsewhere in the Middle East has produced a backlash because they do not usually tally in with initiated women's own subjective experiences and 'harmful effects are the exceptions and not the rule' (Obermeyer, 1999).

> Well, there are some wrong circumcisions which leads to intense bleeding. When others see the bad ones, they will not accept and following illnesses like AIDS, people have seen that they may occur due to circumcision. However, rapid understanding has made some people to stop. When a woman is circumcised, she will not be excited to have sex. Those who are

> not circumcised can be forced emotionally out of their own will. They cannot make two, three, four months without touching a man. If these things were studied well and taken care of by hospitals, things would have been better since they say it is not good because of ill health. Like some dresses, some years, you will see a particular pattern. After some few years, that pattern will disappear. It may reappear after fifteen years, the pattern of the past comes back again. The world can rotate from bad to good and from good to bad. If instruments are clean, safe circumcision can still be good to those who still wish. Sometimes a canoe capsizes in a river, people still continue to go by it. You see a train can derail, people will continue to travel by train. A plane can crash but people will continue to travel by air. We refuse stealing but people still steal (Tambe Robert Agbor 45, Interview of 03/04/06).

In the interview excerpt cited above, the respondent, Mr Tambe Robert Agbor is somehow re-echoing Obermeyer (1999) to the effect that 'harmful effects are the exceptions and not the rule' thereby calling for the need for a re-evaluation of the anti-FC advocacy discourses. He is saying that poorly done circumcisions which lead to excessive bleeding, which are the exceptions but not the rule as well as the advent of AIDS and other diseases has given rise to criticisms. He subscribes to the view that FC dampens sexual anxiety and that if the ritual procedures were medicalized, there will be no problem especially as hospitals will be able to take care of the procedures or to provide biomedical assistance in the eventuality of excessive bleeding and other negative side effects. This of course is contrary to the ethics of WHO and many medical associations. According to him, culture changes as old patterns resurface after a long time and that cultural changes might at times be bad or good. To buttress his point, he makes an interesting comparative analogy between certain mishaps such as a capsized canoe, a derailed train, a plane crash as well as the fact that stealing is condemned, yet some people still continue to steal. Applied to circumcision, there can be no unanimity within a culture and every individual therefore has his or her own choice depending on a cost-benefit analysis framework. On the whole, his argument is based on the principle of exceptionality, that the exceptions, in this case the bad cases are not the rule.

We should however note that accusations of witchcraft are a 'native' explanatory model for the accidents of circumcision among these people (see also, Evans-Pritchard., 1937). The image of these NGOs due to their association with international capital is working against the anti-FC campaigns partly because there is inadequate domestication of the campaign materials, vocabulary and strategies. They are involved in a hegemonic top-down development model given their urban headquarter location, the sporadic nature and spatial geography of their intervention. These factors are further complicated by the rough terrain making even the intervention only seasonal and tied to the trickling down of funds. I argue that due to this lack of consistency, the end result has instead been the production of resistance and contestation.

Despite the tremendous efforts already made by these NGOs such as breaking the silence in which the practice has been shrouded for several years, the main obstacle remains cultural resistance from some segments of the local population as the practice is interwoven with economic, social and political interests. The population's stance may be divided into three interrelated but fluid continuums as I will demonstrate in the next chapter. In the section that follows, I will examine the positions of the other stakeholders: TBAs and circumcisers, the medical corps, local community leaders and members of the Moninkim cult so as to identify and to point out the prospects for internal institutional change in the practice and contestation of FC and then conclude.

4.6 Traditional Birth Attendants (TBAs) and circumcisers

TBAs and circumcisers who carry out the ritual cuttings are part of the local network of internal actors. Although the service is usually for a fee and simultaneous involvement in the feasting that accompanies the procedure, they present themselves merely as performing a cultural duty which was handed over to them. In other words, they assume that they are only performing a cultural role and fulfilling a cultural need and therefore not doing any harm in the process. Most of them said that they were actually 'fixing' the ladies, suggesting a type of surgery meant to repair an ugly body part by making it to be aesthetically appealing. They however have vested interest in the ritual cuttings and usually see an end to it as rendering them unemployed. Like other local agents, it might be said that they tend to see development, rather as a window of opportunity to be exploited (Herdt & Bastiaensen, 2004:875).

Although they have attended seminars and conferences organized by NGOs over the years, they have always publicly vowed to stop the ritual procedures. Most of them have continued with the ritual cuttings thereby maintaining a type of 'double discourse'. Some have however given up the practice usually in the face of negative personal experiences with their own daughters such as over-bleeding. This over-bleeding like all other negative effects, which sometimes occur, is usually attributed to witchcraft, rather than to the fact that they might have inadvertently cut too deep. The training of these TBAs and circumcisers into alternative occupations might be a step forward that can possibly lead to the abandonment of the ritual cuttings. We should however keep in mind that solicitation for their services depends on the availability of children for circumcision, in other words, on a dynamic demand and supply curve- that is on parents who solicit their services. Community consensus and inter-country collaboration with Nigerian NGOs to abandon FC seems to be the only viable solution in sight that will eventually bring about change in the Ejagham area given the people's trans-border location and kinship ties with families in Nigeria. Criminalization of the procedures in Nigeria, a process already underway in some states (Skaine, 2005), might well be circumvented through the loose border crossings.

4.7 The medical corps

They are the translators and implementers of government's health policy at the grass roots. Like the various NGOs, they lack the means with which to effectively penetrate into the hinterlands where sentiments in favour of FC are still very strong. This is the case because although the concept of integrated health services is officially government's pronounced health policy, though characterized by urban monopoly, there is the acute lack of infrastructure and the few that exist are all disease towers lacking even spirit and syringes at times. Furthermore, there is lack of motivation for health personnel which even became worse with devaluation and triple salary cuts which has left most public service workers with poverty level salaries. Health promotion campaigns such as children's vaccination in this region are never thoroughly conducted. In most of the hinterland villages, it is difficult to see a health personnel there partly because of lack of financial incentives and the rough and inaccessible nature of the terrain.

I personally accompanied a team of nurses and other health technicians into the area in June 2006 and they ended up on the way at Ogurang. They pointed out to me that those who were supposed to go further into the hinterlands refused because they were not sufficiently motivated. However, during both prenatal and ante-natal clinic sessions, women are constantly schooled on the harmful effects of FC usually on the most intrusive type which has formed the basis of the anti-FC campaigns for long. The Eyumojock District hospital walls are often littered with posters with these health effects and the prevention of various childhood diseases meant to deter women from engaging in practices that are detrimental to both their health and those of their children. The lone district hospital in the area is mostly staffed by health care volunteers who go for work only when they like since they are not remunerated. Most of them spend their time in the pursuit of other lucrative ventures. To compound matters, most women are too poor and manage, if they can, only to attend prenatal clinics but later give birth at home in the care of TBAs and other relatives, not at the maternity ward of the hospital. The maternity ward of the above-mentioned hospital is almost deserted. This is partly due to the conspiracy between poverty, ignorance and the physical inaccessibility of the health care unit given the long distances to be covered to reach it.

4.8 Local Community Leaders

Structurally, the society under investigation has a segmentary patriarchal political organization meaning that power is diffused and fragmented. This implies that community leaders, be they Chiefs or Quarter heads are equals with the people. In other words, they do not actually command any respect and can therefore not enforce a law against FC because they lack the authority. Although they have always vowed in public to do so, it should however be noted that the Chiefs and community leaders have what I will call both ‘private, personal’ and ‘second discourse’, ‘public voices’. This ambivalence is really a confession of their lack of ‘symbolic power/ violence’ (Bourdieu, 1992). Secondly, they have both personal and communal relationships with almost everybody in the community. Given the people’s trans-border location, a legal ban may be unenforceable since they can always circumvent the law by taking their children for circumcision across the loose border into Nigeria. This is actually one of the most difficult challenges to overcome in the change efforts. When I asked most respondents if they would report their neigbours for circumcising their daughters, most of them laughed, implying that they will not. Some respondents from the interview excerpts in the preceding chapter present the issue of non-circumcision more as a matter of personal choice as some literally vowed to circumcise all their daughters come what may. The disasters of FC usually become public knowledge only when it has gone out of hand since it takes place in the private sphere of an individual’s homestead and not in the public realm.

4.9 The Moninkim cult

Like TBAs and circumcisers, members of the Moninkim cult are another vested interest group in the community. This is because they use the dance as a mechanism to garner scarce resources for themselves from upper class men and others within and beyond the Ejagham locale each time they stage dances. Some have toured various towns and even gone abroad staging in return for a fee from curious onlookers. These monies are used at times by their parents to build houses, sponsor their brothers in school or invested in a trade for the benefit of the initiate.

This association, the very instantiation of traditional patriarchy is actually at the heart and represents all the conflicts and tensions around FC in the community because of both the economics of circumcision and the cultural public performances and accompanying compensations usually garnered by the circumcised. It is the very icon of gendered identity and female personhood in Ejagham society. Most of the Moninkim dancers have become very popular as animators during public occasions for which they are normally "sprayed with banknotes"(ABEMO, 2002). The title of Moninkim carries pride and is a symbol and shorthand for traditional modernity, group identity, ethnic belonging and courage. Dancing is a profession and the already circumcised members actually pointed out that they have nothing to lose now that some people are advocating for non-circumcision. This may imply that they are open to the proposed changes from anti-FC advocates. "Making a woman a Moninkim in those days was like sending her to the university to obtain a degree" (Nkoyo E. Otang, interview of 28/07/06). There is now increasing recognition among the people that there are other ways of 'honouring' a daughter such as by sending her to a formal educational institution. However, my fear is that they may continue to discriminate against uncircumcised members, seeing them as fakes. Dealing with the stigma of non-circumcision is still a key problem in the community as a whole. Some respondents still find it abnormal that a Moninkim should be uncircumcised. But with the ageing of the old Moninkims, the "modern Moninkims" may eventually takeover totally, giving hope that FC can eventually come to an end one day.

There is actually intense debate in the community with regards to the presumed seductive immorality of the dancing costumes of the Moninkims. Some people say it is very immoral given that the bodies of these ladies are always exposed. There is however increasing recognition of the need for the maintenance of the dignity of the female dancers and the people's cultural identity through the dance even without having to circumcise.

There is evidence of the prospect for a change of attitude through deviance. 'Positive deviance' and changes in the nomenclature of the ritual cuttings of FC actually began in Otu village, a village that ABEMO (2002) reports, might be said to be the very bastion and headquarters of FC in the Ejagham area. Almost all females in this village are reported to have been cut and most circumcised Moninkims still in active service come from there. I got reports from this village that the waning of the elaborate celebration of the graduation ceremony began there. This was when one Chief Ekpang who had four daughters to be initiated refused to provide the dynamic but culturally laid down 30 limps of meat and food required for the ceremonies. Thereafter, he is said to have set the rather positive precedence for change in the ceremonial celebrations surrounding the ritual by arguing that each and everyone should henceforth conduct the outdooring ceremony of his daughter within his own household. He further insisted that it should no longer be a communal event involving hundreds, if not, thousands of people and much expenditure.

Conclusion

In this chapter, I have discussed and analyzed the internal political agendas of both internal and external political agents intervening to bring about change in the practice of FC and their various alliances which have instead led to both resistance and contestation of FC among the Ejaghams. The people might be said to be under several fires: calls from local, national, regional and international NGOs, the state and political parties to part with FC. Various internal actors have diverse and conflicting agendas marked by public acceptance to denounce the ritual practices but not keeping to their words because of their own vested interests in the procedures. This is demonstrated by the people's mixed reactions to the anti-FC campaigns through the 'double discourses' some segments often elaborate especially when confronted with the AIDS scourge. I have argued that the interplay of ideologies, differential power to manufacture and disseminate concepts among various stakeholders has led to fragmentation and stalemate in the anti-FC advocacy campaign. This state of affairs has instead reinforced both contestation and resistance to the ritual cuttings. The people's culture "contact zone" location (Bizzell, 1997), places them within a multitude of interconnected power fields. At the local-global nexus, the state alongside national, regional, and international NGOs are in alliance against the ritual cuttings. The state frames the issue and abdicates its functions to NGOs to conduct sensitization and education. The link of these NGOs to transnational NGOs and the health concepts they use present them as agents of neo-colonialism thereby fuelling resistance.

In chapter five, I examine the different, dynamic attitudes and responses of the Ejaghams to the anti-HIV/AIDS and FC fight

CHAPTER FIVE

EJAGHAM RESPONSES TO THE ANTI-HIV/AIDS AND FC FIGHT

In the preceding chapter, I have identified the various stakeholders responsible for both contestation and change in the practice of FC, their agendas and the various alliances they have drawn the Ejaghams into. In line with my power-oriented vision of culture, I will in this chapter examine the different, dynamic attitudes and responses of the Ejaghams to the anti-HIV/AIDS and anti-FC fight. I argue that given the several overlapping "operating units" of power (Adams, 1966, 1975 in Wolf, 2001), their responses shift in line with the power field with which they are confronted thereby producing both resistance and conflict. I will simultaneously attempt to gauge the prospects for internal institutional and socio-cultural change by looking at the interplay between various ideological actors. Basically, I argue here that thanks to the efforts of NGOs, the people have been drawn into dialogue with themselves and with the outside world. And now, there is some sort of general awareness about the risks of FC. In other words, NGO activists have successfully broken the silence that has for long surrounded the ritual cuttings. I also show that the privatization of FC on young girls is clear evidence of simultaneous resistance and contestation.

This chapter is divided into three interrelated parts. In the first part, I examine the people's different dynamic attitudes, by looking at their various positions, arguments for and against FC as well as "neutrality", "mute voices", 'third space positionality'. In the second part, I focus on cultural resistance to FC and the anti-HIV/AIDS discourse as a form of protest against neocolonialism, a reaction to the people's marginal position in a "culture contact zone"(Bizzell, 1997) surrounded by a complex network of powerful state and non-state actors at the national, regional and international scales. I further argue that the very existence of these multiple actors with often conflicting agendas is actually truncating the change efforts as shown by the increasing privatization of FC on younger girls. In the penultimate part, I examine various factors that are militating both for and against change in the FC ritual procedures. Conscious that FC is part of a legalized patriarchal complex suggesting that there is the need for a holistic view of the wider macro social and legal framework so as to understand its interlocking institutions, I argue that the lukewarm attitude of the state has been appropriated by pro-circumcision advocates and has gone a long way to militate in favour of the procedures.

5.1 Conflict and contestation over FC

The issue of FC pits western medicine, scientific rationality and notions of disease and harm against local knowledge, tradition and morality as epitomized by the conflict between progressives who want the eradication of the ritual procedures and conservatives who want the maintenance of the *status quo* on the one hand and on the other suspects/cautious appropriators of both modernity and tradition who at times are in favour of the medicalization of the ritual procedures. Despite the significant efforts of grass root NGOs, some segments of the local Ejagham population are still contesting the side effects of FC. I designate this group who are still subscribing to and who represent the ritual cuttings in the present context as a 'native' therapeutic model against HIV as 'hard-liners'. Contrary to these 'hard-liners', 'soft-liners' want change and the eventual eradication of the procedures, at times, through medicalization. In other words, they recognize the harm done to children and women's health and well being. However, unlike these two groups, groups which cut across both gender and socio-economic classes, another group vacillates between acceptance and refusal of the continuation of FC. They may be called fence sitters, 'soft' 'anti-colonialists-modernists' who can however be won over. Faced with the likelihood of FC transmitting HIV, they at times, like 'hard-liners', subscribe to FC as a moral check against the ravages of the pandemic but at other times, do not. They maintain a somewhat ambivalent posture sometimes subscribing rather to modification. They may be said to be suspect of both "tradition" and "modernity", local and scientific knowledge, and want the cautious appropriation of both and not wholesale appropriation. Stated otherwise, they are still trapped in 'group think phenomena' despite changes over time.

This division is however fluid, showing the multivocality of culture itself as a contested field of action and practice, with no fixed boundaries around any group. This implies that culture is being constantly contested and renegotiated by stakeholders over time. I argue that the multiple positionality around FC and HIV/AIDS should rather be seen in the light of the complex, ambivalent multi-stranded fields of powerful alliances with which the people are confronted. There is on one hand, modernity represented by the Cameroonian state and "its ideological state apparatus" (Althuser,1971) of schools and NGOs, and "tradition" on the other, represented by some dominant segments of the population who are in the process of challenging the latter's "monopoly of symbolic violence" (Bourdieu,1992) and its symbolic power. This "modernity" and "tradition" dialogue is inscribed on women's bodies and appropriated by more powerful actors who at times compete, ally, resist or accommodate (Wolf, 2001) each other depending on the ground circumstances.

5.1.1 Mute voices, for and against FC

NGOs have brought the issue of FC to the attention of national and international policy-makers and created an appropriate forum for open debate and frank talk on the issue. They have also undertaken sensitization on the presumed harmful effects of the ritual practice; but there are still strong sentiments in favour of the practice among some segments of the population in practicing communities. There is the co-existence of mute voices from proponents, opponents and from those opting rather for the medicalization of the ritual procedures. A good majority (75 per cent) of both educated and uneducated men and women among my respondents in various Ejagham villages are however in 'disfavour' of the practice. This might partly be thanks to the educative and health talks given to them by various grass root NGOs intervening in the area. Some men however continue to qualify it as "women's business"- meaning that it is both in and against the interest of the women themselves. These men are re-echoing the traditional divide between the private sphere of the household as women's sphere of authority and influence and the public arena where men are presumed to be at the centre of authority and in total control. This suggests that even within patriarchy, women are able to create some space and leverage for themselves through "patriarchal bargain". In such dichotomous thinking, children are either placed under their mothers to decide for them since mothers have power over them, or are totally erased. Stated otherwise, children have virtually no sphere of authority and influence for the exercise of their own rights and authority such as deciding whether or not to accept the ritual visitations since it is most often their parents in general or their mothers in particular who decide for them. Resistance and contestation to change is however not only found among women but also among men, the young and old alike. It cuts across both gender and generation, and positions in the social structure. It involves socialization and the politics of marriage.

Pro-female circumcision advocates among the Ejaghams frame their claims in terms of anti-colonialism and the maintenance of authentic Ejagham tradition and the honour of the real Ejagham woman. This group frequently invokes modernization and hybridization as negative influences on the moral fabric of their community, a morality that is scripted on women's bodies. They constantly point to the need to uphold sexual morals through FC as a mechanism of maintaining cultural authenticity. They are accordingly being presented and represented as the moral icons of their communities. It is paradoxical that the weaker party is being given control over communal norms even when uncircumcised women's presumed immorality depends on a dynamic sexual demand and supply curve. In other words, men must solicit their sexual services before they engage in sexual intercourse with them even if it is a strategy for them to capture scarce livelihood resources from these men in the form of sweet heart presents.

Two interrelated concepts may explain the state of both contestation and acceptance of FC among these people. These are Jay Gould's (1993) concepts of 'soft-liners' and 'hard-liners' respectively. However, given that some people neither fall into any of these two categories, I will simultaneously use the concepts of 'double discourse' and 'group think phenomena' to capture the people's diverse attitudes towards FC especially within the new institutional context of the AIDS pandemic. Whereas soft-liners are in favour of change, hard-liners want the maintenance of the *status quo* holding that it is the Whiteman who has now come to ask them to stop FC. They see the anti-FC campaigns rather as an imposition of power on them from outside. Some people are however still in a dilemma and prefer to maintain 'a double discourse' especially in the face of the threats and ravages of the HIV/AIDS pandemic. This group may at times decry FC and at other times its members are in favour of the violent ritual cuttings. They seem to be trying to carve out an uncomfortable 'third space' for themselves.

Despite sensitization and education about thc harmful effects of FC, this group of people seem to be facing what kereta (2005:49) with reference to Ethiopia describes as 'the collective action problem' which borders on social stigmatization as individuals will always declare themselves against FC in public discussions but continue to practice it on young babies in private. This, following Habtamu (2002) as cited in Kereta (2005:50) is the case because in African communities, autonomy is defined in terms of an individual's ability to either mobilize or influence social relationships, rather than to act independently of the others. There might therefore be the need here for a Toastan style community declaration to eradicate the practices, which will imply that villages will have to sign a written declaration to that effect and not only seminar or conference room declarations, as has always been the case in the Ejagham area. This project was initiated by the Senegalese NGO, Tostan. It involved persuading stakeholders to institute a convention shift so as to voluntarily give up FC. But when the Senegalese government instituted a law against the ritual cutting, the change efforts were seriously compromised. However, it has so far been one of the few success stories in the anti-FC campaign as the model has been copied, modified and replicated elsewhere with some degree of success.

5.1.2 The double discourse phenomenon

Although almost all mothers with whom I spoke said assuringly that their daughters were not to be submitted to FC any longer, it still seems that deep inside them, they think that abandoning FC will imply that those who have already been circumcised were cheated and violated. Some people made an interesting analogy between a circumcision ceremony and a thrift and loan society. This suggests that to circumcise one's daughter entails local reciprocity. This implies hosting an elaborate ceremonial feast in her honour for the entire community. This shows how interwoven the procedures are to other aspects of culture and that it is not just a health issue *per se*, a stance on which anti-FC activism is usually anchored.

> Anyway, If government says that we should not do it again, we may feel there is a reason. But we do not see the reason. We do not know because even if you give birth to a child and never circumcise her, it will not be good. You took part in the festivities marking the outdooring ceremony of your neighbour's daughter and you are normally expected to organize one in future… (Mr Nji Fidelis,interview of 24/07/06, Araru)

The interview excerpt quoted above announces the social and communal aspects of the ritual ceremony. It implies that when you take part in an individual's circumcision ceremony, you are also expected to circumcise your own daughter(s) one day and to host a feast for all others to enjoy. In other words, they are trapped in a 'group think phenomena' of mutual and obligatory reciprocity and public denial at the same time. Following Borcher (2002) quoted in Kereta (2005:51), 'group think phenomena' refers to faulty decision-making within a group and occurs due to a group's 'cohesiveness' in which case other alternatives are never considered. Under such circumstances, there is the preference of unanimity 'to quality decisions'. Evidence of this 'group think phenomena' will normally include: the rationalization of wrong decisions, holding the group's moral values in high esteem, sharing in stereotypes which underpin a certain decision, failure to express one's misgivings and feelings about a decision, and using tactics to protect the group's presumed reliance on negative information which could unfortunately be contrary to the community's changing values and expectations. Here a group's valued ideals may be said to be working against the interest of the said group by both some insiders and outsiders alike, be they activists or humanists. Although most people in the study area are aware of the presumed harmful effects of FC, some dispute it in the same way that they contest the existence of HIV/AIDS saying that it is the "Whiteman" who has come to say circumcision should stop.

> Whites.....and Western educated people like you say it is not good. Circumcision causes no harm in any way. Whether a woman was circumcised or not made no difference except that while in the fattening room, they were given special foods to eat,.......Women being confined made them reserved but today, a child just jumps out of the house into the streets trying to make life with other children."(PA Etah, Educator,56, interview of 23/03/06).

In the interview excerpt quoted above, the respondent associates the researcher with the anti-FC advocacy camp. He further challenges the harmful effects of circumcision pointing out that it is functional because it makes women reserved. In other words, it is considered to be a 'native' antidote against waywardness and therefore serves as a traditional check on female morality.

> As tradition demands, if they ask me to circumcise, I will do so. My elder sister was circumcised after her first birth but they wanted to circumcise me when I had not yet given birth. She was circumcised 8 days after giving birth. I feel they wanted to circumcise me earlier so that I could start dancing the Moninkim. Moreover, when my elder sister was being circumcised, I was not around (Philo, 21, Secondary school student, interview of 06/20/06).

Philo like most young women in the area already has a child and has therefore literally passed the qualifying exams for circumcision in the past. Despite her secondary school education, she shares a hardened view of culture. It was in her words done to others and she is eagerly awaiting her own turn if her parents so decide. She still adheres into 'group think' by feeling that circumcision is good for her if her parents so desire. She is willing to subordinate her own personal needs for the benefit of the collectivity (family, clan, lineage group, kinship group, village, entire society), and patriarchy by submitting herself to the ritual cutting practice of FC given the high esteem accorded the circumcised in general and circumcised dancers in particular.

> Scientist: As a modern father, I will not want my daughter to be circumcised when she is mature. If circumcision is necessary, she will be circumcised within one week of delivery. You see, when she is given birth to, she should be circumcised immediately, within one week. She will not feel the side effects of circumcision. That will take her naturally if only God blesses and the bleeding stops. As to the non-circumcision of girls which is being called for now, we like it. Because when we are told not to do something, there is a reason behind the prohibition. The best reason for circumcising, I think is to fix a woman. Because in our own tradition, it is understood that you have fixed a woman from that thing (clitoris) growing out. It was like a shame to keep your clitoris intact. Up to now, we are still cutting it. Even my own daughter who is under three years old has already been circumcised and she is fine (FGD session, Scientist, Ogurang Village, 28/06/06).

The informant 'Scientist' appropriates the concept of modernity in the above passage in a rather curious and interesting way. He is actually caught up between the deeply felt need to stick to his culture and subscribes to early circumcisions because to him, the child will neither feel the pains nor the side effects. At the same time however, he likes the anti-FC messages because since it comes from government, showing his willingness to submit himself to the authority of the state, "there must be a reason behind it", a reason that he does not know of course. This informant clearly has an ambivalent attitude towards the anti-FC campaigns: subscribing to and not subscribing to the messages at the same time. His version of modernity implies making procedural adjustments to the ritual cuttings such as the use of a razor blade for each initiate and not for a group of girls as was the case in the past. This to him will do away with the association between FC and AIDS infection/transmission.

> Scientist: When you cut it so that it should not be coming out like a penis, it means you have fixed the woman. But it is only now that people come to say that it is not good to circumcise but we think that it is because of this AIDS problem. In which case, they used one razor blade for a group of girls. But in ancient times, our ancestors reserved one special circumcision knife (for everybody) from generation to generation but with razor blades "one is to one". If there are any other reasons, I do not see them. I am a tradition boy. I was born in the village and although I have been living in

town, I know best. However, women can still tell you about the tradition. But they will not tell you anything than this- to fix women and to curb the rate of sex ambition and thirdly, to look for money so as to keep the Moninkim going during the fattening period.(Co-interview with Drogba, 27 and Scientist, 36, Ogurang village, 28/06/06).

This group of people might be said to hold a hardened view of culture. Others while or seemingly in recognition of the effects on sexuality however maintain that FC is good because it will uphold female morality and honour in the wake of the HIV/AIDS pandemic since they believe that uncut women are highly sexed and will always want to have sexual intercourse at any time. This is another instance of the double appropriation of the harmful health effect paradigm. The anti-FC messages may be said to be working to the contrary in this case- instead re-enforcing the state of contestation and resistance to end the practice. On the other hand, a few respondents however feel that FC instead makes a woman curious to have sex, implying that it does not temper with her sexual desire. To buttress their point of view, they constantly made references to the sexual biographies of some circumcised women in the locality. Herewith an interview excerpt that reflects this stance:

Interviewer: What has been your sexual experience with circumcised women?

Ojong: They are sexually active. To me, it seems that when they circumcise you, it seems they have instead increased the anxiety for sexual intercourse because the girl who was circumcised in 1996, people are complaining that although they cut her clitoris, she is still doing more than those who are not circumcised[having a lot of extramarital sexual activities since she is married].Because she is inside her marital home, neighbours complain that whenever her husband does not sleep with her, there is trouble, may be they have instead increased her anxiety for sex(Ojong Philo,20, interview of 06/20/06,Inukon village).

Madam Mary Ayum, a Boki woman now living with her husband in Eyumojock ran away from circumcision because of the pains. Although she and her husband do not subscribe to the practice because one of her 'step daughters' (given birth to by the husband out of wedlock), almost bled to death, she is still caught up between the pains of FC and the need to preserve sexual morality. She thus maintains an ambivalent attitude towards the ritual cuttings when confronted with the AIDS scourge:

The circumcision that was given to girls in those days cooled down their anxiety for sex (men), the high numbers of uncircumcised girls today are the ones prostituting all over. It should still take place so that sexual anxiety and immorality will reduce (Interview of 20/03/06, Eyumojock).

"Circumcision made our parents to have limits to sex".(Ndifon Abang, 26, Interview of 20/07/06)

Anni, 23 now in high school does not know whether her presumed sexual reservation is due to the circumcision she underwent as a child, which might have dampened her enthusiasm for sex or that is how God made her.

Interviewer: Anni, is circumcision still necessary for girls today with the existence of this AIDS?

Anni: It is still necessary to an extent. According to what I was told, the aim of circumcision is to help reduce the rate of sex in girls [meaning sexual anxiety]. Without that, it is not necessary. God created the clitoris in you and there is no reason to extract it for whatever reason. Some girls are usually qualified by boys as being 100% good. You hear them saying she is not as cheap as that but other girls are said to be very cheap (Interview of 14/03/06).

Many respondents argue that they do not understand the reason behind the anti-FC crusade ("government ban").This seems to suggest that the language of the campaigns is too complicated for the understanding of the ordinary man and therefore does not always reflect their own experiences and sentiments. Most respondents only know that "FC is not good". Most, both initiated and non-initiated respondents alike, contested the harmful effects of circumcision saying that it is a myth and an invention by the Whiteman meant expressly to demonize them and to destabilize their community. They present even their acceptance as imposed and are therefore quietly challenging this same acceptance of the anti-FC advocacy messages by continuing to circumcise their daughters. In other words, there is half-hearted acceptance of the anti-FC campaign messages. The problem might have to do with the fact that unlike in countries like Ethiopia, Egypt and Sudan, the procedure is less intrusive and takes place only once, and not after every birth like in the above-mentioned countries. Furthermore, harmful effects if they are ever experienced take time to manifest and are never seen as an outcome of the circumcision process. They may even be perceived as part and parcel of the routine of being a woman in so called traditional societies. Patients and healers alike see symptoms differently (Kleinman, 1980).

The people's seeming non-comprehension of the anti-FC messages further suggests that the monolithic gospel of eradication that is the focus of anti-FC activism may not be appropriate. This is even more the case especially as WHO (1998) expressly frowns against harm reduction through the medicalisation of the ritual procedures so that they take place in hospitals where care is readily available and where there are ideal hygienic conditions. This organization sees harm reduction rather as an obstacle "against the eradication of this heinous practice". FC practicing communities are left only with one choice-eradication whereas in every culture, people make choices on a cost-benefit analysis framework. Some segments of the local Ejagham population perceive the gospel of eradication as a form of imposition of colonial or neocolonial power on them. They are therefore resisting in both covert and overt ways-sometimes by publicly accepting the anti-FC messages and the need to put an end to the ritual cuttings but at the same time, by continuing the practices in private.

5.2 Resistance as counter-discourse to neocolonialism

The most ardent partisans of circumcision often present their stance as a counter discourse to colonialism and Western hegemony in the production, packaging and dissemination of risk through health concepts. They are determined to hold on to FC as the very last bastion and moral icon of their society. Again, women's health, human and reproductive rights are at stake in this debate in which, as Winter (1994:939) has painstakingly noted, women are merely "political symbols" being appropriated by others for their own selfish interests since it is not really their interests which is at stake but rather other people defining these interests for, and thereby silencing and speaking on their behalf as a way of dominating them.

> As is often the case, the debate concerning these women is less about the women themselves than about the appropriation of women as political symbols. In other words, it is about the use of women as ammunition in a polemic of central concern to their lives, but where the issue at stake is not the women's own interests, but, rather, the consolidation of the powers of others to define those interests (Winter,1994:939).

The position of those who cast FC as a reaction against colonialism and neocolonialism has resonances with the early anti-FC debacle in Kenya (see Kenyetta, 1937) and with the present situation in Egypt where women's bodies have become the battle ground between the government and the fundamentalists.

In Kenya, the fight against clitoridectomy was appropriated by the Mau Mau anti-colonial fighters. In Egypt, while the government wants the eradication of the ritual cuttings, the fundamentalists want continuation, holding that it maintains the sexual dignity of Egyptian women and is therefore a moral check against inordinate sexuality. Like the case in Egypt, the real battle is between modernity and tradition in which case traditionalists resist changes in women's status supposedly as a way of maintaining the women's identity and upholding "authentic" Egyptian values in the process. I will now illustrate this position from my field notes.

> Interviewer: Why is the Moninkim tradition dying away?
>
> Bessong: It is dying away because of the White man's culture. They are out to wipe out circumcision. The World Health Organization is out to wipe out circumcision and secondly, education. With the Moninkim, you would have already given birth to a child, then they circumcise you. You stay at home for quite some time. You begin by rubbing cam wood dye and then come to calabar chalk. Your parents earn respect. They paint and make drawings on your face so as to beautify you (Bessong, interview of 24/03/06).

In the interview excerpt cited above, the informant is saying that neocolonialism has given rise to acculturation and the institution of FC which was a prelude to becoming a Moninkim is threatened leading to changes in the criterion for membership. He further points out that by championing the campaign to eradicate FC through education, WHO, a Western institution whose headquarters can only be found in the West, is a neocolonial institution which is out to demonize their culture and see to its eventual collapse. This is by virtue of its location and the type of presumed contrary health concepts it is promoting. In other words, resistance to FC eradication is a mechanism to resist imposition from this perceived hegemonic health care policy institution. They would therefore want to continue "to fix and honour" their daughters through FC. This informant has an alternative notion of modernity and globalization.

> Interviewer: Please, can you tell me why the Moninkim tradition is dying out.
>
> Bessong: The WHO came here with a story at one time that Female Genital Mutilation is not wanted again. We were trying to accept with them, and accepting it, means that the Moninkim has to start dying out. But pertaining to areas and personalities, this thing came as some sort of, "when you give, I give". My neighbour has circumcised his/her own daughter and due to that aspect, there was a lot of personality conflict with that family. Now that I have my own daughter, so as to acquire pride, I will circumcise her. Now, WHO came and we were trying to listen to them with one eye and one ear, putting another ear to village and family personality [relationships]. Now, coming back again, we were looking at

its action to be the political aspect of it. So, we decided that we should not die out from our own culture, only to follow WHO, whose headquarters could only be in America [Switzerland] while we in Africa, are diminishing our own culture. Then, we were doing that as some sort of stealing aspect. Now as of the year 2000, we were not listening to them again because looking at them there, they were still following their own culture, and keeping their own cultural tradition intact. While pushing our own children to inculcate their values and culture, inculcate western lifestyles. That is why we want to believe that if my own neighbour is doing this, having the priority in our area, I should also do it. That is why we don't want to fall out with the Moninkim tradition.

Abang: You understand? We can not joke with tradition, you understand? Not until now that government or the Whiteman has brought us some feedback, that no more circumcision. But to us, we still continue with it because there is no harm over it. To such a person.... It is just like a debt you owe. You gave it yesterday, I am supposed to give it back today, and you understand it. That is why circumcision can never end in our clan.

Ayamba: But now, most of these things we are doing here, the Americans always come in to tarnish our own culture in certain ways/aspects while they are practicing their own culture privately. You see, like the Whites, we don't know whether they have been doing circumcisions or not or anything of the sort. But when they just come that we do not want this, we the Africans, what is sweet to us, we cannot just pull out from it. I think you see, so what the Whiteman/ Western world is saying that we should fall out from this circumcision, I think, the African man cannot just absorb it immediately. Because, we are used to it and what the Western world is used to, we cannot deprive them from that and so it becomes a problem. We falling out immediately from their own rights and even government over us. So that is why all these things they are saying that we should fall out from circumcisions, Moninkim, all this and that we cannot just fall out immediately. We want to see their own culture and to go into their own culture and to do research inside their own culture before we can start falling out of our own culture. Somebody cannot just come and be saying that "Look you are a thief, I don't want a thief" and then, you just start absorbing it. But though it is a bad thing, but then, but then, there are certain aspects that if somebody, if your master, comes and says don't do this, you assess the master. If the master is a drunkard, if he says don't drink, don't do this and that, assess him and copy from him. That is why we have never gained the culture of the whites or the western world. And so whatever the rights they have been giving us, we just absorb it immediately. That is why we are still holding on to our rights and to our culture. This aspect of circumcision, we cannot just abandon it because when the whites, when they come here, we cannot just take them and use them immediately. But when the whites come here, they can use us immediately. Why? We have to begin asking questions (FGD, Ekoneman-Awa, 23/08/06).

The next informant, Bessong, cited above, is in line with the first respondent. He states that their apparent resistance as manifested by their half-hearted acceptance of the anti-FC messages, a nice illustration of their claim of lack of reciprocity, has to do with the fact that the messages are only meant to demonize them, they are not based on truth. Here, he raises the issue of alternative truths, positionality, multiple realities and multiple conceptions of health. It should be noted that in this context, WHO is used as shorthand for biomedical ideas, Western health concepts and its agents-health care personnel, NGO activists as well as the government. Stated otherwise, everybody who is against FC is seen as representing and propagating the ideas of WHO. Some people are resisting these agents, their agendas and programmatic approaches because of the reciprocal social functions of FC ceremonies: "give and take", "gift and counter gift", pride and recognition which give it clear resonances with potlatch ceremonies. A total end will therefore in his view, lead to personality conflicts and squabbles between those who have already given-circumcised, confined, organized and celebrated elaborate feasts for their daughters, and those who will as a result, not return what they consumed from others. The issue at stake here really has to do with fulfilling psychological and social needs of FC if the change initiatives should be successful, must be resolved. It is however, not certain if the organization of large scale public feasting ceremonies to formally end circumcision will work. However, it seems plausible that the presumed cultural break can be achieved through the creation of an institution for initiating girls without cutting them but with all the feasting as a way of absorbing the psychological shock that will be created say through a legal ban. The success of this strategy again really depends on community consensus to end the ritual cuttings.

One other key issue in the second interview excerpt quoted above is that the people are listening to the WHO messages with regards to the presumed harmful effects of FC, "only with one eye and ear"(Bessong). He might be saying that the messages do not reflect their own local situation. They see it more as a component of the politics of neocolonial domination through the negation of their culture. In other words, the messages are only meant to erase them from their culture. The very location of WHO's headquarters is again invoked here and the organization is presented as being merely another outpost of neocolonialism meaning that the covert aim of anti-FC activism is to uproot the people from their culture- a culture inscribed on women's bodies. Here, the very modernity advocated by the West is represented as a threat to the moral fabric of the people's communal values as children are supposedly uprooted when they inculcate Western lifestyles and values. This is again part of the effects of the trappings of the "group think". Read very closely in another way, the anticolonialism discourse is a reaction to the people's marginality within a "culture contact zone" (Bizzell, 1997) between the global forces of western capitalism represented by WHO, the Cameroonian state, regional institutions, local NGOs and all those against FC including educated individuals like this ethnographer.

In the above passage, Bessong again points out that criticism is a one way traffic apparently showing the cultural dominance of the entire West over the rest of the world in general but towards Africa in particular. The West frames and determines the concepts to be used for the debate, a debate such as over the issue of FC in which they occupy a rather marginal position. He expresses the wish that they still have to critically assess the messages disseminated through the anti-FC campaigns before absorbing them and taking a position on the issue. Stated otherwise, change will come about from within only when they see the advantages in the alternative values and practices with which they are presented and which is being imposed on them. He says that accusations of the harmful effects of FC are not founded and should therefore be grounded in some sort of comparative, empirical data. In other words, we should question the moral authority of the person who wants a particular order of things. He presents the Western world, "Whites" in this regard as using Africa for their own ideological interests. This finding is clearly in line with the gulf between Western and African feminists (see among others, Abu-Lughod (2002), Mohanty (2002), Lazreg (1998), Spivak (1998), and Sylvester (1995). He also asks for reciprocity. He has a very relational view of it, a projection from local reciprocity rules.

Bessong further attributes the presumed psychosexual effects of FC such as the loss of sexual interest to genetic heritage within a family, which might lead to the transmission of the gene of hypersexuality from parents to children. He goes forward and cast FC as being rather a local antidote to halt the spread of the HIV/AIDS, a disease, he believes is only imposed on Africans and reportedly, has neocolonial undertones "We the blacks have to go into research.....before we can start absorbing the message"(Bessong). He brings us back here to the presumed demonisation of African systems of sexuality in the wake of the AIDS scourge by colonial writers, which the likes of Gausset (2001) and others have taken issue against. He equally debunks the initial hypothesis with regards to the AIDS virus which attributed the source of the disease, to a yet unknown country in Africa, a position that led Africa to become the cradle of the disease, stigmatizing both the continent and its people in the process.

Seemingly challenging the 'hardened' view of culture as cast in stone as held by some analysts, he reports that they are modifying FC unlike their ancestors who used the same pen knife called *okarang* on several initiates at the same time by using "one blade per individual". Such analysts hold that so called "traditional societies" are impermeable to change. With regards to HIV/AIDS, he points out that the "Blackman" is genetically stronger when compared to the Whiteman who is said to be weak and can therefore easily be infected by HIV. According to him, before the coming of the Whiteman and his subsequent invention of AIDS, "the Blackman" had been living his life like that.

Interviewer: Do you feel that there is a difference between a woman who is circumcised and one who is not circumcised?

All answer "yes" in unison.

Bessong: We have been told that a woman who is circumcised has lost sexual curiosity unlike a woman who is not circumcised (All: "That is the difference"). But then, all these things come about according to genetic heritage. You can come from a family, mother whose gene is so active, and you are circumcised but the gene you have inherited cannot stop you from that. That is why such aspects cannot be defined.

Interviewer: With the coming of HIV/AIDS, do you still find circumcision relevant?

Bessong: Circumcision could be relevant. Because with the HIV, we have not gone into research and we have not come to the research of HIV, so we can never conclude as to whether the cause of HIV lies in circumcision. But we are doubting and suggesting that from this, we can abstain from such aspects but then, we are not really out of it. Because the factual aspect is not… the scientists have not come and we the blacks, we have never gone into research but we have been hearing only from the whites who started introducing this aspect of HIV to us. So, we the blacks have to go into and come out with research findings before we can start absorbing the message.

Interviewer: But they say that you people use roasted blades, roasted okarang, no anaesthesia and that this can lead to HIV infection through circumcision.

Bessong: That is their own story.

Agbor: Who told them so?

Bessong: Let me come. He is just giving us a message. Let us discuss this point.

Otang: Circumcision means what? The Whiteman is a dull man.

Interviewer: Cutting the clitoris.

Otang: They want to tell me that a man goes to circumcise a female?

Bessong: Monsieur, monsieur, don't say that I have cut you short. What is there is that what is pertaining to those instruments we were using in those days, is just like when you eat and do not clean your hands. When you greet me with your hands and as I am going, when taking my hands on to my nose, I get the message of what you have eaten. It is just like transmitting the same disease when you use the same blade or okarang or anything, then you use it on another person, the message on the okarang you used on the other person can be transmitted onto another person. That is why the fear is moving. But let us absorb one thing that… the black man has been living before the Whiteman came with this idea about AIDS. The black man has been living and now if the Whiteman wants to tarnish or to stop this act, we should know the culture of the Whiteman first before him coming to our own culture to even tarnish other things

Etah: Do not learn your own and forget about the other man's own. Let us forget about the Whiteman's culture and continue with ours. And continue with our black man's culture.

Nkoyo: The white man is a very stupid man. Why are they coming to confuse us?

Fidelis: He is not stupid. He is just telling you to go and do research in your own area. Why not go and do research?

Abang: Most of these illnesses come from the Whiteman. We do not have AIDS in this village. With us here, we don't have AIDS. We have ossung, etati, all those things which are anti-AIDS. The Whiteman is so soft, that is why he is being attacked by AIDS.

In the above interview excerpts, the discussants point out that they are careful with the instruments used for ritual circumcisions because of their awareness that various diseases can be transmitted from one initiate to the other if the same instrument is used on or by several initiates at the same time. This might seem to suggest that the debate orchestrated by the association between the transmission of HIV through the ritual cutting of circumcision has led to modifications. They further point to the presumed resistance of the Black man unlike the Whiteman in the face of disease even before the advent of the AIDS pandemic. They are presenting a counter- discourse as to the origin of various illnesses, a likely reaction to the African origin of the AIDS myth. Moreover, they are saying that cultural borders between Africa and the West should be opened up for each camp to freely enter and study the other. They seem to be protesting here against Western dominance in the production and subsequent circulation of knowledge about cultural 'others'.

5.3 Multiple actors, different agendas

Apart from the people's spatio-temporal connections with the outside world, they are flanked by several, overlapping and interconnected power fields. At the local-global nexus, we have the Cameroonian state. The state in alliance with national, regional and international NGOs, is against the ritual cutting of FC. However, the state because of partisan considerations only frames the issue and abdicates its functions to these NGOs to conduct sensitisation and education at the grass root level. Within the local Ejagham community, there is wide division. Some segments of the population are with the state-NGO alliance (modernity). While some individuals are against the ritual cutting practice of FC and therefore subscribe to tradition and to continuity. Another group of individuals are still in a dilemma particularly when they are faced with the HIV/AIDS threat. This group appropriates both modernity and tradition simultaneously. At times, they forward FC as a useful, native therapeutic response to the HIV/AIDS threat. At other times however, they are against FC because of its violence and negative heath effects. Some moderates among their fold are instead opting for harm reduction through the medicalization of the ritual procedures. This group of internal ambivalent actors may be said to maintain a "double discourse". Tradition is at times contested in response to modern pressures and at other times, modernity is appropriated. In other words, they vacillate between maintaining FC because of its presumed functional value, particularly its supposed ability to sap women's anxiety to enjoy sexual intercourse and the need for change because of the ritual's harmful health effects with the former shortcoming inclusive.

The outcome of the people's interaction with other forces therefore shifts in response to power fields through time. This is explained by "the several operating units of power" (Adams, 1966, 1975, cf, Wolf, 2001). Stated otherwise, there are multiple capillaries and ways of subverting power through resistance. In the most enclaved regions, people often asked me the question of how the government will know whether or not their daughters have been circumcised. They further questioned how the police will reach the area given its enclaved nature so as to arrest them for circumcising women. The following interview excerpt captures this fact:

> Interviewer: Don't you think that if a road network were to pass here, the police can easily arrest you?
>
> Madam Ndom: Arrest us? For our tradition? Do you mean to tell me that those police officers do not have their own tradition? Insofar as our tradition is concerned, there is no police. Even if there is a main road here, we will still circumcise our daughters. If you circumcise your child at home, how will the police know? Do they announce it over radio, over television? You have seen my female children, how do you know whether or not, they have already been circumcised. Unless they are smeared with cam wood dye or calabar chalk, you cannot know (Egbe Ngon, Interview of 31/07/06, Babi)

The informant quoted above, presents the people's marginalization and neglect by the state in the sharing of development resources as an obstacle to state intervention in the practice of their culture, with FC inclusive. For instance, they pointed out and it could be observed that they lack basic necesities such as a road network, potable water, electricity and a modern hospital facility among others . She further states that the construction of a road network will not deter them from continuing to circumcise women because the ritual cutting takes place within the private sphere of the household and not in the public realm.

However, the people readily go in for whatever material enticements they are offered by the dense network of local NGOs and their external allies intervening against FC in exchange for an end to the ritual cuttings. Thereafter, they continue with the ritual cutting practices.

> Interviewer: But now government is against female circumcision, what is your reaction?
>
> Ngon: Even if government is telling us to abandon female circumcision, we cannot do that because it is our own tradition. And circumcision helps us as we are poor. We have no roads, we have nothing. If you put your daughter in the fattening room, the small money that comes in will permit you to buy soap, maggi cube, kerosene, palm oil and because we have no other work, circumcision helps us. (Ngon, Interview of 20/06/06,Ogurang).
>
> We cannot abandon female circumcision because it is like our own activity; it is like our own occupation. It helps us. Although government has asked us to stop circumcision, we cannot unless they give us a road. Because as I have returned from the farm like this, with cassava, there are no people to buy because everybody has. But if there was a road network here linking us to the outside world, people will come and buy. It is for the same reason that we are not able to send our children to school- because of poverty. If a road comes here, people will come and buy our products (Interview, Agbor,24/06/06,Okurikang).
>
> If the government wants to stop (female) circumcision, they must do something to help the women. They will agree.
>
> (Mr James Inyang,interview of 03/05/06, Babong)

The above cited interview excerpts demonstrate that circumcision is intertwined with poverty and that the need to uphold this 'age-old tradition' has led to socio-cultural resistance to the abandonment of the ritual mutilation practices. This is the case because of the presumed economic benefits of the ritual ceremony. The Ejaghams therefore present both poverty and underdevelopment as justification for their resistance to change. However, it seems to me that using the economics of the ritual procedures as justification for its continuation put to question the wisdom of reducing its complexities, nuances and ceremonialities to poverty alone. NGOs in the Ejagham area have used this 'gift exchange strategy' for decades. This has been without any significant fall in the number of girls undergoing the ritual cutting since earlier circumcisions is now the norm. In fact, neonates are increasingly being cut so as to stifle resistance at maturity. Both the ritual practice of FC and anti-advocacy campaigns have become "strategic fields of power".

> Interviewer: Why is government refusing female circumcision?
>
> Scientist: It is like a conspiracy. The Western world is telling us that this thing [female circumcision] is not good. There are however people whose experience shows that it is good. And since government depends on them [western donors] to have money, there is nothing the government can do. They have to tell us to stop circumcision. All NGOs working against female circumcision depend on government finance. They say this thing is risky, we say this thing is fine. The other person says this thing is bad. It is like bargaining with somebody who has more powers than you.
>
> Interviewer: Why is the government abolishing female circumcision?
>
> Jeannette: Because the Whiteman has told us to stop. If it was in those days, we cannot abandon it. Time changes and things change (Interview of 18/07/06,Ogurang).

A close reading of the interview excerpts quoted above suggest that the Ejaghams interpret calls for the criminalization of FC as an imposition of power on them by the 'Whiteman' with the conniviance of the government. Although they simultaneously recognize the government's subscription to international norms, they are accusing the state of complacency with the 'Whiteman'. The interview excerpts further suggest that the government has monopoly over "symbolic violence" (Althusser, 1971) but is under the superior power and gaze of the international system to enact and implement anti-FC legislation. Even when the people feign ignorance of any law restraining them from practising FC, they however recognize the government's monopoly of 'symbolic violence'. The point is that from their own perspective, the social benefits of circumcision far outweigh a legal ban. FC has clear reminiscences to a thrift and loan society. This system of communal reciprocity implies that when one takes part in an individual's circumcision feast, s/he is expected to circumcise his/ her own daughters and to host a feast for others to enjoy. The most important consideration is the social aspect of the ritual and not the actual physical cutting. This is better examplified by the increasing privitization of ritual FC on young girls at tender ages, an issue that I now turn my attention to below.

The increasing privatization of circumcision on younger girls beginning from as early as a few weeks after birth is one of the outcomes of the 'double discourse phenomenon', one of the several strategies of resistance against the anti-FC campaigns and multiple power fields in which the Ejaghams are embedded. It is in fact a mechanism of ensuring that children are circumcised before they come of age, enjoy sex and start contesting the ritual cutting practice under the influence of the ''Whiteman'': the Cameroonian state and NGOs at multiple scales. This shows that ''perpetrators'' still see the need for 'fixing girls' and that the anti-FC campaigns have rather been counter-productive as it has instead reinforced the need for circumcision as a local panacea to the HIV/AIDS pandemic. Perpetrators, I argue, are appropriating the harmful effects, particularly the fact that FC is said to decrease sexual anxiety in girls and can therefore prevent them from being wayward. It is widely claimed that circumcised women are sexually reserved and less demanding. This dovetails with the perception of hardliners that FC can save as a 'native' therapeutic model against the ravages of the HIV/AIDS pandemic. In other words, they seem to be arguing that the benefits of circumcision far outweigh its disadvantages. Even the notion of health security is being doubly appropriated. The modernist paradigm sees FC as a threat against human security, the bodily integrity and the human rights of the initiates. Here competing notions of security and risk are at play. On the one hand, traditionalists see the ritual cuttings as a social security mechanism that provides 'social protection' against HIV/AIDS infection, integrates the initiate into the social security network of her community since it secures for her social acceptance, guarantees marriageability thereby bringing benefits to patriarchy. It therefore serves as a social security scheme. I must also point out that although FC is done as a cultural obligation and as a mark of parental love, it is a violation of the human rights, bodily integrity and health security of the initiates. Although some people gave me to understand that they prefer circumcising children because they will not feel the pains and side effects, I suspect that their real intention is to thwart resistance at this tender age given the 'double discourse' between acceptance to change through eradication and the need for modification through medicalization which suggests the continuous perceived saliency of FC among some segments of the Ejagham population. We should note here that parents are only custodians of rights on behalf of children. These children are increasingly at risk since FC takes place within the private sphere of the household making it almost impossible for the state to intervene and punish perpetrators and their accomplices. As if to ridicule government threats, respondents persistently asked to know how government will become aware that their daughters have been circumcised.

> You have seen my female children, how do you know whether or not they have already been circumcised. Do we announce it over radio, over television? Unless they are rubbed with cam-wood dye just like a woman in the fattening room. Everybody has a choice but for me whether police or no police, I must circumcise all my daughters before they grow too big and start claiming rights (Erica Bassey, interview of 26/06/06, Ogurang)

Closely related to this point is the appropriation of the concept of individual/community rights and choice by some people within the Ejagham community. This point of view is ably illustrated by the following interview excerpt:

> When I just came here and was staying down there, a woman gave birth to a baby. Her child was circumcised and the very next morning, the child died. They did not report to the police. It is their culture and it was their child. How will they tell the police?(Mami Celina , interview of 07/03/06, Eyumojock).

The respondent cited above points to a conspiracy of silence between family members because of their failure to bring the case of a dead occasioned by circumcision to the attention of the forces of law and order. She further invokes both individual and cultural rights as justifications for such acts of complicity.

> If instruments are clean and safe, circumcision can still be good to those who still wish. At some times, a canoe capsizes in a river, people still go by it. You see a train can derail, people will still continue to travel by train. A plane can crash but people will continue to travel by air. We refuse stealing but people still steal (Tambe Robert, 03/04/06, Eyumojock).

In the interview excerpt cited above, the respondent opts to continue with FC practices through the medicalization of the procedures. He further points out that despite the various health risks that FC entails, some people are still submitting their daughters to the ritual practices. Like the former respondent, this informant's statement partly highlights the issue of individual/community rights and choice with regards to whether or not to circumcise one's daughter exposing an irreconcialable chasm between parental and community rights on the one hand and individual and children's human rights on the other. One other issue that he highlights is that people are willing and will decide to take risks notwithstanding the cost. In other words, the burden of liability or the duty of care does not fall on passengers using an available means of transport alone. If people are not allowed to travel, canoes, trains and planes should not be made. Here, the legal concepts of contributive negligence, non feasance and mal feasance clearly come into play to justify the fact that although FC is risky, people have a choice.

It might be stated here that social and cultural change always involves contradictions as demonstrated by the 'double discourse' phenomena manifested through simultaneous recognition of the harm done to women and children through FC and the need to tighten control over female sexuality using FC because of vested interests among certain internal stakeholders. While the youths are increasingly seeking satisfying love relationships and see FC as an obstacle, their parents and elders see them as breaking away from the laid down criteria for appropriate spouses. Some parents because of their inability to dictate to their children, have adopted an attitude of resignation while others have rejected their children's spouses from non-circumcising groups. On their part, some of these youths given their financial power have decided to stay with their 'foreign' partners despite their parent's opposition because their spouses are uncircumcised and will most often, indulge in extramarital sexual intercourse. It can be stated here that the increasing independence of the youths thanks to their western education and urban jobs has led to the loss of control over them, their resources and labour by their parents. These profound changes in their lifestyles, values and orientation have led to different ideas concerning spousal choice, marriage and sexuality. Most youths want partners with the same orientation, level of education, life-style and taste. They are more concerned about partner compatibility and not the instrumental criteria of elders such as the prospective spouse's ability to work on the farm, to be kind and to be entertaining to extended family members among others. There is a cultural shift from collective to individual destiny, from 'Us' to 'I', from collectivism to individualism. What this implies is that FC as a way of giving up individual needs and aspirations for the welfare of the collectivity is no longer the case. Social mobility beyond the village nexus thanks to education and employment will eventually lead to the gradual disappearance of long term distinctions and differentiations based on birth between free-born and slaves. It should be recalled that FC like membership in various secret societies, was one marker of this distinction although its diffusion from the upper class to the entire Ejagham community was a way of identifying with the mainstream. Increased access to resources and independence in decision-making, will impact on the cultural continuity of FC and how its contradictions are being perceived. For instance, people who abhor circumcised women may get married to them out of love. Some males may even get married to them without knowing they are circumcised. We should note that the elders, most of whose wives are already circumcised have maintained an attitude of resignation, pointing out that they love their already circumcised wives and there is nothing they can do.

Having discussed the different appropriations of the harmful effects of FC and the privatization of the ritual cutting on neonates this far, I shall now turn my attention in the next section to the issue of romantic love, another ambivalent framework for contestation, resistance and change. Thereafter, I will examine the factors working both for and against change in the ritual procedures and then conclude.

5.4 FC as Virtuous cut: Romantic Love

One issue that has animated debates and led to contestation and conflict is the assumption that FC impedes female sexuality and is an obstacle to the consummation of romantic relationships. This has led to intense and widespread sexual networking among some initiates while others do not know whether or not their lack of interest in sex is because of their circumcision status. Both conservatives and progressives alike, especially within the context of the HIV/AIDS pandemic, have appropriated this ambivalent framework for both resistance and contestation. The most important outcome however has been the surge of sentiments and the loss of control by parents and elders over the youths, women and their sexuality. The youths are increasingly placing affection and personal compatibility as top priority among criteria in choosing marriage partners and even those who continue to use the instrumental criteria of prudence are behaving romantically within those limits, a transformation that lies at the centre of the relationship between romantic love and community control (Shorter, 1976:148). It should be stated here that FC by subordinating individual for collective needs transforms women into productive and reproductive units by depriving them of sexual emotionality through the ritual cutting as part of the patriarchal control complex. In line with the politics of marriage, FC is a social mechanism for transmitting property and status from one generation to another. The sexual reservation of women guarantees paternity and thus tends to achieve this aim in the eyes of traditionalists. On the other hand however, personal happiness and individual self-development are becoming increasingly the criteria for choosing a marriage spouse among the youths, thereby pitting them at conflict with the elders since the former seem to care less about the 'posterity business'. Property is being replaced with sentiment and then with sex as the bond between man and wife (Shorter 1976:7). Stone

(1977) has pointed out that marriage is an economic, productive and reproductive undertaking rather than an emotional relationship. As a mechanism for transmitting property, sex becomes justified only by the need to propagate the species. There is in fact, the collapse of the 'chain of generations' which serves no larger moral purpose for adolescents and the moral authority of parents and elders as 'moral entrepreneurs' over children and women has waned. Children have totally different aspirations from those of their parents and elders who unlike in the past are unable to influence their children's choice of spouses. The young generation is increasingly breaking free from traditional concerns and following their own emotional and sexual inclinations (Anderson, 1980:53-54) as evidenced by changing attitudes to sexuality, which can be read partly as evidence of the surge of romantic sentiments. Personal choice and expressive considerations are replacing instrumental criteria as the main basis of spousal selection.

I conceptualize love and sex as at times independent, but interrelated power fields. Sex should be seen as intertwined with power and both as convertible currencies that merge into one another. 'Sex may lead to power, through the conduit of seduction. Power is also a basis for obtaining sex, whether by force or lubricated with money and what it can buy' (Therbon, 2003:1). Following Shorter (1976:14-16) romantic love is 'the capacity for spontaneity and empathy in an erotic relationship'. Spontaneity, he goes on, 'represents the rejection of traditional, community-imposed forms in interpersonal matters' and 'romance is the vehicle of self-exploration and self-development' among couples. Empathy and spontaneity are key components of a wide gamut of human relationships but only become romantic love in erotic relationships. In their quest for sexual fulfilment, the youths are increasingly seeking erotic relationships and some of them see FC as an obstacle to the attainment of their objective.

Although from a biomedical paradigm FC is said to temper sexual initiative, only a few initiates gave experiential 'evidence' to this point of view. Some of the initiatees even appropriate the fact that it tempers with sexual anxiety for the promotion of their own interests and for their own self-agency. The testimonies that follow were recorded during an anti-FC advocacy seminar in Eyumojock on Friday, April 28th, 2006 and complemented with follow up individual in-depth interviews.

> I have been circumcised with effect. I have advantage over you. The advantage I have is that I do not have cause to be easily tempted for a man. So, I was going to secondary school as we were students, when I got a boyfriend and my friends too had boyfriends. When there were occasions when there was the need for sex, or anything my friends will refuse but

> once the boys started touching them, there was no way.[They had to give in and offered themselves for sexual intercourse] .But for me, since I had been circumcised, no matter what my boyfriend could say [or do]. That is how I succeeded to sail through education without getting pregnant. A man could not touch me at any minute and I just become tempted and give in to his sexual demands.
>
> Moderator: What is your advice?
>
> Benedicta: All victims [of female circumcision] should not regret it because it has already passed but anybody who has not undergone it and because of the disadvantages, should not (Benedicta Obam, 38 years old, initiate, graduate and politician).

The above initiate's testimony is ambivalent but she maintains that her circumcision was beneficial to her as it made her capable of withstanding sexual requests and seductions from her boyfriends unlike her mates who when cajoled and pressured, normally gave in apparently because they were uncut. She believes that it was because of her circumcision, ("virtuous cut") that she was able to sail through secondary school without getting pregnant. She now has three children. Interestingly, she however advises those who are still uninitiated not to submit themselves to the ritual visitation and those who have already been ritually cut not to regret because they cannot do anything about it any longer.

This informant's viewpoint seems to resonate with Abusharaf's (2000, 2001) notion of FC as a 'virtuous cut'. Her respondents reported that they have an agency over sex with their husbands and that unlike uncut women, can use it to get most of whatever they want from the latter by refusing to have intercourse. Abusharaf (2000, 2001), and EL Dawla (1999) independently report that their informants present the ritual as a symbol of their power. In other words, they are able to use their circumcision status to garner scarce resources from their husbands and to get their voices heard. Similar emic contextual personal accounts have equally been rendered by Ahmadou (2001), Njambi (2004) among others. The presence of the clitoris in the view of radical Western feminists seems to be a symbolism for women's political power since by lacking it, African women are said to lack agency and need to be 'saved'. But as Abusharaf (2000, 2001) and EL Dawla (1999) show, women use their ''Bottom power'' (circumcision status) as a source of "tactical power"(Wolf, 2001) by being able to resist sexual demands from their husbands and in the process to get them to do what they like. The recent adoption of FC by girls among the Sara partly attracted by the feasting and pleasure they derive from the public ritual celebrations, is an interesting ethnographic curiosity. They mobilized the necessary material resources and recruited a circumciser by themselves. They did it despite refusal by significant social others in their community and in the process declared their own self-autonomy by institutionalizing and bureaucratizing the procedures (see Leonard, 2000). They may be seen as vectors of 'negative change'

The Freudian concept of penis envy seems to be appropriate here. Following Sigmund Freud, males at puberty manifest the desire to take over their mothers from their fathers and become jealous of the former. At the same age, girls are said to be eager and sexually jealous of their fathers and want to take them from their mothers.

> I have my own experience, which I want to share with you young people, my senior brothers and sisters. Nearly everything put up here, seems I am picturing myself. So, at the age of four, when I knew nothing in this world, I was circumcised. I cannot really recall the pains I went through. But what I experienced was that I bled profusely and was rushed to a medical facility [hospital] by my mothers because they could not handle the situation at home. The blood overflowed in such a way that they could not handle. I was too young. And because I was circumcised, it brought me some serious effects- my vagina became completely closed, I mean sealed. I was no longer like a woman. I could not urinate again. They had to rush to a woman in Nigeria to come and carry out a traditional treatment on me using coco leaves….struggling to insert it so that it could open up my vagina. You can imagine the pains. So, for months, she did that. At that time, I was in primary one. The rule was that nobody had to touch my hair, nobody had to shave me while I was undergoing the treatment. The hair remained like that while I was going through that treatment… until my vagina started opening gradually. So, for the first time when I saw blood like a woman [meaning first menses] it pained me a lot. I mean, it pained me a lot. It seemed I was eating the earth with my teeth. I took it that like a woman it was normal to have such menstrual pains. So, I went to secondary school with my friends, I knew nothing about a man until I wrote the ordinary level certificate examination. I had not even known what a man was any way. I was never even moved in any way. When I saw a man, it moved me in no way. So, in the village here, I was given a certain name-that I am /mpiay/.I do not know how to interpret it in English. It is an animal in the bush that does not have a vagina. That is how I was being called. My mother started swearing that anybody who calls her daughter that name will face her personally. That is because I had no urge for sexual activities. It did not mean anything to me. It had no use to me.
>
> Until……When I was about to give birth, I was going to the maternity (for prenatal care).Each time I was sent back to the doctor and not to the midwife. They complained that my pelvic bones had joined and will cause me problems during delivery. Each time I went to the clinic, the doctor struggled to send his hands inside me, there, so as to expand it. At the time when I had to deliver, MA Bea told me that she had to do me forced

delivery if not, the child might struggle and might die in the process. I said whatever she said I knew nothing. After that long labour, she had to do me forced delivery. She carried out forced delivery on me and after that forced delivery just as Mami was complaining here- that you have to use hot water to heal the wounds, I preferred tablets and injections. After that, I came to realize that I had body itches, in my vagina. I explained it to my elder sister and she said it was sugar sugar. I asked her what sugar sugar was. I went back to the hospital and lab tests were conducted and I got a long list of prescriptions to be bought and taken. All that has been written on the board I am reading and cross-examining myself point by point. For me, there is no advantage in undergoing female circumcision, apart from the advantage that our co-coordinators have pointed out-namely, money making. Apart from that, there is no advantage. My brothers and sisters who have not gone through that experience, please, do not try it (Anna Mkpot, 28 years old).

Anna's interview excerpt quoted above shows that she encountered excessive bleeding. In fact, her vagina almost closed and her parents had to seek therapy from a TBA. The treatment entailed inserting a solid substance into her vagina to open her up and the prohibition that nobody should touch her head while she was undergoing this therapy. Then later on in life when she became pregnant, she suffered from lengthy labour because of her small vagina and the fact that she has a small pelvic necessitated forced delivery. She is however silent as to how she became pregnant since she "hated" men which would have certainly permitted for a much more rigorous analysis.

Interviewer: Do you feel that your circumcision has affected your sexual response in any way?

Anna: Weah, you see, I was circumcised at the tender age of four and I cannot know the difference and everything seems to me to be normal, as If I was born like that. Whether it reduced my sexual anxiety or not, I cannot tell (Anna Mkpot, 28 years old)

Like the first respondent quoted above, Anna seems to attribute her self-declared sexual reservation at school to her circumcision status. She was stereotypically compared to "mpiaye"- an animal in the people's ethno-botanical universe whose flesh is prohibited for consumption by women in general and pregnant women in particular. This animal is said to have a very small vagina. When pregnant, this animal falls from a tree at the moment of giving birth and the vagina opens for its young ones to come out. Given this characteristic of the animal's behaviour, it is believed among the Ejaghams that if a woman consumes its flesh, she will suffer from lengthy labour before giving birth. This animal metaphor like many others, was one way of enforcing the symbolic gender control of women by prohibiting them from consuming certain food items. Taken from a Bourdian perspective, prohibited food items for women are symbolisms of masculine power.

The third respondent, Madam Eret, on her part testifies in the interview excerpt below that she usually loses sexual appetite at the beginning of every pregnancy. She could stay with her husband for three weeks without making love to him. She hated sex. However, a closer reading of her testimony against the grain seems to suggest that whenever she was not pregnant, she liked having sex. Unfortunately, several attempts to get her husband's own side of the story did not yield any fruit. She like Anna and Benedicta, attributes her 'dislike' for sex at the verge of every pregnancy to her circumcision status. She points out that a woman's refusal to offer sexual intercourse to her husband could send him out into the arms of other waiting women. This could in the long run eventually lead to matrimonial breakdown because of his wife's inability to render him sexual services. She has nevertheless given birth to five daughters.

> I salute you my children. I have something too to say. All this while that you have been coming and talking to us about circumcision, it is now that I am realizing something. When I got married to my husband too, I and my husband could stay for three weeks like that. Whenever he wanted sex, I did not like it mostly when I was at the beginning of another pregnancy. I did not even want him to touch me. I just did not have the appetite for such a thing. It is now that I am realizing it as they are saying it because I was circumcised. I was circumcised after my first born. To us, when you gave birth to a girl child, a first daughter, and did not circumcise her, therefore you do not value her. So, I was with my brother in Kumba and my father was insisting that I should come and give birth in the village so that I should be circumcised. I came although I was afraid. At that time, they circumcised us by scrapping and removing everything [from inside the vagina] altogether. I and my husband could stay for two weeks and he will not be talking to me only because of that, but I did not know the reason. So, I am rather very happy because you have enlightened us......we have to know what we had done. At times, your husband could abandon you and continue going out with other women because, what he is looking for, you cannot provide. What he wants, he is forced to go out so I think even those who think that circumcision is a manifestation of love, I think there are other ways of showing love for our daughters, not through circumcision. I have not circumcised any of my children (Informant has five daughters). I am begging you my children not to submit yourselves to female circumcision (Madam Eret, 40 years old).

What is worthy of note from these testimonies is the fact that the first and third respondents had no sexual experiences before their circumcisions unlike the second respondent. The former were circumcised while they were children unlike the latter who encountered the ritual visitation when she had already given birth to her first child as the cultural routine demanded. Her testimony is silent as to her sexual experiences before circumcision. What the above case studies show apart from bleeding and pains which most initiates reported, is that the experience of harmful effects usually comes later on in life and may be taken as part of the natural cycle of a woman's life. To Anna for instance, she thought that painful menstruation was part of womanhood. The anti-FC advocacy messages may however be said to have psychologically conditioned initiates that they do not enjoy sex, that they are suffering from 'lack' which might lead to both contestation and change. This seems to confirm Obermeyer's (1999) conclusion that "harmful effects are the exceptions and not the rule". In the wake of early calls for democratization and good governance in Cameroon, a vaccination campaign targeting women of childbearing age in the Western Grassfields region, an opposition stronghold, was discursively termed a government "sterilization campaign". This led to the psychological conditioning of most women that they had been sterilized and in a bid to test their fertility, most of them resorted to inordinate sexuality. The end result was huge and constantly mounting cases of unwanted pregnancies. Sexually transmissible diseases (STDs) including the AIDS virus spread like wild fire in the Sahara desert in the process and the area is today partly topping the national AIDS prevalence chart.

Whether or not FC is antithetical to women's sexuality depends on the extent of the cutting and whether or not the woman already has sexual experience before her submission to the ritual visitation with which to compare her sexual life after circumcision against. This finding however does not expunge the fact that FC is a violation of international human rights and a form of child abuse and gender-based violence. This subordination of an individual's needs and pleasure is supposed to be for the good of the collectivity. There are of course, other variables that determine whether a woman reaches orgasm or not: the man's sexual performance and ability, the degree of love between the couples, and her/his mood at the time and many more. To compound matters, there are many constellations of sentiments within any given (Shorter, 1976) sexual relationship. Intensive comparative psychological evidence is still desperately needed on this point.

Although FC, independently or alongside other factors may compromise the fertility of a woman, infertility among the people is attributed among other causes to the handiwork of witches and wizards who might have 'mystically eaten up' the womb of a woman out of jealousy. This might be in a bid to settle scores with either herself, her family, or with her husband for his failure to pay the culturally laid down bride price. Some people however perceive a woman's infertility as predetermined by God. In other words, it is God's will that some women will not give birth. The mechanism through which witches and wizard are said to cause infertility is worthy of illustration. The following excerpt from an interview with a witchdoctor, Ajim, is in order here:

> Interviewer: Now, tell me how and what witches and wizards do to ensure that some women do not give birth.
>
> Interviewee: Right now, this is a woman (pointing to Nkoyo). To bewitch her so that she does not give birth, we have the right to send another woman who has a prick (penis) to sex her mystically. Once she sexes her, she has dirtied her womb and we do not want her to marry you. It might be that one of her boyfriends has instructed us to prevent the proposed union between her and this man who has come to conduct interviews. From there, we will send one girl. We have a girl amongst us, who makes love to other women through witchcraft. We equally have a girl only for black star, another one who is only a town crier and a girl who defends medicine and a male who is in charge of other operations. So, if we want to make you useless, we remove your womb. We then mount a wrappen and insert there. You will normally continue to see your menses but you can never take in (Ajim, interview of 03/06/06, Inukon village)

However, the biomedical causes of infertility or sub fertility are related to untreated or poorly treated venereal diseases, which are rampant in the area. I observed a lot of sexual networking usually involving a multiplicity of partners between both the young and the old alike. Elderly men engage in sexual intercourse with young ladies with the aim of re-energising their sexual energies whereas the "young babies" are enticed by the prospects to harvest and grab something from these elderly men. These old men ("sugar daddies") believe among others that these young and energetic ladies are still intact, do not have ''large vaginas'', coupled with the unfounded believe that the latter are not carriers of HIV/AIDS.

But ironically, it has been well documented that it is rather young men and women in their prime productive ages that are mostly affected by the HIV/AIDS pandemic. Since condom is discriminatively and circumstantially used with these multiple partners, there is the likelihood of the spread of diseases. Most men and women alike said that they do not often use condoms with their regular partners as a mark of trust, love and fidelity. They may only use condoms with them to avoid pregnancy. Unlike with regular sex partners, some said they use condoms usually with those who might be suspected to be infected or with those they do not actually love but are curious to capture scarce life sustaining resources from. A few women however told me that they are capable of testing whether a man is infected or not by physically squeezing his penis with their hands before inserting it into their vaginas. If the man shows signs of feeling pains, he is infected. What they did not say however was whether they would refuse him intercourse at this sensual and emotionally ladden moment or insist that he wears a condom and what the consequences will be if he refuses. Ironically, it is common practice in neighbouring towns around the area for women in commercial sexual encounters to insist that the man who wants unprotected sex should pay above the normal price, usually twice the laid down but negotiable price. This sounds like buying death at a higher price. But given the women's lack of power to negotiate safer sex, and the preference of most men "to go live"- perceiving condoms as a foreign object meant to reduce sexual pleasure, a sign of lack of love, trust and a license for infidelity, there is the likelihood of the rapid spread of STDs including AIDS in the community. Disease, Kleinman (1980) maintains, find their social and cultural origins in people's living and working conditions.

In keeping with the complex set of cultural understandings informing FC, some of the people constantly argue that FC does not impede conception. In other words, it serves the interest of patriarchy insofar as it provides a "native" cure against infertility, sub fertility and helps to keep women in matrimonial service. After all, patriarchy depends on social and biological reproduction for its survival and perpetuation. The fact that FC is a fertility enhancing ritual among the Ejaghams is another tacit protest and counter discourse to the health effect paradigm that dominates the anti-FC campaigns. An exemplary excerpt follows:

> ....but now people are talking of no circumcision for females. Those things do not disturb reproduction. Sometimes, some women in those days when I was a child without reproducing became pregnant while confined. The government does not want circumcision. However, here in Ejagham we still do it despite the coming of AIDS. Witches and wizards too can take advantage of it. HIV/AIDS campaign also targeted Female circumcision through radio messages (Regent Chief of Okurikang, interview of 20/04/06).

The informant quoted above is of the opinion that FC is functional because it instead stimulates a woman's fertility whereas the second respondent quoted below holds that it facilitates the birthing process and makes the woman's private to be aesthetically pleasing, odourless, attractive and "unfrightening" to the male partner.

> When a woman is circumcised, even when she wants to give birth, she does not find it difficult. But when not circumcised, on many occasions, it is difficult and we see that. Some men who look at the private of women, find the woman's clitoris as long as a stick. It becomes very long and even bends and at times, it is not even nice to be looking at it. At times, it looks discouraging and unsightly, not even good to look at it but it is odourless when it is circumcised (Warrior,35, traditional healer, 23/03/06, Eyumojock).

The presumed functional value of FC among certain segments of the Ejagham population now leads us to explore the influence of FC to the establishment of both sexual and erotic relationships. On the overall, the major finding here is that romantic love among partners takes precedence over everything.

The presumed psychosexual effects of FC, particularly fridigity, were hinted at indirectly by a few informants. As I have argued above, this is another double-edged sword discourse, which has instead enhanced the position of partisans of the ritual procedures, the very cardinal point on which anti-FC advocacy is based at the same time. Painful penetration is considered to be another obstacle which might prevent a couple especially a cut woman from enjoying sex. This might partly be a result of a man's failure to sufficiently arouse a woman before penetration or the unpreparedness of such a woman to receive a man in bed. I will illustrate these two points immediately with interview excerpts from my field notes before proceeding on. Informants who hold this view include Madam Ashu Glory, 40 years old, a resident of Ndebaya. She recalls that in answer to a controversial question on the harmful effects of FC which they forwarded to a sensitization seminar meant to discourage the ritual practice, they were told that:

> ...a woman who has not been circumcised takes a man more easily than a woman who has been circumcised. But I do not know. She receives a man more easily in bed than a circumcised woman. It seems that some important parts have been removed from a circumcised woman. That is what our delegation to Eyumojock came back with as a reply to our question.
>
> Interviewer: Did you believe that message?
>
> Respondent: I believed it whether it is true or false because it has already entered the records. We have made progress from the past. We are now talking about new things. We are now in the modern world. We are no

longer comparing things with the past because the things that our mothers and fathers were doing, we can no longer do today (Madam Ashu Glory, 40, interview of 03/06/06).

The phrase "more easily' in this informant's statement seems to suggest having intercourse without pains since painful penetration is usually outlined in the laundry list of adverse side effects indiscriminate of the type of circumcision undergone or whether it is repeated after every birth as is the case in some practicing societies. However, the respondent's subscription to the message is rather because ''it has been documented''. In other words, it is rather the power to produce, package and disseminate information particularly health concepts, a part of modernity which is influencing her to believe the message. She submits that times have changed and this modernity to her implies a total break away from things of the past, one of which was FC. She nevertheless underscores the willingness to be part of the changing times, part of the new modernity through the abandonment of FC.

> Ajim: They were circumcising because small children had the anxiety to go after men because their bodies were overcharging. They were having a lot of sexual stimulation. When circumcised, they kept away from men. But once a girl is circumcised, they run away from men. You can come across a fully mature girl who will have no interest in sex. This explains why she might not accede to your wishes.
>
> Interviewer: What is your experience with uncircumcised women?
>
> Ajim: My experience is that you can touch a circumcised woman for a long time before she becomes excited to make love to you unlike an uncircumcised woman who immediately you touch her, gives in spontaneously.

A frigid woman is however believed to pose a problem by some pro-FC advocates once a man is already under heat because he will need to stimulate her for long so as to get her ready for eventual penetration. This respondent is saying that the aim of circumcision was to thwart children's anxiety towards sex. His interlocution quoted above suggests that his preference for uncut women borders on his fear of the presumed sexual powers of uncircumcised women due to their presumed hypersexuality. I argue that forms of human sexuality are socially constructed and variable.

One bone of contention between pro and anti-FC advocates has to do with marriage to initiatees. When I questioned both the young and the old, the former were fiercely against any union with a circumcised girl whereas the latter were in favour possibly because most of their wives have already been circumcised and there is virtually nothing they can do about it. Twenty six years old Richard, for instance stated that:

> A circumcised woman is not as God made her. She does not attract me at all because she has been devalued from her original state. I do not have that anxiety, that love, that interest towards that particular woman who is circumcised.

The respondent Richard seems to harbour some of the sexual prejudices against circumcised women such as their presumed insatiable desire for sex. He is one of those seeking a fulfilling sexual life for both himself and his partner and sees FC as a cheat on women's sexuality. However, 10 per cent of my respondents were of the opinion that it does not really matter as to whether or not a woman is circumcised. What is of particular interest to them is rather the love between the couples. One possibility for change in the practice of FC is deviance to any of the multiple perceptions harboured by various segments of the population about both circumcised and uncircumcised women, which has fragmented the anti-FC campaigns in significant ways. 'Positive deviance' is in reality, one way of appropriating the modernity discourse and project where the body of women is the discursive turf among both 'modernists' and 'traditionalists'. I will argue that 'positive deviance' through marriage to uncircumcised women by men who 'fear' the presumed hypersexuality of circumcised women to those who still hold that view can eventually break the seeming deadlock between 'hard-liners' and 'soft-liners'. I recorded anecdotal cases of a few men who had disowned their wives when they returned after their first births from their in-laws already circumcised. They are said to have individually insisted that they wanted their wives as they were before they got married to them. In other words, these men might be said to be aware of the sexual impact of FC. While such instances may well serve to deter other parents from circumcising their daughters thereby leading to an end to the ritual cuttings, it could as well lead to earlier circumcisions now that children are being increasingly circumcised at far tender ages.

I have thus exposed various attitudes towards the ritual practice of FC. I have demonstrated that the advent of AIDS has led to argumentation producing resistance and contestation to change, a conflict that cuts across various segments of Ejagham society. The anti-FC messages based on pathology have been appropriated by both partisans of FC and anti-FC advocates particularly within the new institutional context and the reinvigorated debates set in motion by the AIDS pandemic. 'Hard-liners' are now increasingly framing their stance in terms of anti-colonialism and the preservation of cultural authenticity. They have successfully appropriated the AIDS discourse to reinforce resistance, 'fence-sitters' on the other hand are generally ambivalent about change- maintaining a somewhat 'double discourse' (resisting and simultaneously subscribing to changes). The 'fence-sitters' are at times against FC when they cast the harmful effects against the presumed benefits and some people among them are open to change through medicalisation. Unfortunately, in their 'culture contact zone' (Bizzell,1997) and marginal location, they have been given only one alternative by the international hegemonic health care superstructure that privileges biomedicine which is to summarily eradicate the ritual cuttings. Positionality of course, is dynamic over time as responses to modernity equally vary across space, groups, time and fields of power.

In the next section, I will examine the factors both for and against change in the FC ritual procedures. Conscious that FC is one of the constitutive elements of a legalized patriarchal complex, I begin with an examination of the macro-social and legal structure and the erasure of women's voices.

5.5 Factors for and against change in the practice of FC

The macro socio-legal context of Cameroon within which the Ejaghams are found is characterised by institutionalised patriarchy and women's ''erasure''. I argue that this has contributed to the lukewarm attitude of the government. With no specific set of laws in place against the ritual cuttings, individuals are appropriating the legal vacuum, a key component of the institutionalized patriarchal complex that is common to both Cameroonian and Ejagham societies.

5.5.1 Statecentric structural factors

The legal system of Cameroon like that of other African countries is characterised by socially institutionalized patriarchal domination. The law is gendered in favour of men, though not in men as a class. I am in line with feminist scholars such as Lazreg (1988), Spivak (1988) and Mohanty (2002), among others who disparage the generalization of male sexual politics all over the world which presents women as universal victims. As already documented by numerous feminist scholars, eg Parpart & Stuadt (1988), Mbilinyi (1983), Swant (1985) with specific reference to Tanzania, nation-states like Cameroon are inherently gendered in their constitution and objectives. Section 27(1) of the Southern Cameroons High Court Law 1955 for instance, provides that "The High Court shall observe and enforce the observance of every native law and custom which is not repugnant to natural justice, equity and good conscience nor incompatible with any law for the time being in force, and [that] nothing in this law shall deprive any person of the benefit of any such native law or custom". The Cameroon national chapter of the International Federation of Female Lawyers (FIDA) (1999) however reports that under Cameroonian customary law, the wife is defined as the property of the husband. With specific reference to the case of *Achu v. Achu*, the organization frowns against the court's ruling. The verdict reached by the court was that "customary law does not countenance the sharing of property, especially landed property between husband and wife on divorce. The wife is still regarded as part of her husband's property". To compound matters, estate letters of administration are invariably issued only to male relatives and not to the widow and children of the deceased. Most often, exclusion from property inheritance usually results in the expulsion of the widow from the marital home of her late husband. This is particularly the case when a widow refuses to remarry from within her late husband's kinship group. The Cameroon Chapter of the IAC has rightly characterised this inheritance law as a 'harmful traditional practice'.

As a matter of fact, Cameroonian laws are a sort of conspiratorial system in which elite men cling to power at the exclusion of women and young men, promoting their masculine self-interests, framing political and economic development agendas that only reinforce their own authority (Hodgson, 2001:150) and benefit only them. Modelled loosely after both the French and English legal systems, the Cameroonian state invokes both, but mostly, French and to a lesser extent, British case holdings as precedents. Like the earlier colonial legal system which it is an exact duplicate, it however makes recourse to "customary law" whenever possible. As Chanock (1982) incisively demonstrates for Northern Rhodesia, "customary law" was a collaboratively produced conspiracy by both elders and colonial administrators who distilled the normative rules in each 'culture' that could be learned, recorded and applied to specific cases. In the process, the elders selectively offered only partial, interested versions of customary law so as to consolidate their hold over both women and young men. By so doing, they reified specific decisions reached on each case usually depending on extenuating circumstances such as previous exchanges and kinship ties. They later got colonial administrators to enforce these laws that strengthened their positions at the detriment of women and young men alike. This legal dualism, "Decentralized despotism" (Mamdani, 1996:109) is a reflection of two distinct, but related, forms of power: the centrally located modern state and the locally organised Native Authority who dispensed customary law consolidating their non-customary power. Yet, the 'customary' like the notion of culture itself has remained a contested field. As Ranger (1983:212) points out, imperial European respect for 'tradition' predisposed them to look favourably 'upon what they took to be customary in Africa', mirroring inflexible European neo-traditions. They were composed of unchanging sets of recorded rules and procedures in a period of flux. These invented traditions provided the 'aristocracy of color' with authority and confidence to act as vectors of social change, agencies of 'modernization' when applied to Africans (see Ranger, 1983: 221)

Mamdani also takes issue with the colonial presumption of an implicit and unchanging consensus over the customary. He notes that 'instead of a traditional consensus about custom, it signified a time of rapid change and much contest over the customary'(1996:110). The 'customary' is therefore opened to constant reinterpretation in the light of the often shifting interests of the elders and the state gerontocracy.

In the colonial bipolar judicial system, there were courts of chiefs and headmen for natives. The intermediate category was made up of tribunals staffed by white officials called Commissioners in British and Commanders in French territories. They listened to appeals from chief's courts but were charged with the general administration of native populations. In the postcolonial state context, chiefs have been co-opted as an arm of the modern administration and are often called upon to give cultural evidence in the adjudication of disputes particularly in instances where there is the need to appropriate 'tradition'. Through this process of co-optation, they like the elders, have lost their authority. Global and regional structural, economic and social changes have further weakened their already diminished authority. They have lost control over strategic resources such as land, which now largely belongs to an alien power, the postcolonial state. Simultaneously, they cannot command the labour of the youths, most of whom forced by poor economic circumstances back at home in the rural environment have migrated to the cities in search of white collar jobs. In other words, the elders lack both the economic and social capital of the present generation and have lost their authority over children and women because they cannot provide for them. The above structural, economic and social changes have led to deep rooted conflicts of generation between the youths on the one hand, who rely on scientific knowledge and the elders on the other who rely on tradition as the source of their authority.

I have earlier argued that the Cameroon government's failure to match rhetoric with action as demonstrated by the non-criminalization of FC is due to political considerations. The minority tribes practicing FC are the electoral fiefs of the ruling CPDM government. Furthermore, there is no distinction between the government and the ruling party. This has made it almost impossible for the minority opposition political parties in parliament to push for appropriate legislation to criminalize FC because it seems the government will be "sacrificing" its votes in the process even when it always wins the elections even before they are organized. Whereas the government has joined the international modernist normative order represented by international organizations: WHO, nation states, feminist organizations, human rights groups, women's health advocates on the importance of the eradication platform showing the interaction of local political discourse with international discourse against FC and other practices that negatively affect the health of both women and children, its engagement has been half-hearted as it has not yet enacted a specific law against FC. I am in line here with the observation by Boyles and Preves (2000) that the functional relevance created by the enactment of similar laws and policies by state parties has however combined to affect levels of contestation. This is because of power imbalances in the international system. States like Cameroon are simultaneously with and against international activism as they are caught up between political expediency, the protection of minority rights and international human rights norms. The state therefore maintains an ambiguous, pendulum-like posture because human rights as a precondition for obtaining much needed international aid was tied to FC eradication and the improvement of the status of women and children by the American State Department in the early 1990s.

I will argue however that although the institutionalization of criminal sanctions can be a right step forward in the fight against FC and other degrading HTPs, it should not be too hasty. It must be based on community consensus and consultations without which it will not work particularly as FC takes place within the private sphere of individual households in practicing communities. The law can actually be a double-edged sword. On the one hand, it can legitimize the efforts and position of grass root activists and local community leaders. According to Kercta (2005:57), in situations where laws are enforced, they may create incentives for change in the behaviour of individuals. On the other, where they fail, resistance will follow. Colonial attempts, be it in Egypt, Kenya or the Sudan backfired woefully because of local resistance to the perceived imposition of an external norm. Criminalization however sends a clear message to society that FC is a violation of a girl's right and is punishable. (See also Antanazzo, 2000, Fotheringham, 2004, Grande,

2004., Dorkenoo and Elworthy, 1992). Boyle and Preves (2000) make note of the importance of law in eradication efforts in these words:

> Law is a key ingredient in the social construction of reality. For example, African countries anti-FGC policies bolster the perception of an international consensus to eradicate female genital cutting and are viewed as an institution by international activists to work within countries to eradicate the practice. In this way, laws have real consequences in fuelling eradication efforts, regardless of whether local individuals are actually prosecuted under them (Boyles and Preves, 2000:706-7).

Legal prohibition shows the supremacy of the constitution over culture but conflicts with the cultural rights of individuals making it impossible for them to internalize the law. The law becomes a mere sign post. It is resisted and can create both resentment of the government and the interfering outsiders. This is because FC is usually practiced by minorities within specific state boundaries. Criminalization puts the state in an uncomfortable situation whether to respect minority rights and sentiments, or to trample on them outrightly and be accused by human rights groups for violation of cultural rights. Such a situation will clearly put human rights groups in a limbo as to the appropriate course of action to take.

Kereta (2005:57-58) enumerates three sets of factors for the likely failure of a hastily or forcefully imposed legislation against FC in the countries of Africa. First and foremost, she points to the weak state structures and law enforcement mechanisms in Africa, which is even further accentuated by the lack of resources and the fact that the customary laws supporting FC are unlikely to support legislation to outlaw such cultural practices.

The second obstacle in her view is the fact that in kinship-based societies, behavioural change at the individual level is difficult to achieve. Group consensus will therefore certainly play a pivotal role in changing the *status quo*. In other words, without the community's approval which the individual is part of, the law will be unenforceable and will become an idle sign post. This implies that taking legal action against one's relatives may produce far graver social consequences than the penalty that is eventually dished out to the defendant if s/he is found guilty.

The third obstacle to criminalization according to her, has to do with the minority factor. The institutionalization of a criminal law against FC can fuel ethnic animosities and might instead hinder the change efforts while exposing change agents and activists alike to the wrath of the population like the case in Sierra Leone suggests. The Economist (1999) rightly noted that "When the entire community participates in the criminal activity, it is impossible to enforce the law without mass terror". Rahman

& Toubia (1998) in the same vein have introduced an interesting perspective to the discussion on the efficiency of using criminal sanctions when they make note of the fact that:

> "When FC/FGM is common among one ethnic group and not another, enacting and applying a criminal law could fuel ethnic animosities" (Rahman & Toubia, 1998).

On his part, Mackie (2001:278) captures his misgivings and doubts about criminalization and points up the difficulties therein thus:

> If some outsider tells you that you are a bad person because of some family tradition you follow, and you follow this tradition because you are a good person, then will you abandon the practice and thereby confirm the outsider's ignorant judgment that you are a bad person? I think not. Legal prohibition that is not the expression of local popular will on the subject is ineffective, if not undemocratic (Mackie, 2001:278)

What is clear from the above discussion is that if the people involved in the practice are convinced through education and sensitization but not through the threat of criminal sanction or coercion, the timely introduction of a criminal law could be a step ahead in the right direction. Since change is already underway, the people's wholehearted support to the efforts of change activists can pave the way for the eventual introduction of a law to sustain this change. However, a poorly and hastily introduced law can backfire, truncate the emerging social consensus, lead to social rifts and drive the practice underground (The Economist, 1999).

5.5.2 The harmful health effect paradigm of anti-FC campaigns

The overemphasis on harmful effects, the very reductionist pillar of the anti-advocacy campaign messages seems to have actually derailed the change efforts in the Ejagham area thereby reinforcing both contestation and resistance. The educative and sensitization materials and concepts are usually distilled from those tailored on the most intrusive aspects of the ritual practices in places like the Sudan, Ethiopia and Egypt with seemingly inadequate cultural contextualization. While contestation and resistance shows the existence of competitive concepts of modernity, health, disease and disease symptoms, like between doctors and patients, the presumed harmful effects usually forwarded by activists most often do not tally in well with the experiences of most initiates. This might be explained by two interrelated plausible reasons. In the first place, these harmful effects take place only over time and may not be immediately noticeable by the initiates themselves or attributed to these circumcisions. Secondly, harmful effects seem to be the exceptions and not the rule. Usually, witchcraft provides a contrary, alternative explanatory paradigm when the circumcision of an initiate fails and complications such as excessive bleeding and even death set in. Two interview excerpts are illustrative here.

> Well, there are some wrong circumcisions which lead to intense bleeding. When others see the bad ones, they will not accept and following illnesses like AIDS, people have seen that they may occur due to circumcision. However, rapid understanding has made some people to stop. When a woman is circumcised, she will not be excited to have sex. Those who are not circumcised can be forced emotionally out of their own will. They cannot make two, three, four months without touching a man. If these things were studied well and taken care of by hospitals, things would have been better since they say it is not good because of ill health. Like some dresses, some years, you will see a particular pattern. After some few years, that pattern will disappear. It may reappear after fifteen years, the pattern of the past comes back again. The world can rotate from bad to good and from good to bad. If instruments are clean, safe circumcision can still be good to those who still wish. Sometimes a canoe capsizes in a river, people still continue to go by it. You see a train can derail, people will continue to travel by train. A plane can crash but people will continue to travel by air. We refuse stealing but people still steal.(Tambe Robert Agbor 45, interview of 03/04/06).
>
> Honourable: Many NGOs are flying about talking about circumcision. Generally, they say female circumcision kills cells. Look at this finger, if you cut it, blood will automatically flow. The same blood will flow if your leg is cut. So these wounds we used to have with cutlasses in the bush does not kill our white blood cells. They don't kill any cells except that it blends the interest for sex. You understand?
>
> Interviewer: Are you sure it blends the interest for sex?
>
> Honourable: I don't know because I am not at the same time having the two. Automatically, if you have a clitoris, you will believe what they are saying. And then somebody who is circumcised will say oh, had it been I was having a clitoris, I will be having more sexual interest oh....One person not having clitoris cannot be that same person to differentiate the two. Who knows whether what they are saying is not just propaganda or reality? (Interview, Eyumojock, with Honourable Benedicta, 03/04/06).

This finding resonates well with Abdullahi's (1989) suggestion that the language of the campaigns is complicated and beyond the comprehension of the target population because of the apparent reduction of the complex symbolism of the ritual to health alone.

5.5.3 FC as functional native response to HIV/AIDS

It is rather ironical that despite the likely associations and relationships between circumcision and the transmission of the AIDS virus to initiates if one and the same instrument is used on several individuals without sterilization or if the circumciser wounds herself in the process when any of the initiates is an HIV/AIDS patient, some people in the community still see FC as a rather useful "native" tool against the virus. There however seems to be some degree of awareness by these circumcisers as most activists and the circumcisers themselves reported using one blade per initiate and the use of anaesthesia as a pre-emptic measure against the likely transmission of diseases from one initiate to the other and to themselves.

Nevertheless, despite these modifications in the nomenclature of the ritual cuttings partly as a reaction to criticisms bordering on the hygienic conditions under which the cuttings take place; FC remains violence and a threat to the bodily integrity of the initiates and their human rights. Seemingly re-echoeing the fact that the ritual cuttings can lead to psycho-sexual dysfunction and frigidity, some hardliners see this particular harmful effect to be rather functional for the maintenance of female sexual morality and the stemming of the tides of the AIDS virus as they constantly pointed out that it helps reduce promiscuity and therefore curbs the sexual anxiety of women even when prostitution depends on a demand and supply curve, on poverty and inequality. Their argument is however weak as the HIV can still be transmitted through unprotected heterosexual intercourse since poverty has seriously weakened women's ability in the area to negotiate for safer sex. Whereas some argued that it limits a woman's anxiety for sex, some initiates totally expunged such a view as well as the other presumed harmful effects.

Atabe: No, people are complaining that….I don't see any relationship between circumcision and HIV/AIDS. Those who are circumcised, are they not flirting more than those who are not circumcised?

Ojong: I know that those who are not circumcised flirt but will you tell me that those who are circumcised do not also flirt? All of them flirt equally.

Interviewer: Is it true that they lack the anxiety for sex?

Atabe: I don't know. I am not a man to test them. All burst into laughter.

Interviewer: Since you were circumcised, in what ways has your circumcision affected your life?

Atabe: It has affected my life in no way because first of all, we are reasoning today that if you are circumcised, if you are not careful, you cannot give birth to children. But I was circumcised before I ever saw my menses. I have since then continued to see my menses, given birth to my three children. I see nothing disturbing me. I have continued to have nice and enjoyable sex with my husband, very good for sixteen years at this material moment [that we are talking]. If my husband says oya, (Laughing).Let us go [and have sex], we will. Smiling. I see no good reason in it. I felt that it was lack of circumcision that made a woman to have interest in sex but now, the thing or not [meaning circumcision or no circumcision], you still want to have sex, do what you are supposed to do. Laughing.

5.5.4 Modernization and intercultural contact

Whereas elders condemn the uncritical adoption of western value systems and lifestyles by the youths, these youths are questioning the very traditional rationality that deprived them in matters of knowledge with regards to sexuality and in other domains of social life. This is due partly to the influence of formal education. By imbibing scientific knowledge, they are now able to question and challenge the wisdom of tradition as the very vestige of both an outdated and pristine past. With regards to FC, most adults said children are increasingly contesting the custom and some are even ruling out the prospects of getting married to cut women whereas a minority instead stereotypically presents a cut woman as being rather difficult to satisfy sexually in bed.

Modernization has equally fuelled resistance in the sense that some parents have vowed to circumcise all their daughters whereas a large majority to forestall contestation in future have resorted to earlier circumcisions when the infants are barely neonates. Although they say that it is because the children will not feel pains, the main reason is to forestall contestation under the presumed influence of the Whiteman when they eventually come of age.

> The Whiteman has come and told them that it is not nice, it is painful and they have started contesting it (Ndifon Abang, 26 years old).

A further modernizing influence in the Ejagham community is the adoption of Christianity by a large majority of the people although some still practice religious syncretism- both Christianity and their traditional religion at the same time. Church leaders have been part and parcel of the anti-FC crusades. Most Christians and even lay individuals with whom I spoke invoked the Bible or God as being against female and not male circumcision.

> The tradition of circumcision is not good because God does not like it. Two captains cannot be in the same ship. If I decide to be a house girl [house help], I have to serve only one man. God who made woman the way she is was not a fool [that is with a clitoris] (Mami Born Again, interview of 18/03/06)
>
> A circumcised woman is not as God made her. She does not attract me at all because she has been devalued from her original state. I do not have that sexual anxiety, that love, that love towards that particular woman that is circumcised. (Richard, interview of 03/05/06, Eyumojock)

A few informants (5 per cent) however disparaged the sermons of the church against presumed negative cultural practices such as polygyny and belonging to any cult within the culture and vowed they would live and die as diehard advocates of tradition. This group sees the church merely as one of the agents of the Whiteman probably because missionaries brought Christianity to Africa from Europe.

It might be stated here that contact and interaction with the outside world has played a preponderant role both in breaking the culture of silence in which FC was shrouded in the recent past and in changing people's orientation about the traditional cultural motivations informing the ritual practice. Some of the people have got married to women from tribes that do not circumcise women while others have travelled and have had sexual escapades with uncut women. This cultural contact has worked both ways- produced both resistance and contestations at the same time. But most of the youths with whom I spoke do not really care whether their potential spouse is circumcised or not, what matters to them as they told me is the love binding the two parties. This particular finding seems to suggest that "positive deviance" in getting married to uncircumcised women will eventually lead to the abandonment of FC in the not too far away future and the uncircumcised will no longer be stereotyped and mocked at. The few who were still against marriage or sexual intercourse with uncircumcised women may eventually have no choice but to join the majority. Interestingly, none of the men reported having sexual difficulties with their partners because they were circumcised. However, with increasing circumcision of children usually at tender ages, the men might not even be aware that the very ladies they are considering to be uncut might have already been cut. Asked about his reaction to the government ban against FC, one respondent had this to say:

> Even before the government came in, some of us had seen that it was not good. Because while we were growing up, we have interacted with other civilizations. I happened to have exchanged view points on this subject with a Dutch woman. I was the first to ask her whether she was

> circumcised. She told me, she was not circumcised. I asked her why? She told me it was not proper, not good, that it is total destruction. You are denying a woman her normal sexual satisfaction, which is not permitted even by God. But I went further to ask several questions such as "How do you feel when you meet with a man with that your long thing like that and it is disturbing?. She said no, it does not matter. It is God's creation and he knows why he did it… But sexual satisfaction depends on that, she told me (George, 35 years old, quarter head, interview of 23/03/06, Eyumojock).

This informant points out that contact with other societies has shaped their perceptions, a new perception about the psychosexual dangers of FC. But at the same time, he is ambivalent as he has already been socially conditioned by significant social others into believing that "circumcised women do not enjoy sex". He therefore maintains a somewhat "double discourse" as he continues to represent uncut women as easy preys to sexual manipulations through mere stimulation since to him, the presence of the clitoris in a woman "spurs her into sexual activities", it absence will therefore restrict her and permit her to maintain her dignity. Here again women's bodies and their sexuality have become the social slat on which behavioural norms are written and enacted.

Conclusion

In this chapter, I have examined the varied and often shifting attitudes of the Ejagham people towards ritual FC within the new institutional context of the HIV/AIDS pandemic. There is wide division over FC among the people. Some segments of the population are subscribing to the alliance between the state and its allies (modernity). While others are against, another group of people are in a limbo when faced with the HIV/AIDS threat presenting the ritual cuttings as a "native" therapeutic response. This internal group of ambivalent loose actors may be said to maintain a somewhat "double discourse" as tradition is at times contested in response to modern pressures and at other times, modernity is appropriated. This implies that the outcome of their interaction with other forces therefore shift in response to different power fields through time. I have further shown that one of the outcomes of this multiplicity of actors and their conflicting agenda is the increasing privatization of FC on younger girls. At the same time, the youths are opting for self-fulfilling romantic relationships and see the FC ritual as an impediment. I have also examined the factors militating in favour of and against, creating contestation, resistance and conflict to the FC ritual cuttings.

The next chapter is a summary of my findings and some recommendations for the fight against FC and HIV/AIDS.

CHAPTER SIX

SUMMARY OF FINDINGS AND CONCLUSION

This study set out to qualitatively investigate actors' interaction in the heightened fight against HIV/AIDS and FC among Ejagham clans in Southwest Cameroon. The aim was to search for openings that allow for an alliance of local cultural practices and modern medicine to emerge through the dialogic balancing of local and international interests, the harnessing of local and scientific knowledge. What is clear is that NGO intervention should not be the imposition of another power on the people. The nomenclature of the ritual and categories of initiates has changed dramatically over time with earlier initiations now the rule. This is obviously one of several responses to the anti-FC campaigns. At the same time, the people are increasingly using a fresh blade for every initiate unlike in the past when one special knife, *okarang* was used on several initiates. They are therefore responding to the criticism of the ritual cuttings which partly borders on hygiene and the prospects of transmitting HIV. The fattening period too has waned as some of the people are realizing the necessity for girl children to attend school rather than to be exclusively trained as housewives. Despite modernization and the adoption of procedural changes, the ritual has remained. The major findings that emerge from this study can be summarized as follows:

The key anthropological finding that emerges from this study is that FC is a polythetic cultural category, not merely a health issue. It is intertwined with the whole cultural political economy of the Ejaghams. Under patriarchy where there is the dominance and magnification of male power through monopoly over property and where family and kinship serve as mechanisms for allocating labour, appropriating and distributing its revenues, FC becomes a crucial 'pars pro toto' for a complex of rituals and arrangements that are intended to 'fix women' and teach them, as if in a 'loan and thrift society', subordination and suppression of her own needs for the benefit of the family, kinship and patriarchy as evidenced by the high esteem enjoyed by the Moninkim dancers. This social arrangement has been kept in place by conditions of poverty, underdevelopment and dependence as well as by local gendered discourses of respectability, honour, and reciprocity among kin and community. Women use ritual FC as a "patriarchal bargain" –a powerful tool for negotiating with patriarchy in this system of inequality.

Anti-HIV/AIDS interventions by both the state and NGOs misses the point by focusing on health alone whereas it is increasingly becoming a human, social, gender rights and development issue. As a polythetic cultural complex, its methods can be modernized, rationalized and sanitized but its resilience has to do with the functions that it serves to gendered femininity and female personhood and its reproduction over time. State and NGO actions that adopt the pathological model and cast FC as 'harmful' have instead pushed it into the private sphere and children are increasingly being circumcised at far too tender ages so as to circumvent resistance.

The advent of the AIDS pandemic gave rise to a 'patriarchal' moral panic against female sexuality, promiscuity and prostitution- an outcome of the articulation of the African kinship system, patriarchy, female dependence, feminized poverty and commercialization- a situation that led to the emergence of a 'conservative' party that advocates FC as a mechanism of keeping women in matrimonial service. This group rejects arguments against FC made by biomedical actors and turns the AIDS crisis into the case for rather than against FC. Within the institutional context of AIDS, FC became an ambivalent framework for resistance, conflict and debates between partisans and opponents. On the one hand, FC advocates present the ritual cutting as a useful, "native" anti-dote against the scourge of the pandemic because FC is believed to temper with women's sexuality and is therefore seen as a functional physical and moral check on inordinate sexuality. On the other hand, anti-FC advocates present it as fuelling the spread of the HIV because the bloodletting that the ritual cutting entails can lead to the spread of diseases, with HIV/AIDS inclusive between participants. This has even led some people within the local population to be opting instead for the medicalisation of the procedures so as to do away with the harmful effects, particularly its association with HIV transmission. This finding shows that by reducing the complexity and nuances of the ritual cuttings to health alone, anti FC activism has instead produced a backlash marked by both contestation and practice.

Inter-tribal marriages with members of non-circumcising tribes and romantic love relationships beyond the purview of the traditional patriarchal orbit has led younger lovers to be increasingly seeking mutually satisfying love relationships for which FC is often seen as an impediment. Most young men are unwilling to take a circumcised spouse because she has reportedly been 'devalued' through ritual FC. This implies the need for total transformation in the political economy of sex and marriage and not in 'health 'alone.

The major contribution that this study claims to make to knowledge is the need to look at local level processes through an analysis of actors' multiple positioning, resources and their linkages to and alliances with other actors. This implies that local processes are rooted in wider fields of power and are affected by local, national, regional and international forces at various scales. This calls for the need to look at the intertwinement between local and global economic, social and historical processes in the study of health and other cultural issues. Such "critical junctures perspective" in health calls on us to foreground local ethnography within the extralocal context of larger historical processes and flows- that is, in terms of connections in space (and in and out of a place/ in and out of a group, the relations through time, the internal and external relations of power and dependency (see among others Kalb and Tak, 2005 and Singer, 1986). This perspective traces resistance, contestation and practice from below while taking note of circumstances in the larger social, political and economic context since each society's history is just a part of the larger history and struggle of humankind.

As far as the anti-FC and anti-HIV/AIDS interventions are concerned, I have directed attention to the fact that change should not necessarily imply doing away with one culture to impose another. Rather, it should be in the interest of the people and not against them. For this to happen they must be engaged and their perspectives and needs attended to for them to be able to absorb the culture shock that a hastily imposed change can bring about. This calls for an all encompassing approach to change that takes cognizance of multiple needs. FC is more than just about health; it fulfils social, cultural and psychological functions calling for the need to put in place appropriate mechanisms that will fulfil these aims. The socio-cultural and political economic context is very important in any change effort and the mere copying and replication of what works elsewhere might backfire and instead lead to a backlash as the anti-FC and anti-HIV/AIDS interventions suggest. In addition, this study has exposed several shortcomings and constraints affecting these interventions. The language and materials used in the anti-FC and anti-HIV/AIDS campaigns by intervening NGOs for instance, is based on risk and pathology reflecting the most intrusive types of the ritual cutting of FC and the assumption that the society has remained in a pristine state, which is clearly not the case. Activists do not adequately domesticate the health concepts used for the campaigns. This shows that they are merely a transmission belt for the spread of perceived 'strange health concepts'. They are further linked to a network of powerful international stakeholders making the local population see them as agents of a sort of colonialism. Furthermore, NGO actors are disunited. Their activities are seasonal given their urban headquarter location, while the road network is deplorable. Their location impacts negatively on the spatial geography of the anti-HIV/AIDS and anti-FC activism.

These findings can help government officials and grass root NGOs in Cameroon to make informed decisions with regards to policy and intervention against FC and AIDS in particular and rural development in general. In keeping with the main objective of this study, namely to find ways for an alliance between local cultural practices and modern medicine so as to foster dialogue and to reconcile both local and international interests in the anti-FC and anti-HIV/AIDS campaigns in Cameroon, I now propose some recommendations on how the problems identified in the study can be resolved. These suggestions will focus on the HIV/AIDS and anti-FC interventions.

6.1 Recommendations and perspective for better anti-FC and anti-HIV/AIDS interventions

6.1.1 On NGO activism against FC and AIDS

This study exposed several shortcomings and constraints of the anti-HIV/AIDS and anti-FC campaigns. While some can be attributed to the government's lack of political will in grass root development in general and in the fight against AIDS and FC in particular, others are a result of the NGOs' intervention strategies. This is the case with the type of universalizing health concepts they use which turns to alienate the people and do not reflect their experiences. The urban location of these grass root NGOs and their relationship with transnational stakeholders further present them as agents of the latter. Research has to respond with information based on local ethnography of stakeholder's interaction with each other and with the local population on how to solve these problems. The suggestions in this section therefore relate to circumstances over which these NGOs do not have some control, that is, what they can do without much external help particularly from the government. While it is true that even in the presence of no specific laws criminalizing FC, the government has been able to frame the terms of negotiations and allow grass root NGOs to conduct sensitization, these NGOs like local community leaders and activists are disempowered. Since the Chiefs and elders have virtually no power, the eventual enactment of a specific set of anti-FC legislation must be based on community consensus without which its implementation will be resisted. The earlier circumcisions which are increasingly taking place today support this view.

- Intervening NGOs need to form an alliance among themselves and to work in close collaboration with the government towards the eradication of FC.
- They should avoid the various reductionist approaches that have characterised their intervention over the years. While FC might be incompatible with women and children's reproductive health, human rights and well-being, reducing the whole procedure to health misses the point. Health is just a sub component of a much larger and complex whole. There is clearly the need here to identify the ritual's embeddness with other aspects of culture such as networks of reciprocities which is enacted through the communal feasting that often accompanies the ritual ceremony.
- The tendency to reduce FC to poverty has worked both ways. While on the one hand, it articulates the need to empower women and especially circumcisers through the creation of alternative income generating activities, on the other, practitioners often take whatever they are offered and therefore see the perpetuation of the practice as a smokescreen and a bargaining tool with which to constantly garner scarce livelihood resources from these NGOs. Some NGOs on the other hand, use empowerment through the provision of alternative sources of livelihood as a ruse to garner resources from donors that never reach the grass roots. This situation calls for a multipronged approach that respects community sentiments and is based on consensus and for NGOs to be accountable to the local masses and not only to their funders.
- An alternative rite of passage with all the symbolisms, connotations and ceremonialities of FC but without the actual physical cutting might be appropriate way of halting the ritual cuttings.
- My field observations showed that the various NGOs working in the Ejagham area have largely targeted only women thereby giving men the impression that it is "women's business". This is quite unfortunate because men wield a lot of power within households and are key stakeholders in decision making within their individual families in particular and in the community at large.

Although the government of Cameroon has signed and ratified several treaties for the protection of women and children's rights, this is not enough. The government must match words with action by transforming its obligations into concrete action so as to bring benefits to its people. This implies the need for national-level actions and policies to ensure adherence with various ratified treaties in this domain. Apart from consulting with the people and eventually enacting a specific set of appropriate legislation against FC, such an action would represent a clear commitment to the protection of women and children's rights and could empower the developing local social movement to intensify the fight against the ritual practices. Since internal cultural stakeholders are already debating the issue of FC, it might be said that social change is well underway and with political backing from the state, the process of debating and successfully passing a law could accelerate change. However, a poorly timed and hastily introduced law could backfire by truncating an emerging social dialogue; causing social rift and eventually driving the practice underground (The Economist, 1999). There is the further need for the government to repeal all existing laws that are incompatible with the health and well-being of women and children such as the law that forbids women from inheriting property, ban on information with regards to contraceptives, and labour and recruitment related discriminatory practices against women.

- The government should further provide various grass root NGOs and health personnel with the necessary resources for the fight against HIV/AIDS and FC. Given the enclaved nature of the area, there is the need for a good road network, potable water, modern health care facilities and rural electrification among others. The lack of communication infrastructure in particular has impacted negatively on the spatial geography of the intervention against FC and AIDS making these interventions to be only seasonal. Without a good road network, it will be impossible to implement a law if and whenever it is eventually enacted. The most important challenge to the anti-FC and anti HIV/AIDS fight is the people's trans-border location. This calls for both inter-governmental and inter-country collaborative efforts by NGOs in both Cameroon and Nigeria.
- There is clearly the need here for intersectoral collaboration among various government departments: Justice, Community development, Women and Family Ministry, Public Health rather than the usual reductionism of the ritual procedures' complexity to health alone

by various government departments. The government's poverty alleviation strategy should clearly tackle issues such as FC.

- The government further needs to introduce human rights and reproductive health education at all levels of the national school system: nursery, primary, secondary, high school and at university and in teacher training and vocational education institutions. The content should reflect the cognitive, affective and action aspects of learning. In other words, the target audience should be drilled on their rights and responsibilities and the rights and obligations of others. This could also be disseminated in local lingua franca through in-service courses and over radio and television. Educational materials discouraging harmful traditional practices such as breast ironing and FC should also be included in curriculum development materials.

These policy interventions should be pro-active. Local NGO activists should sharpen analytical and advocacy skills so as to ensure gender-equity and to hold the state party responsible for its commitments towards women and children's rights in international law. They should form coalitions and stop working as secretive, dissociated groups. Gender equity advocates in Egypt have rightly advised that "the challenge is not only one of opposing harmful traditional practices or mobilizing around rights but of publicly deconstructing the ideological and social system-rooted in age-old gender divisions-that make those practices acceptable and sometimes, even desired" (EL Dawla et al, 1998:110). Such a possibility for deconstruction is clearly offered by the growing public awareness over the risk of infection with HIV, although some people still contest the existence of the pandemic, attributing HIV/AIDS related deaths to witchcraft.

6.2 Limitations to the study and prospects for further research

This study provides a mere snapshot of transformations in the institutions of Moninkim and FC and the global fight against these institutions which is based on culture as "risk factor". Although the research has attempted to highlight critical issues related to the interventions and how actor's interaction has truncated the change initiatives thereby producing a backlash marked by both contestation and practice that constitute huge areas of research in their own right, it is obvious that I have not reached the bottom of possible explorations that can be made of issues investigated. For example, the exclusion of the factors that led the Bayangs, the Ejagham people's eastern neighbours to give up FC in the 1950s even when the anti-HIV/AIDS and anti-FC campaigns were yet to begin have not been explored. This is clearly evidence of internal change when a society without any outside influence decides to rethink certain aspects of its culture. Moreover, the efficiency of the "gift approach" practiced by intervening NGOs against FC is still to be investigated in its own right. My own observation shows that by trying to lure participants away from FC by offering them alternative sources of livelihood instead turns to foster the ritual cutting practices, by producing resistance as the people are aware that FC is money and that NGOs are taking advantage of the custom for their own aims.

Given its limited scope and focus on the Ejagham area alone, it is important to recognize the limits and generalisability of the findings and proposals. The recommendations do not pretend to explain fully all misconstrued or unknown facts (or provide answers to all burning questions) regarding FC and the relationship between actors. Any suggestions towards enhancing and refining the arguments in the light of future developments in studies of FC would be heartily welcomed. It is nevertheless, hoped that useful insights have been provided to add up to our understanding of how actors' interaction in health education, local development projects, their relationship with each other, the power fields they occupy and how community members perceive them have been provided to boast our understanding of how such interventions work, and that this study will contribute immensely to health education in general and to the anti-FC and anti-HIV/AIDs fight in the Ejagham area in particular.

It is also envisaged that lessons learnt might be dissimilar to other situations elsewhere, both in terms of local contextual constraints impeding the change initiatives and in the ways that they affect social change efforts. For instance, a multi-pronged and collaborative approach among various stakeholders: government departments, grass root NGOs in both Cameroon and Nigeria is absolutely necessary. Any reductionism of the multiple embeddedness of the ritual of FC in local social structures and institutions will backfire.

LIST OF ABBREVIATIONS

ACAFEM:	Cameroon Association of Female Medical Doctors
ACAFEG:	Association For the Fight Against Female Genital Mutilation
AIDS:	Acquired Immune Deficiency Syndrome
CDHS :	Cameroon Demographic and Health Survey
CEDAW:	Convention for the Elimination of All forms of Discrimination against Women
CIA:	Central Intelligence Agency
CRR:	Cross River Region
BLCC:	Bakweri Land Claims Committee
CMA:	Critical Medical Anthropology
CPDM:	Cameroon People's Democratic Movement
FC:	Female Circumcision
FIDA:	International Federation of Female Lawyers
FGD:	Focus Group Discussion Session
FGM:	Female Genital Mutilation
FGS:	Female Genital Surgery
GTZ:	German Technical Co operation
MINASCOF:	Ministry of Women's Affairs
HIV:	Human Immuno Deficiency Virus
HTPs:	Harmful Traditional Practices
IAC:	Inter-African Committee for the fight Against Harmful Traditional Practices
ICPD:	International Conference on Population and Development
IMF:	International Monetary Fund
NGO:	Non-governmental Organizations
SAP:	Structural Adjustment Programme
SDF:	Social Democratic Front
STD:	Sexually Transmissible Diseases
STI:	Sexually Transmissible Infections
UN:	United Nations
US:	United States
USD:	United States dollar
UNICEF:	United Nations Children Emergency Fund

UNPF: United Nations Population Fund
WHO: World Health Organization
YDC: Youth Development Centre

BIBLIOGRAPHY

Abasiattai, B, M. (Ed).1990. *A History of The Cross River Region of Nigeria. Enugu:* Harris Publishers.

Abusharaf, M, R. 2000. Revisiting Feminist Discourses on Infibulation: Responses from Sudanese Feminists. In: Shell-Duncan, B & Hernlund, Y (Eds) *Female ''Circumcision'' in Africa, Culture, Controversy and Change*. London, Lynne Reinner.

—. 2001. 'Virtuous Cuts: Female Genital Circumcision in An African Ontology'. *Differences: A Journal of Feminist Cultural Studies. Volume 12(1): 112- 140.*

ABEMO.2002. Report on Legal Awareness Programme in Ejagham Community, Buea, Cameroon.

Abu-Lughod, L. 1993. 'Writing Against Culture' *In R.G Fox (ed). Recapturing Anthropology.* School of American Research Press, Sante Fe. pp. 137-163.

Achebe, C. 1969.*Things Fall Apart.* New York: Faucet Crest.

Adendorff, F. 1998. 'The functions of code-switching among high school teachers and students in KwaZulu and implications for teacher education' in: K. Bailey and D. Nunan (Eds*) Voices From Classroom,* Cambridge: Cambridge University Press.

Adongo, P et al.1998. "Female Genital Mutilation: Socio-cultural Factors that Influence the practice in Kassena-Nankana District, Ghana". *African Journal of Reproductive Health.* Editors: F.E Okonofua and R.C Snow. Vol. (2)2:24-36.

Ahlberg,M, Njau, W et al. *2000. 'Gender* Masked or Self-inflicted pain : Female Circumcision, Eradication and Persistence in Central Kenya'. *African Sociological Review, 4(1): 35-54.*

Ahlberg et al.2004. "It's only tradition': making sense of eradication interventions and the persistence of female 'circumcision' within Swedish context''. *Critical Social Policy.* Vol. 24(1): 50-78.

Ahmadou, F. *2000.* Rites and Wrongs: An Insider/Outsider Reflects on Power and Excision. In*:* Shell-Duncan and Y. Hernlund. (Eds). *Female 'Circumcision' in Africa: Culture, Controversy and Change.* Boulder, Colo: Lynne Rienner.

Ajaga, N.1999. 'Empirical Evidence of the Spread of HIV/Aids in a rural area in Cameroon (Africa)'. *African Anthropology:* Journal of the Pan-African Anthropological Association.Vol.VI (1):32-54.

Alexandra, R. 2000. *Culture and Pedagogy,* Oxford: Blackwell Publishers.

Allman, J, Geiger, S. et al. (Eds). 2002. *Women in African Colonial Histories.* Indiana: Indiana University Press.

—. 2001. "Rounding Up Spinsters: Gender Chaos and Unmarried Women in Colonial Asante'' In: Hodgson, J, McCurdy, A.S. (Eds)*"Wicked Women and the Reconfiguration of Gender in Africa''*. pp.130-148. Heinemann.

Aljaafreeh, A, Lantolf, J. 1994. 'Negative feedback regulation on second language learning in the zone of proximal development', in: *S.* Magnam and J. Lantolf (Eds*). Modern Language Journal, 78 (4): 465-483.*

Almroth, L, Almroth V, et al. 2001. 'Male Complications of female genital mutilation'. *Social Science and Medicine*. Volume 53(11): 1455- 1460.

Althaus., A.F., 1997. Female Circumcision: Rite of Passage or Violation of Rights? *International Family Planning Perspectives.* Vol., 23(3): 130-133.

Anderson, P. 1998. ''Confidentiality and Consent in Qualitative Research". British Sociological Association Network 69:6-7.

Anderson,M.1980.*Approaches to the History of the Western Family*, 1500-1914. London: Macmillan.

Anjezza, S. 2005. Modern Beauty: A Case Study of Female Identity among Female University Students In Elbasan, Albania. MA Dissertation. Central European University, Hungary.

Antanazzo, M.2000. 'Problems with Criminalizing Female Genital Cutting'. *Peace Review*. 15(4): 471- 477.

Althusser, L. 1971. *Ideology and Ideological State Apparatuses. (Notes toward and Investigation. Lenin and Philosophy and Other Essays*). New York: Monthly Review.

Amaduime, I. 1987. *Male Daughters and Female Husband, Gender and Sex in an African Society*. London: Zed Books.

Appadurai, A. 2004. 'The Capacity to Aspire: Culture and the Terms of Recognition'. In: Vijayendra Roa and Michael Walton(eds).*Culture and Public Action*. Stanford University Press.

Apena, A. 1996. Female Circumcision in Africa and the Problem of Cross-cultural Perspectives. *Africa Updates* 3(2): 7-8.

Appiah, A. 1992. *In My Father's House. Africa in the Philosophy of Culture*. New York, Oxford: Oxford University Press.

Ardener, E. 1996. *Kingdom on Mount Cameroon. Studies in the history of the Cameroon Coast, 1500-1970*. Providence, R.I: Berghann Books.

Ardener, E.S. Ardener and W.A Warmington. 1960. *Plantation and Village Life in the Cameroons: Some Economic and Social Studies.* London: Oxford University Press.

Argyrou, V. 2005. *The Logic of environmentalism: anthropology, ecology and postcoloniality*. London: Berghahn.

Arrey, T.1995. Form and Content of Dirges in Ejagham. Postgraduate Dissertation. Higher Teacher's Training College, University of Yaounde, Cameroon.

Assaad, M, B. 1980. 'Female Circumcision in Egypt: Social Implications, Current Research and Prospects for Change.' *Studies in Family Planning* (11): 3-16.

Austen, A.R. 1983. 'The Metamorphoses of Middlemen: The Douala, Europeans and the Cameroon Hinterland ca. 1800- ca. 1960. *The International Journal of African Historical Studies*. Vol. 16(1): 1-24.

Baer, H, A.1982. On the Political Economy of Health. *Medical Anthropology Newsletter,* Vol.14 (1), 1982,1-2+13-17.

—. 1997. *Medical Anthropology and the World System: A Critical Perspective*. London: Oxford University Press.

Bailey, R, Muga R, Poulusse, R. 2000. 'Trial Intervention introducing male circumcision to reduce HIV/STD infections in Nyanza Province, Kenya'. Baseline Results. *International Conference on AIDS* (Abstract No. MoOrc196).

Bailey RC; Neema S; Othieno R, 1999."Sexual behaviors and other HIV risk factors in circumcised and uncircumcised men in Uganda." *J. Acquir Immune Defic Syndr.* Nov 1;22(3):294-301.

Barkty, BSL.1990.*Femininity and Domination: Studies in the Phenomenology of Oppression.* New York: Routledge.

Bastiaensen, J, De Herdt, T. 2004. 'Aid as an encounter at the interface: the complexity of the global fight against poverty'. *Third World Quarterly*, Vol. 25(5):871-885.

Bebbington, A. 2004. 'NGOs and Uneven development: geographies of development intervention'. *Progress in Human Geography* 28 (6): 725- 745.

Beck, U, Ritter, M. 1992.*Risk Society: Towards a New Modernity*. Sage. London.

Bettina,S.,Henlund,Y. (eds). 2000. *Female 'Circumcision' in Africa: Culture, Controversy and Change.* Boulder: Lynne Rienner Publishers.

Bizzell, P. 1992. 'Contact Zones and English Studies'. *Cross-Talk in Composition Theory*. Urbana, Illinois, NCTE.

Bishop, J, P. 2004. 'Modern Liberalism, Female Circumcision, and the Rationality of Traditions. *Journal of Medicine and Philosophy.* Vol. 29(4): 473-497.

Bloemenkamp, K., Farley, TMM. 2000. Male circumcision and risk of HIV infection in Sub-Saharan Africa: a systematic review and meta-analysis, *AIDS* 14(15): 2361-2370.

Boddy, J. 1982. 'Womb as Oasis: Pharaonic Circumcision in Rural Northern Sudan'. *American Ethnologist* (9): 682-98.

Bonner, K. 2001. Male circumcision as an HIV control strategy: Not a "Natural Condom". *Reproductive Health Matters.* Vol. 9(18):143-155.

Bonchuk, O.M. 1997. International Boundaries And Divided Peoples: A Case study of Boki and Ejagham Communities in the Cross River Area, 1884-1994. Unpublished PhD Dissertation. Department of History. University of Calabar, Calabar, Nigeria.

Borchers, T. (2002). Groupthink. Morehead State University. Retrieved 24 March 2003 from http://www.abacon.com/commstudies/groups/groupthink.html.

Bordo, S. 1993. *Unbearable Weight: Feminism, Western Culture, and the Body.* Berkeley CA: University of California Press.

Bourdieu, P.1977. *Outline of A Theory of Practice.* Trans.Richard Nice. Cambridge. Cambridge University Press.

—. 1994. 'Rethinking the State: Genesis and Structure of the Bureaucratic Field'. *Sociological Theory*, 12(1): 1-18.

Boyle, E. H and Preves, E. S. 2000. 'National Politics as International Process: The Case of Anti-Female-Genital Cutting Laws. *Law and Society Review*, Volume 34(3): 703-736.

Burawoy, M. 1998. 'The Extended Case Method'. *Sociological Theory* 16(1): 3-33. March. American Sociological Association.

—. 1991. *Ethnography unbound : power and resistance in the modern metropolis.* Berkeley: University of California Press.

Bloemenkamp K, Farley T, M. 2000. HIV and male circumcision. World Health Organization Internal Document. February.

Bonner, K. 2001. 'Male Circumcision as an HIV Control Strategy: Not a 'Natural Condom'. *Reproductive Health Matters,* Vol. 9(18) :1-13.

Bryman, A. 1988. *Quantity and Quality in Social Research*, Unwin Hyman.

Bryman, A, Wawick, D, P. 1988. 'On methodological integration in social research', in: M. Bumar and D. P. Warwick (Eds) *Social Research in Developing Countries*, New York: John Wiley.

Buchfinder, S, Heagerty, P, Mayer, K et al. 1998. 'Risk factors for HIV seroconversion in a contemporary cohort of high risk men who have sex with men.' (MSM). International Conference on AIDS, 12:411 (Abstract No. 23350).

Burns, R. 2000. *Introduction to Research Methods*, 4th Ed, Sage.

Buruma, I.2006. *Murder in Amsterdam.The Death of Theo van Gogh and the Limits of Tolerance*. London: The Penguin Press.

Burton, D. 2000. 'The use of case studies in social science research', in: D. Burton (Eds). *Research Training For Social Scientists*, Sage.

Caglar, A.1997. "Hyphenated Identities and the Limits of "Culture".In T.Modood and P.Werbner (eds). *The Politics of Multiculturalism in the New Europe*. London and New York: Zed Books.Pp:169-185.

Campbell, *C*. Foulis, C. A et al. 2005. ''I Have an Evil Child at My House'': Stigma and HIV/AIDS Management in a South African Community. *American Journal of Public Healt*h. Vol. 95(5):808-815.

Castel, R.1991. 'From Dangerousness to Risk. Governmentality', in Burchell G, Gordon C. and Miller P.eds. *The Foucault effect: Studies in Governmentality with Two Lectures by and an Interview with Michel Foucault*. Chicago : The University of Chicago Press.

Caldwell, J.C,P. Caldwell, and P.Quiggin.1989. The Social Context of AIDS in Sub-Saharan Africa. *Population and Development Review* 15(2):185-234.

Charrad, J.P. 1994. *The Nation and Its Fragments, Colonial and Postcolonial Histories*. Princeton: Princeton University Press.

CIAF.1994. "Etude Sur les Mutilations Génitales Féminines au Cameroun'' (document inédit).

Civil Military Alliance.1996. "Spirit of Harare Prevention Efforts". Major Regional Seminar on African Military HIV/AIDS. *Alliance Newsletter*.1996. April. 2(2).

Chanock, M. 1982. "Making Customary Law: Men, Women and Courts in Colonial Northern Rhodesia.'' In Margaret J, H and Marcia, W (eds). *African Women and the Law: Historical Perspectives*. Boston: Boston University Press on Africa, VII.

Chiabi, E.M. 1986. "The Nigerian-Cameroonian Connection: A Study of the Historical Relationship and Its Effect on Anglophone Cameroon'. *Journal of African Studies* 13(2): 59- 68.

Chatterjee,P. 1993. *The Nation and Its Fragments.Colonial and Postcolonial Histories*. Princeton, NJ: Princeton University Press.

Clifford, J.1997.'Spatial Practices: Fieldwork, Travel and the Discipline of Anthropology. In: A.Gupta and J. Ferguson.(Eds). *Anthropological Locations*. Berkeley: University of California Press.Pp.185-122.

—. 1988. On Ethnographic Authority. In: J.Clifford. *Predicaments of Culture*. Cambridge: Harvard University Press. Pp.19 51.

—. 1986. Introductions: Partial Truths: In: Clifford, James and Marcus, George. (eds).*Writing Culture. The Poetics and Politics of Ethnography*.Pp1-26. Berkeley: University of California Press.

Cohen, D. 2004. The Uncertainty of Africa in an Age of Uncertainty. Paper Presented at the History Department, University of KwaZulu-Natal, April 30.

Coutler, A, Magee, H. 2003. *The European Patient of the Future*.Open University Press

Cutrufelli, M.R. 1983. *Women of Africa: Roots of Oppression.* London: Longman.

Colson, E. 1971. 'The Impact of the Colonial Period on the Definition of Land Rights'. In: Victor Turner (ed), *Colonialism in Africa.* Cambridge: Cambridge University Press. pp. 221-251

Comaroff, J & Comaroff, J. (eds). 1999. *Civil Society and the Political Imagination in Africa. Critical Perspectives.* University of Chicago Press.

Cocks, P. 2001. Gluckman and the Critique of Segregation in South African Anthropology. 1921-1940. *Journal of Southern African Studies*. Vol. 27(4): 739-756.

Cook, L. S, Koutsky, L. A, Holmes K. K. 1994. Circumcision and sexually transmitted diseases. *American Journal of Public Health, 84(2):197-201.*

Cook, R. J, Dickens, B. M. et al. 2002.'Female Genital Cutting (Mutilation / Circumcision): Ethical and legal Dimensions. *International Journal of Gynecology and Obstetrics*. Vol. (79): 281- 287.

Cowan, J.K, Benedicte, M. and Wilson, A.R. (Eds). 2001. *Culture and rights: Anthropological Perspectives.* New York: Cambridge University Press.

D'Costa LJ, Verncauteren G. 1986. Retrospective seroepidemiology of AIDS virus infection in Nairobi populations (Communication 51, In: program and abstracts of the 2nd International Conference on AIDS., Paris.

D'Costa LJ., Plummer FA et al. 1985. Prostitutes are a major reservoir of sexually transmitted disease in Nairobi, Kenya. *Sex Transition Disease*, 12:64-67.

Daly, M. 1978. 'Gyn/Ecology'. Boston, MA: Beacon Press.

De Herdt, T. Bastaiensen, J.2004. Aid as an encounter at the interface: the complexity of the global fight against poverty. *Third World Quarterly, Vol. 25(5):871-885.*

Dellenborg, L. 2004. 'A Reflection on the Cultural Meanings of Female Circumcision. Experiences from Fieldwork in Casamance, Southern

Senegal': Signe, A. (Ed). *Re-thinking Sexualities in Africa*. Sweden: Almqvist &Wiksll Trycker, AB. pp. 79-94

Dembour, M.B. 2001. 'Following the Movement of a Pendulum: Between Relativism and Universalism'. In: *Culture and Rights: An Anthropological Perspective*. (eds). Cowan, K, Jane Dembour, M, Wilson, R, Richard. Cambridge: Cambridge University Press. pp. 79-120.

Denzin, N. K, Lincoln, Y.S. 1994. *Handbook of qualitative Research*, Sage.

D'Epie, A.1982. Language of Traditional Medicine in Bakossi: A Study in the Power of Language. PhD Dissertation. Department of English, University of Yaounde, Cameroon.

Douglas, M. 2004. 'Traditional Culture-Let's Hear No More About It' In: Vijayendra Roa and Michael Walton (eds). *Culture and Public Action*.Stanford University Press.pp.59-84.

Douglas, Mary. 1966. *Purity and Danger: An Analysis of the Concepts of Pollution and Taboo*. London: Routledge and Kegan Paul.

Dorothy, E. S.1987. *The Everyday World as Problematic: A Feminist Sociology*. Boston: Northwestern University Press.

Dorkenoo, E. and Elworthy, S. 1992. *Female Genital Mutilation: Proposals for Change*. London: Minority Rights Group.

Duffield, M. 2001. 'Governing the Borderlands: Decoding the Power of AID'. *Disasters* (25) 4:269-378.

Dugger, C.W. 1996. ''New Law Bans Genital Cuttings in the United States: Violators Could Face Five Years in Prison''. New York Times, 12, Oct.P.1A.

Eade, D.1997. *Capacity-Building. An Approach to People-Centered Development*. Oxford: Oxfam Publication.

Ebot, W.A. 1986. Language in Traditional Diagnosis: A case study of the Language of Obhassi-Njom as an example of the use of language in specific context. In: *Annals of the Faculty of Letters and Social Sciences*, University of Yaounde, Cameroon.

Eckstein, H. 2000. 'Case Study theory in political science', in: R, Gomme, M, Hammersley, and P. Foster (Eds) *Case Study Method*, Sage Publications.

Edwards, A, Talbot, R. 1994. *The Hard-pressed Researcher*, New York: Longman.

Effiom, C.2001. ''Presentation of World Situation of Female Genital Mutilation with Emphasis on Cameroon''. Personal Communication. Inter-African Committee for the Elimination of Harmful Traditional

Practices against the Health and Well-being Workshop, Yaounde 14-17th May.

Egan, T. 1994. ''An Ancient Ritual and A Mother's Asylum Plea''. New York Times, March 14, 1994: A 25.

Ekpo, I. A. 1985. Trade and Religion in a west African City State: the Ekpe Society of Old Calabar, Unpublished MA Thesis, Howard University.

El Dawla, A,S.1998.'The Political and Legal Struggle over Female Genital Mutilation in Egypt: Five Years Since the ICPD'. *Reproductive Health Matters*. Volume 7(13): 128- 136.

Elliot, C. 1987. Some aspects of relations between North and South in the NGO Sector. *World Development* (15)(Supplement).:57-58.

EL Tom, A. 1999. 'Female Circumcision and Ethnic Identification in Sudan With Reference to the Beri of Darfur'. *Geojourna*l 46: 163-170. Kluver Academic Publishers, Netherlands.

Eret, O.S. 2005. The Obhassi-Njom Institution of the Ejagham People: A Case study of Mbakem Village. MA Dissertation. Department of Anthropology and Sociology. University of Yaounde 1,Cameroon.

Escobar, A. 1984. Discourse and Power in Development: Michel Foucault and the relevance of his work to the Third World, *Alternatives*, 10 (10):659-682.

—. 1991. Anthropology and the development Encounter: The making and marketing of development anthropology'. *American Ethnologist*, 18 (4):658-682.

—. 1995. *Encountering Development: The making and Unmaking of the Third World.* Princeton NJ: Princeton University Press.

Evans-Pritchard, E.E. 1937. *Witchcraft, Oracles and Magic Among the Azande*, London: Oxford University Press.

Equality Now.1991. Cameroon's Submission to the UN Human Rights Committee.67th Session.

Eyongeta, C.1998. Performance and Communicative Aesthetics of Moninkim Songs. MA Thesis. Department of English. University of Yaounde, Cameroon.

Eyongetah, T, Brian, R. (nd). *A History of the Cameroon*. London: Longman.

Eyo, E. (ed). 1986. *The Story of Old Calabar. A Guide to the National Museum at the Old Residency,* Calabar. Calabar: National Commission for Museums and Monuments.

Fakuyama, F. 1992. *The End of History and the Last Man*. New York: Free Press.

Fanon, F. 1963. *Wretched of the Earth*. New York: Grove.

—. 1965.*Studies in a Dying Colonialism or a Dying Colonialism.* New York: Oxford University Press.

Fanso, V.G. 1989. *Cameroon History for Secondary Schools and Colleges: The Colonial and Postcolonial Periods*(Vol. 2). London: Macmillan.

Fisher, W. F. 1997. Doing Good? The Politics and Antipolitics of NGO Practices. *Annual Review of Anthropology.* Vol. (26): 439-464.

Fisiy, C.F. 1992. *Power and Privilege in the Administration of Law: Land Reforms and Social Differentiation in Cameroon.* Leiden: African Studies Centre.

Fotheringham, M. 2004. 'Culture Clashes: Balancing Local and International Interests in Ending Female Genital Cutting Practices'. *Lydon B. Johnson Journal of Public Affairs.*XVI (spring):72-84.

Forde, D. (ed). 1956. *The Efik traders of old Calabar.*Oxford: Oxford University Press.

Ford, C. D. 1937. 'Land and Labour in a Cross River Village in Southern Nigeria'. *Geographical Journal* 90: 24-51.

—. 1950. "Double Descent Among the Yako' In: *African Systems of Kinship and Marriage.* Edited by Radcliffe-Brown and Daryll Ford. London: Oxford University Press.

—. 1951. *Marriage and family Among the Yako in South- Eastern Nigeria,* London: The International African Institute.

Foster, GM, Anderson, BG. 1978. *Medical Anthropology* New York: John Wiley and Sons.

Foucault, M.1979.*The History of Sexuality.* Vol.1.An Introduction. London: Penguin.

—. 1979.*Discipline and Punish: The Birth of the Prison.* New York: Vintage.

—. 1986.*The Care of the Self. The History of Sexuality.* New York: Vintage.

—. 1994.*Society Must be Defended: Lectures at the College de France,* 1975-1976.London: Allen Lane,The Penguin Press.Volume 1.

Garett, L. 2005. 'The Lessons of HIV/AIDS'. *Foreign Affairs.* 84 (4). July/August, Internet). www.foreignAffairs.org/2005/4.html. Last accessed May 9th,2005.

Gausset, Q. 2001. AIDS and cultural practices in Africa: the case of the Tonga (Zambia). *Social Science and Medicine.* 52: 509-518.

Gerry, M. 1996. 'Ending Footbinding and Infibulation: A Convention Account. *American Sociological Review*, Vol. 61(6): 999- 1017.

Gherardi, S, Turner, B. 1987. *Real Men Don't Collect Soft Data,* Quaderno, Department of Social Policy; Trento University.

Gibbens, R, and Reimer, B. 1999. *The Politics of postmodernity*. London: Sage Publications.

Giddens, A. 1987. *The Nation –State and Violence*. California: University of California Press.

—. 2000. *Contemporary Critique of Historical Materialism.* California: University of California Press.

Gledhill, J. 2004. 'Neoliberalism', In: David Nuget and Joan Vincent, *A Companion to the Anthropology of Politics: A Reader in Ethnography, Theory and Critique*. Blackwell Publishers.

Gluckman, M. 1940. "Analysis of a social situation in modern Zululand". *Bantu Studies*, 14:1-30.

Goldman, R. 1998. *Circumcision: The Hidden Trauma.* Vanguard Publications.

Gould, J, S.1993. 'American Polygeny and Cranometry before Darwin: Blacks and Indians as Separate Inferior Species': Harding, S. (ed.) *The Racial Economy of Science: Towards Democratic Culture.* Bloomington: Indiana University Press. Pp. 84-115.

Gupta, A & Ferguson, J. 1992. 'Beyound Culture: Space, Identity and the Politics of Difference'. In: A. Gupta and J. Ferguson (eds) *Culture, Power, Place, Explorations in Anthropology.* Durkham: Duke University Press.pp.31-51.

Gramsci, A. 1971. *Selections from the Prison Notebooks.* New York: International Publishers.

Grande, E. 2004. 'Hegemonic Human Rights and African Resistance: Female Circumcision in a Broader Comparative Perspective'. *Global Jurist Frontiers.* 4(2): 1-21.

Green, E., Jurg, A., Dgedge A. 1992. Sexually transmissible diseases, ethnomedicine and AIDS in Africa. *Social Science and Medicine*, 35(15):261-281.

—. 1993. Sexually transmitted diseases, AIDS and traditional healers in Mozambique. *Medical Anthropology* 15: 261-281.

Green, C, E. 1999. "Engaging Indigenous African Healers in the Prevention of AIDS and STDS" in: *Anthropology in Public Health: Bridging Difference in Culture and Society*. pp 63-83.Editor Robert A. Hahn. New York: Oxford University Press.

Green, E. 1994. *AIDS and STDs in Africa:bridging the gap between traditional healers and modern medicine*.Boulder Co and Oxford, Westview Press.

—. 1995. The Participation of African traditional healers in AIDS and STD prevention programmes. *AIDSLink*, 36:14-15.

—. 2000. African Men, Circumcision, HIV/AIDS and Anthropology, Paper Presented at the American Anthropological Association. Annual Meeting, 11/18/00, San Francisco.

—. 2000. "The Male Circumcision and AIDS Issue." Anthropology News Vol.41(1) Jan. 2000, p.22

Green, M. 2003.'Globalizing Development in Tanzania: Policy Franchising through Participatory Project Management, In: *Critique of Anthropology*. Vol. 23(2):123-143.

Gressenguet, G. et al. 1997. HIV infection and vaginal doucing in Central Africa. *AIDS*, 11:101-106

Gruenbaum, E. 'The Movement against Clitoridectomy and Infibulation in Sudan'. *Medical Anthropology Quarterly* 13(2): 4- 11.

—. 1991. 'The Islamic Movement, Development, and Health Education: Recent Changes in the Health of Rural women in Western Sudan'. *Social Science and Medicine*. 33 (6): 637- 45.

—. 1996. The cultural debate over female circumcision: The Sudanese are arguing this one out for themselves. *Medical Anthropology Quarterly*, 19:455-475.

—. 2000. *The Female Circumcision Controversy: An Anthropological Perspective*. Philadelphia, PA.: University of Pennsylvania Press.

Guha, R. 1999.Elementary Aspects of Peasant Insurgency in Colonial India.Duke University Press.

Gupta, A. & Ferguson, J. 2001.*Culture, Power, Place. Explorations in Critical Anthropology*.Durham and London: Duke University Press.

Gomme, R, Hammersley, M, Foster, P. 2000. *Case Study Method*, Sage Publications.

Government of Cameroon.1998. Plan d'action National pour l'Elimination des Mutilations Génitales Feminines.Yaounde, Cameroun.

—. 2005. Third Cameroon National Demographic and Health Survey. National Printing Press.Yaounde, Cameroon.

Guba, E. G, Lincoln, Y,S. 1988. 'Do inquiry paradigms imply inquiry methodologies ?', in: D. M. Fetterman. (ed.) *Qualitative Approaches to Evaluation in Education, The Scientific Revolution*. New York: Praeger.

Fisher, J. 1993. *The road from Rio: Sustainable Development and the Non-governmental Movements in the Third World.* Wesport, CT: Praeger.

Fisiy, C.F. 1995. 'Chieftancy in the modern state : An institution at Cross Roads of democratic Change. *Paideuma*. 41: 49-61.

Habtamu, W.2002. 'The Contradictions between the proclaimed and the practiced in human rights in Ethiopia: blaming cultures and victims for the violations'. Unpublished Paper.

Hahn, A.R. 2003. (Ed). *Anthropology in Public Health: Bridging Difference in Culture and Society*. New York: Oxford University Press.

Harris, R. 1972. 'The History of Trade at Ikom'. *Africa* 43.

Hammersley, M, Atkinson, P. 1983. *Ethnography: Principles and Practice*, Tavistock.

Hayes, R. O. 1975. 'Female Genital Mutilation, Women's Roles, and the Patrilineage in Modern Sudan: A Functional Analysis.' *American Ethnologist* 2: 617-33.

Henry, L et al. 2004. Networks:Transnational Agents of Development. *Third World Quarterly*, 25(5):839-855.

Hernlund, Y and Shell-Duncan, B (Eds). 2000. *Female 'Circumcision' in Africa: Culture, Controversy and Change*. Boulder,CO: Lynne Reinner.

Heron, B. 2004. ' Gender and Exceptionality in North-South Interventions: Reflecting on Relations. *Journal of Gender Studies*. Vol. 13 (2):117-127.

Hirozawa, A.2000. 'In Sub-Saharan Africa, Circumcised Men Are Less Likely Than Uncircumcised Men to Become Infected With HIV. *International Family Planning Perspectives*, Vol. 27(2): 102-103.

Hirsi, A.2007.*Infidel*. New York: Free Press.

Hobsbawn, E, Ranger, T (eds). 1983. *The Invention of Tradition*. Cambridge University Press.

Hodson, L. D, McCurdy, A. S. 2001. *"Wicked Women and the Reconfiguration of Gender in Africa*. Heinemann.

Hosken, F. 1979. The Hosken Report: Genital and sexual Mutilation of Females. Lexington MA:WIN Women's International Network News.

—. 1995. 'Stop Female Genital Mutilation: Women speak, facts and actions'. Lexington, Massachusetts. *Women's International Network News*.

—. 1995. *Stop female genital mutilation. Women speak, facts and Actions*. Lexington: Massachussetts.Women's International Network News.

Hountondji, P. 1983. *African Philosophy: Myth and Reality*, Bloomington: Indiana University Press.

Homan, R. 1991/2002. *The Ethics of Social Research*. London.Longman.

Howard, R. E. 'Occidentalism, Human Rights, and the Obligation of Western Scholars'. *Canadian Journal of African Studies*. Vol. 29(1): 110- 126.

Hrdy, B. D.1987. Cultural Practices contributing to the transmission of human immunodeficiency virus in Africa. *Reviews of Infectious Diseases* (Chicago)., Vol. 9(6):1109-19.

Hunter, D. J. 1993. 'AIDS in Sub-Saharan Africa: the epidemiology of heterosexual transmission and the prospects for prevention. *Epidemiology* 4(1) : 63- 72.

Ibbawoh, B. 2002. Between Culture and Constitution: Evaluating the Cultural Legitimacy of human rights in African States. *Human Rights Quarterly*. 22(1): 838-860.

Igoe, J. and Tim K. (eds). 2005. *Between a Rock and a Hard Place: African NGOs, Donors and the State*. Durham: Carolina Academic Press.

Islam, M, M., Mosleh, U. 2001. 'Female Circumcision in Sudan: Future Prospects and Strategies for Eradication'. *International Family Planning Perspectives*, Vol. 27(2): 71-76.

James, SM and Robertson, CC.2005.(Eds). *Genital Cutting and transnational sisterhood. Disputing US Polemics.* University of Illinios Press.

Jeater, D.1993. *Marriage, Perversion, and Power. The Construction of Moral Discourse in Southern Rhodesia 1894-1930*. Oxford: Oxford Studies in African Affairs.

Jentsch, B. 2004. 'Making Southern realities count: research agendas and design in North- South collaborations'. *International Journal of Social Research Methodology*, Vol. 7 (3) 259- 269.

Joko, M. 2007. 'Access to economic justice in the common law jurisdiction in Cameroon'. Open Society Institute. Africa Governance Monitoring and Advocacy Project, AfriMAP. Working Paper.

Jones, H, Diop, N. et al. 1999. 'Female Genital Cutting Practices in Burkina Faso and Mali and their Negative Health Outcomes. *Studies in Family Planning*, Vol. 30(3): 219-230.

Jones, G.I. 1956. 'The political organization of Old Calabar' In: Darill Forde (ed). *The Efik traders of Old Calabar*. Oxford: Oxford University Press. Pp 116-160.

Jones, G.I. 1963. *The Trading States of the Oil Rivers*. Oxford University Press.

Joyce, P. 2001. 'Governmentality and Risk: Setting Priorities in the New NHS'. *Sociology of Health and Illness*. 23(5): 599-620.

Kalb, D and Tak, H. 2005. *Critical Junctions: Anthropology and History beyond the Cultural Turn.* New York: Berghahn Books.

Kalb, D. 2006. 'Uses of Local Knowledge' In: Robert, E. Goodin, Charles Tilly. (Eds) *The Oxford Handbook of Political Science. The Oxford*

Handbook of Contextual Political Analysis. London: Oxford University Press. Pp.578-599.

—. 2004.On the Cheap. *Focaal.* Number 43(1) v-vi.

Kapoor, I. 2004. 'Hyper-Self – reflexive development? Spivak on representing the Third World 'Other'. *Third World Quarterly.* Vol. 25(4): 627-647.

Kempadoo, K. 2004.*Sexing the Caribbean: Gender, Race and Sexual Labour.* London: Routledge.

Kemshall, H. 2002. *Risk, Social Policy and Welfare (Introducing Social Policy)*.First Edition.London: Open University Press.

Kennedy, M. 1979. 'Generalizing from single case studies', *Evaluation Quarterly*, 3(4), pp. 661-678.

Kenyatta, J. 1937. *Facing Mount Kenya.* London: Zed Books.

Kelly, R., Kiwanuka, N., et al. 1999. "Age of male circumcision and risk of prevalent HIV infection in rural Uganda". AIDS, Feb25.,13(3):399-409.

Kereta, K. 2005.Female Genital Mutilation as a human right violation: The case of Ethiopia. *MA*. Thesis. University College Dublin, Ireland.

Kirby, D, Waszak, C et al. 1991. Six School-Based Clinics: their Reproductive Health Services and impact on Sexual Behaviour. *Family Planning Perspectives.* Vol. 23(1):6-16.

Kleinman, A.1980. *Patients and Healers in the Context of Culture. An Exploration of the borderline between Anthropology, Medicine and Psychiatry.* Berkeley. University of California Press.

Klouman, E., Manongi., R. et al. 2005. self-reported and observed female genital cutting in rural Tanzania, associated demographic factors., HIV and sexually transmitted infections. *Tropical Medicine and International Health*, 10:105-115.

Koso-Thomas, O. 1987. *The Circumcision of women: A Strategy for Eradication.* London England: Zed Books.

Kouba, L, J, and Muasher, J. 1985. 'Female Circumcision in Africa'. *African Studies Review 28: 95-110.*

Kun, K. E. 1997. 'Female genital mutilation: the Potential for increased risk of HIV infection. *International Journal of Gynecology and Obstetrics, (59): 153- 155.*

Kratz, C, A.. 1994. *Affecting Performance: Meaning, Movement and Experience in Okiek Women's Initiation.* Washington, DC. Smithsonian Institution Press.

—. 2002. 'Circumcision Debates and Asylum Cases: Intersecting Arenas, Contested Values, and Tangled Webs'. In: *Engaging Cultural Differences: The Multiculturalism Challenge in Liberal Democracies.*

Eds. R. Shweder, M, Minow and H, Markus. New York: Russell Sage Foundation Press. pp. 309- 343.

—. 2003. 'Circumcision, Pluralism, and the Dilemmas of Cultural Relativism'. In*: Applying Anthropology: An Introductory Reader.* Edited by Aaron Podelefsky and Peter J, Brown. New York: McGraw Hill Publishers, pp. 269- 280.

Konings, P. 1993. *Labour Resistance in Cameroon: Managerial Strategies and Labour*. John Currey Publisher.

Kreiss, J.K., Hopkins., S.G. 1993. The Association between Circumcision status and immunodeficiency virus Infection among Homosexual Men. *The Journal of Infectious Diseases.*Vol. 168(6):1404-1408.

Larsen, U, Yan, S. 2000. 'Does Female Circumcision Affect Infertility and Fertility? A Study of the Central African Republic, Cote D' Ivoire and Tanzania'. *Demography. Vol. 37(3): 313- 321.*

Larsen, O, Okonofua, F, E. 2002. 'Female Circumcision and Obstetrics Complications. *International Journal of Gynecology and Obstetrics'. Vol. (77): 255- 265.*

Lazreg, M. 1988. 'Feminism and Difference: The Perils of Writing as a Woman on women in Algeria'. *Feminist Studies, Vol. 14(1): 81- 107.*

Law, L.2000. *Sex Work in Southeast Asia. The Place of Desire in a time of AIDS.* London: Routledge.

Lerner, G.1986. *The Creation of Patriarchy.* New York. Oxford University Press.

Leonard, L. 1996.Female Circumcision in Southern Chad: Origins, Meanings and Current Practice. *Social Science and Medicine 43(2): 255-63.*

—. 2000. 'Interpreting Female Genital Mutilation: Moving Beyond the Impasse', *Annual Review of Sex Research 11: 158- 91.*

Les droits des femmes en métier de santé reproductive au Cameroun. Rapport Alternatif. 1999. Centre pour le droit et les politiques en matière de santé reproductive (CRLP) et Association camerounaise des femmes juriste (ACAFEJ).

Lightfoot-Klein, H. 1989. *Prisoners of Ritual: An Odyssey into Female Genital Circumcision.* Binghampton, NY: Howorth Press.

Limunga, F.E. 1999. The Literature of Initiation Rituals of the Lyengu Female Secret Society among the Bakweri of Cameroon. Postgraduate Dissertation. Higher Teacher's Training College, Yaounde, Cameroon.

Lincoln, Y, Guba, E. 1985. Naturalistic *Inquiry*, Beverley Hills, CA: Sage.

Lohman,L.2005.'WhatNext?Activism,Expertise,Commons'http://www.globalpolicy.org/globaliz/econ/histneol.htm. [Last accessed January 8, 2008].

Lupton, D. 1994. *Medicine as Culture: Illness, Disease and the Body in Western Societies*. London: Sage Publications.

Lowndes CM et al. 2008. West Africa HIV/AIDS epidemiology and response synthesis: implications for prevention.Washington, DC, World Bank.

MacGaffey, W. 1996.'Husbands and Wives'. *Transition*, No, 71: 122-130.

McCurdy, S.A. 2001. ' Urban Threats: Manyema Women, Low Fertility, and Venereal Diseases in Tanganyika' in: Hodson, L. D, McCurdy, A.S. (Eds). "*Wicked Women" and the Reconfiguration of Gender in Africa*. Heinemann. pp. 189- 211.

Marcus, G.E. and Clifford, J. (eds) .1986. *Writing Culture: The Poetics and Politics of Ethnography*. Los Angeles and Berkeley, CA: University of California Press.

Marcus, G.E. and Cushman, D. .1982. Ethnographies as Texts. *Annual Review of Anthropology*. 11: 25–69.

Marcus, G.E. and Fischer, M.M.J. 1986. *Anthropology as Cultural Critique: an Experimental Moment in the Human Sciences*. Chicago, IL: University of Chicago Press.

Mackie, J. 1996.'Ending Footbinding and Infibulation: A Convention Account. *American Sociological Review*, 61(6):999-1017.

Manyi, M. 1994. Sociopolitical Impact of Ejagham Integration into Cameroon. MA Dissertation, History, University of Calabar.

Massay, D. 1993. Power-geometry and the Progressive sense of place. In Bird, J. B., Putnam, T, Robson, G. and Tickner, L. editors, *Mapping the futures: local cultures, global change*, London: Routledge. PP. 56-69.

Mbacke, et al. 1990. Prevalence and Correlates of Female Genital Mutilation in the Kassena-Nankana District, Ghana''. Editors: F.E Okonofua and R.C Snow. *African Journal of Reproductive Health*. Vol.2 (2):13-22.

Mbilinyi, M.1988.''Runaway Wives in Colonial Tanganyika: Forced Labour and Forced Marriage in Colonial Rungwe District 1919-1961.'' *International Journal of Sociology of Law* 16(1):1-29.

Mbiti, J. 1975. *African Religions and Philosophy*. London: Harcourt, Heinemann.

McIntyre, D. 1980. 'Systematic observation of classroom activities', Educational Analysis, 2(2), pp 3- 30.

Mcknight, J. 1986. Politicising Health Care. In: *The Sociology of Health and Illness*. Peter Conrad and Rochelle Ker, eds.pp.10-23. New York: St Martins Press.

McNamee, M, Bridges, D. 2002. *The Ethics of Educational Re*search, Blackwell Publishing.

McNamara, N, Morse, S. 2004. 'Voices from the AID 'Chain': the personal dynamics of Care'. *Social and Cultural Geography*, Vol. 5(2): 253-270.

Malcolm, L.W.G. 1925. "Notes on the Seclusion of Girls among the Efik at Old Calabar"MAN, XXV,p. 113-114.

Malinowski, B. 1922. *Argonauts of the Western Pacific*. New York: Dutton.

Mamdani, M.1996. Citizen and Subject. Contemporary Africa and the Legacy of Late Colonialism. Princeton: Princeton University Press, New Jersey.

Manderson, L.2004. 'Local Rites and Body Politics'. Tensions Between Cultural Diversity and Human Rights'. *International Feminist Journal of Politics*. 6(2): 285-307.

Mason, C. 2001. 'Exorcising Excision: Medico- Legal Issues Arising From Male and Female Genital Surgery in Australia'. *Journal of Law and Medicine (Australia),* Volume 9(67) 1: 58- 69.

Miles, Huberman, M. 1994. *Qualitative Data analysis. An Expanded Source Book*. Sage Publications.

Miscouna, S.1998. Les Mutilations Génitales Féminines Chez les Arabes Choa du Logone et Chari(Cameroun).Mémoire de fin de formation d'inspecteur des Affaires Sociales en vue de l'obtention du Diplôme de L'ENAM. Yaounde,Cameroun.

Mishra VR et al. (2007). HIV infection does not disproportionately affect the poorer in sub-Saharan Africa. *AIDS*, 21 (Supp. 7):S17–S28.

Missiroli, A. 2005. (Ed) 'Disaster, Diseases and Disruptions: A New D-Drive for the EU' Challot Paper Number 83. Institute For Security Studies. [Internet] 20th February 2007. Available from http://www.challiot/chai83.pdf.

Muizarubi, B et al.1991. Targeting Truckers in Tanzania. *AIDS and Society*, April/May: 4.

Morgan L. 1987. Dependency theory in the political economy of health: an anthropological critique. *Medical Anthropology Quarterly,* June; 1(2):131-154.

Moses S, Plummer FA, et al.1994 "The association between lack of male Circumcision and risk for HIV infection: a review of the epidemiological data."*Sexually Transmitted Infections* 1994; 21: 201-10.

Mohan, G. 2002. The disappointment of Civil society: the politics of NGO intervention in Northern Ghana. *Political Geography* (21): 125-54.

Moses S, Plummer FA, et al.1994 "The association between lack of male Circumcision and risk for HIV infection: a review of the epidemiological data. *Sexually Transmitted Infections* 1994; 21: 201-10.

Moore, H.1996.'The Changing Nature of Anthropological Knowledge: An Introduction'. In H, Moore(ed)*The Future of Anthropological Knowledge*. London: Routledge. pp1-15.

Mohanty, C. T. 2001. "Under Western Eyes" Revisited: Feminist Solidarity through anti-Capitalist Struggles. *Signs, Journal of Women in Culture and Society* , Vol. 28(2): 499- 533.

Mosse, D. 2006.'Anti-Social Anthropology? Objectivity, Objection, and the ethnography of Public policy and professional communities. *Journal of the Royal Anthropological Institute*, 12(4):935-956.

National Intelligence Council.2002.The Next Wave of HIV/AIDS: Nigeria, Ethiopia, Russia, India and China. Washington.

Naanen, B.B.1991. "Itinerant Gold Mines": Prostitution in the Cross River Basin of Nigeria, 1930-1950'. *African Studies Review*, Volume. 34 (2): 57- 79.

_____. 1988. "Economy and Society in Eastern Nigeria, 1900- 1966: A Study of the Problems of Development and Social Change". PhD Dissertation, Dalhousie University.

Narman, A. 1997. Development Thinking: Bridging the Gap between Theory and Practice. Geografiska Annaler . Series B, *Human Geography* Volume 79(4): 217-225, Current Development Thinking.

Nici, N.1987.'Selling her kiosk':Kikuyu notions of sexuality and sex for sale in Mathare Valley, Kenya. In Pat Caplan (ed) *The Cultural Construction of Sexuality*. London: Tavisko Publications Ltd. Pp.194-217.

Ness, D. and Brechin, S.1988. 'Bridging the Gap: International Organizations as Organizations'. *International Organizations.* 42: (2): 245-273.

Nnaemeka,O. 2005 (ed). *Female Circumcision and the Politics of Knowledge: African Women in Imperialist Discourses.* Westport, Conn: Praeger.

Ndifor, T. K.2004. A Study of Teacher's Feedback Practice and Its Relation to Student Learning in the Context of Three Secondary Schools in English-Speaking Cameroon. Phd Dissertation, Faculty of Education, University of Cambridge.

Ngwa, M.A.1999. Orature in Performance: A case study of the Takumbeng Female Secret Society among the Mankon people of the Northwest Province, Cameroon. Postgraduate Dissertation. Higher Teacher's Training College, Yaounde, Cameroon.

Niger-Thomas, M. 2001. 'Women and the art of Smuggling' *African Studies Review*, Vol. 44(2): 43- 70.

Njambi, N, W. 2004. 'Dualisms and female bodies in representations of African female circumcision'. A feminist Critique. *Feminist Theory*. 5(3): 281-303.

Njoh, A.J. 2002. Development Implications of Colonial Land and Human Settlement Schemes in Cameroon. *Habitat International*, (26): 399-415.

Njua, N.1999. 'Differential Responses to Disappearing Transitional Pathways: Redefining Possibility among Cameroonian Youths' *African Studies Review*, Volume. 46(2): 13-36.

Nkiru, N. The Epistemological Challenge of Motherhood to Patriliny. [Internet] Last accessed 10th January2006 at http://www.jendajournal.com/issue5/nzegwu.htm.

Noah, M.E. 1980. *Old Calabar. The City State and the Europeans*. Scholars Press Nigeria.

Nkongho,A.1999.'The Poetry of Female Circumcision Rituals Among the Ejaghams of Cameroon''.Postgraduate Dissertation. Higher Teacher's Training Diploma (ENS Yaounde).

Nkwi P, Nyamongo, I, Ryan, W.G. 2001. *Field Research Into Socio-Cultural Issues. Methodological Guidelines*. Centre For Applied Social Science Research and Training, Yaounde.

Nyamongo, I. 1995. 'Anthropology: A Social Science in the Control of HIV Transmission in Africa'. *African Anthropology. Journal of the Pan-African Anthropological Association*. Vol. II(1): 45-58.

Nzegwu, N. 2006.'The Epistemological Challenge of Motherhood to Patriliny'. Jenda: *A Journal of Culture and African Women's Studies. Issue* 5, Last Consulted 10/01/2008 at www.jendajournal.com .

Nzima, M et al.1996. A targeted intervention research on ntraditional healers perspectives of sexually transmitted illness in urban Zambia. *Société d'Afrique and SIDA*, 13:7-8.

Nzyuko,S. 1991. Teenagers along the Trans-African highways. *AIDS and Society*, July/August: 10.

Oberleitner, G. 2005. 'Human Security: A Challenge to International Law?' *Global Governance* 11(2)185-203.

Obermeyer, C.M.1999. On Cutting Women's Genitals. Female Genital Surgeries, Reproductive Health and Sexuality: A Review of the Evidence. *Reproductive Health Matters*. Vol. 7(13)112-119.

—. 1999. The Known, the Unknown and the Unknowable about Female Genital Cuttings' *Medical Anthropology Quarterly* (13): 1-28.

Obiora, L, O. 'The Little Foxes that Spoil the Vine: Revisiting the Feminist Critique of Female Circumcision'. In: (ed) Oyeronke Oyewumi ,*African Women and Feminism. Reflecting on the Politics of Sisterhood.* Trento,NJ: Africa World Press. Pp . 197-230.

Ong, A. 1998. Feminism and the Critique of Colonial Discourses. *Inscriptions* 3(4):79-93.

Onor, S.O. 1994. *The Ejagham Nation in the Cross River Region of Nigeria*, Ibadan: Kraft Books Limited.

Orubuloye et al.1994. 'The role of high risk occupations in the spread of AIDS: truck drivers and itinerant market women in Nigeria'.pp. 88-100. in *Sexual Networking and AIDS in Sub-Saharan Africa: Behavioural Research and the Social Context.* Eds I.O Orubuloye, John C. Caldwell, Pat Caldwell and Gigi Santow.Health Transition Centre: The Australian National University.

Oyewumi, O.1997. *The Invention of Women. Making Sense of Western Gender Discourses.* University of Minnesota Press.

—. 2001. Ties that (Un)Bind: Feminism, Sisterhood and Other Foreign Relations. *JENDA: A Journal of African Women and Culture.*Vol(1):1

—. 2003. (ed).*African Women and Feminism. Reflecting on the Politics of Sisterhood.* Trento,NJ: Africa World Press.

—. 2005. *African Gender Studies. A Reader.* New York: Palgraves Macmillan.

Oja, C. 1994. Cooperation between modern and traditional health practitioners in the struggle against HIV/AIDS in Botswana. Report.

Ojang, S,O. 1992. Ejagham Nationality in the Cross River Region of Nigeria: A Case Study of Its Origin and Development to 1900. Department of History. University of Calabar: Calabar , Nigeria.

Onyille, B, O. 2000. 'Abang Dance: Radiance From the River and the Ifik Ideal of Feminity' *Ijele: Arts ejournal of the African World.* 1525-447X: Consulted online at http: www. Africaresource.com/ ijele/vol.1.1/onyile.html. 10/18/2006.

Padersen, S. 1991. 'National Bodies, Unspeakable Acts: The Sexual Politics of Colonial Policy Making'. *Journal of Modern History* (63):647-680.

Parpart, J and Staut, K.Eds.1989. *Women and the State in Africa.* Boulder, Colo: Lynne Reinner.

Pateman, C. 1991. "God Hath Ordained to Man a Helper" in: Hobbes, *Patriarchy, and Conjugal Rights, In Feminist Interpretations and Political Theory.* (Eds) Mary Lydon Shanley and Carole Paterman. Cambridge: Polity Press. Pp. 53-73.

Petras, J and Veltmeyer, H. 2001. *Globalization unmasked: Imperialism in the 21st Century* . London. Zed Books.

Pemunta, NV. 2001. The Social and Cultural Aspects of healthcare delivery: A Case study of Client's perspectives on indigenous medicine in Yaounde, Cameroon. In African Anthropology and the Challenges of the 21st Century. Paul Nchoji Nkwi, ICCARST Monograph Series, Pp.62-72.

—. 2007. Health and Development: HIV/AIDS and the Double appropriation of the discourse of Human Security by Practitioners of female circumcision and Development NGOs in Cameroon". *Journal of Human Security*. Vol.3(1):pp.45-61.

—. 2009. Multiple Identities: Gender, Power and the Production of Anthropological Knowledge. *Anthropology Matters*. Spring, Vol. 11(1) http://anthropologymatters.com.

—. 2010. Intersubjectivity in Ethnographic Research. *Qualitative Research Journal*. Vol.10(2):38-54.

Pemunta, NV. Fonmboh, NM. 2010. "Experiencing Neoliberalism from below: The Bakweri Confrontation of the State of Cameroon over the Privatization of the Cameroon Development Corporation" *Journal of Human Security*.Vol /(1):38-53.

Piot P, Greener R, Russell S (2007). Squaring the circle: AIDS, poverty, and human development. *PLoSMedicine*, 4(10):e314.

Pottier, J, Bicker, A & Sillitoe, P. (eds). 2003.*Negotiating Local Knowledge. Power and Identity in Development.* London: Pluto Press.

Postma, W. 1994. NGO Partnership and Institutional Development: Making It Real, Making it Intentional.' *Canadian Journal of African Studies*. Vol. 28(3): 447- 471.

Programme of Action of the 1994 International Conference on Population and Development (Chapters 1-VIII). *Population and Development. Review*, 1995. Vol. 21(1): 187- 213.

Rahman, A, & Toubia, N. 2000.*Female Genital Mutilation: A guide to Laws and Policies Worldwide*. New York: Zed Books.

Ranger, T. 1983. "The Invention of Tradition in Colonial Africa", in *The Invention of Tradition,* ed. Eric Hobsbawm and Terence Ranger. Pp. 211-263.

Reynolds, P.D.1982.*Ethics and Social Science Research*, Prince Hall. Eaglewood Cliffs N.J.

Richens J, Imrie J, Copas A. 2000. Condoms and seat belts: the parallels and the lessons. *Lancet* ;29:400

Rhoda, H. 1995.'Female Circumcision-Is there a Legal Solution? *Journal of Social Welfare Law*, (6):323-333.

Robert, H. 2001. 'Disciplining the Female Aboriginal Body: Inter-racial Sex and the Pretence of Separation' *Australian Feminist Studies*, Vol. 16(34): 69- 81.

Romanucci-Ross, Moerman, E. et al.1991.*The Anthropology of Medicine: From Culture to Medicine.* New York.

Rose, N and Miller, P.1992.Political Power Beyond the State".*British Journal of Sociology.43: 1,173-205.*

Rossi, B. 2004. Revisiting Foucauldian Approaches: Power Dynamics in Development Projects. *Journal of Development Studies.* Vol. 40(6):1-29.

Röschenthaler, U.M. 1998.' Honoring Ejagham Women'. *African Arts*, Spring, Vol. XXXI, No. 2(38-49).

—. 2006. 'Translocal cultures: The slave trade and cultural transfer in the Cross River region'. *Social Anthropology*, 14: 1, 71- 91. European Association of Social Anthropologists.

—. 2007. *Purchasing culture. The dissemination of association and cult agencies in the cross river region.*London: Free Press.

Rudin, H.R. 1958. *Germans in the Camerouns, 1884-1914.* London: Claredon Press .

Ruel, M.1969. *Leopards and Leaders. Constitutional Politics among a Cross River People.* London: Tavistock Publications Limited.

Russell, B. 1988. *Research Methods in Cultural Anthropology.* California, Sage Publications, Inc.

Sachs, W (ed). 1992. *The Development Dictionary: A Guide to Knowledge as Power.* London: Zed.

Said, E. 1978. *Orientalism.* New York: Pantheon.

—. 1993. *Culture and Imperialism.* New York: Vintage.

Salamon., JA., Hogg R., et al. 2006. The case for expanding access to highly active antiretroviral therapy to curb the growth of HIV epidemic. *Lancet* .368:531-536.

Salamon., R. 1999. Circumcision, infection par VIH et age. *Transcriptase* 76-15-16.

Seidlin, M., Vogler., M. Et al. 1993. Heterosexual transmission of HIV in a cohort of couples in New York City. *AIDS.*, 7:1541-54.

Schoepf, B.1992.Sex, gender and Society in Zaire. *in Sexual Behaviour and Networking: Anthropological and Socio-Cultural Studies on the Transmission of HIV*, ed. T. Dyson. Liege:Derouaux-Ordina. Pp.358-368.

Scoones, I, Thompson. J. 1994. 'Knowledge, Power and Agriculture-towards a theoretical understanding in I. Scoones and J.Thompson (eds) *Farmer First: Rural People's Knowledge, Agricultural Research and Extension Practice*. London: Intermediate Technology Publications. pp. 16-32.

Schofield, J. 2000.'Increasing the generalisability of qualitative studies', in R. Gomme, M, Hammersley and P. Foster (Eds). *Case Study Method*, Sage Publications. pp. 69-97.

Seccombe,W.1993.*Weathering the Storm.Working Class Families from the Industrial Revolution to the Fertility Decline*.London:Verso Books.

Sewell, B. 1985.Ideologies and Social revolutions: Reflections on the French Case. *Journal of Modern History* 57:57-85.

Sewell.,W.H.jr. 1996."Three Temporalities: Toward an Eventful Sociology" In: *The Historic Turn in the Human Sciences*,(ed)Terence J. McDonald.Ann Arbor. University of Michigan Press.

Sterk, J.P. 1998. *A dictionary of Gade (Nigeria)*. Reimer, Berlin

Shorter,E.1976.*The Making of the Modern Family*.London: William Collins &Sons Co Ltd.

Shweder, R. 2005. "What About Female Genital Mutilation? And Why Understanding Culture Matters in the First Place". In: *Engaging Cultural Differences: The Multiculturalism Challenge in Liberal Democra*cies. Eds R. Shweder, M, Minow and H, Markus. New York: Russell Sage Foundation Press. Pp. 217-251.

Sillitoe, P, Bicker, A & Pottier, J.2002. *Participating in Development. Approaches to Indigenous Knowledge*. London: Routledge.

Singer, M, Baer, H. 1995.*Critical Medical Anthropology. Critical Approaches in the Health Social Sciences*. Baywood Publishing,Inc.

Singer, M. 1986. Developing a Critical Perspective in Medical Anthropology. *Medical Anthropology Quarterly*, 17 (5): 128-129

Silk, J. 2004. Caring at a distance: Gift Theory, aid chains and social movements. *Social and Cultural Geography*, Vol. 5(2):229-251.

Simon, A, Boyer, E. 1974. *Mirrors for Behaviour III: An Anthology of Observation Instruments*, 3rd Edition, Penn: Wyncote.

Skaine, M. 2005. *Female Genital Mutilation: Legal, Cultural and Medical Issues*. Jefferson,N.C:McFarland.

Skocpol, T. 1985. 'Bringing the State Back in: Strategies of Analysis in Current Research' in P. Evans, et al. Eds. *Bringing the State Back*. Cambridge University Press. New York.

Steady, F. C.1987. African feminism: A worldwide Perspective. In *Women in Africa and the African Diaspora*. Ed. Rosalyn Terborg-Penn, Sharon Harley and Andrea Rushing. Washington, D.C: Howard University Press. pp31-57.

Strydom, P. 2002. *Risk, Environment and Society*. Buckingham: Open University Press.

Smelser, J.N. 1992. 'External and Internal Factors in Theories of Social Change' in (Eds) *Social Change and Modernity*. Hans-Haferkamp and Neil J. Smelser. Berkely: University of California Press.ucpc 1992.http:ark.cdlib.org/ark:13030/ft60000785/

Smith, M., 2005. *'Into Cerberus' Liar: Bringing the Idea of Security to Light'. British Journal of Politics and International Relations. 7(4): 485: 508.*

Smith, D. 1987. *The everyday World as Problematic: A Feminist Sociology*. Toronto: University of Toronto Press.

Sogge, D. with Biekart, K. and Saxby, J.1996.Compassion *and Calculation: The Business of Private Foreign Aid*. London and Chicago,IL: Pluto Press and Transnational Institute.

Some, M, P.1986. *Of Water and the Spirit.Ritual, Magic and Initiation in the Life of an African Shaman*.London: Penguin Books Ltd.

Sowande, F.ND. ''Introduction to Mythology and Folklore'', *Black Lines*, pp. 8-15.

Spaulding, J. 1992. 'The Value of Virginity on Echo Island, 1860-1866'. *The International Journal of African Historical Studies*, Vol. 25(1): 67- 83.

Spivak, G. 1988. Can the Subaltern speak?, in: C. Nelson and L. Grossberg (eds), *Marxism and Interpretation of Culture*. Chicago, IL: University of Illinois Press. pp 271- 313.

Stake, R. 1995. *The Art of Case Study Research*, Sage.

Strydom, P. 2002. *Risk, Environment and Society*, Open University Press, Buckingham.

Swantz, M.L.1970. *Ritual and Symbol in Transitional Zaramo Society with Special Reference to Women*. Lund, Sweden. Almqvist and Wiksell. Scandinavian Institute of African Studies.

Sylvester, C. 1995. Africa and Western feminisms: world traveling and the tendencies and possibilities, *Signs,* 20(4), pp 941- 976.

—. 1999. Development Studies and postcolonial studies: disparate tales of the 'Third World', *Third World Quarterly,* 20 (4):703- 721.

Talbot, .P.A. 1910. 'The Land of the Ekoi, Southern Nigeria, *Geographical Journal* (36):637-56.

—. 1912, 1946. *In The Shadow of the Bush. With Illustrations and a Map*. New York: George H. Doran Company.

—. 1967. *Some Nigerian Fertility Cults*. London: Frank Cass and Co. Limited.

Tangwa, G. 1998. 'Circumcision: An African Point of View'. In: *Sexual Mutilations: Medical, Legal and Ethical Considerations in Paediatric Practice*. Proceedings of the Fifth Symposium on Sexual Mutilations.

Editors George C. Denniston, Frederick M. M. Hodges, Marilyn F. Milos. New York: Springer Publishers. Pp. 183-195

Thomas, C, 2000. *Global Governance, Development and Human Security*. Plato Press. The United States.

Tierney, J.1990. . 'AIDS in Africa: Experts study the role of promiscuous sex in the epidemic'. *New York Times*. October, 19:A10.

Therborn,G.2004. *Between Sex and Power. Family in the world,1900-2000*.London: Routledge.

Turner,V. 1970. *The Forest of Symbols. Ithaca*: Cornell University Press.

—. 1992. *The Ritual Process: Structure and anti-Structure*. Chicago Il: Aldine Publishing Company.

Toubia, N. 1995.*FGM: A Call for Global Action*. New York: Rainbow Publishers.

Towsend, J,G. and Towsend, A,R. 2004. Accountability, Motivation and Practice: NGOs North and South'. *Social and Cultural Geography*. Vol. 5(2): 270-283.

Van Gennep, A.1966. *The Rites of Passage*. Translated by Monika B. Vizedon and Gabrielle L. Caffee. Chicago, IL: The University of Chicago Press. (Original Work first published 1909).

Van Onselen. C. 1982. *Studies in the Economic and Social History of the Witwatersrand 1886- 1914*, Vol. 1: New Babylon. Hallow Essex: Longman.

Von Reyn, C.F.1990.Epidemiology of HIV Infection in Africa, *AIDS and Society*.April/May:3:8.

Walby, S. 1990. *Theorising Patriarchy*. Oxford: Basil Blackwell.

Waly, J.C. 1997.'Searching for "Voices": Feminism, Anthropology, and the Global Debate Over Female Genital Operations. *Cultural Anthropology*, Vol. 12 (3), August. 405- 438.

Walker, A.1992. *Possessing the Secrets of Joy*. Harcourt Brace Jovanovich.

Walker, A. and Parmar, P. 1995. *Warrior Marks*. Harcourt Brace Jovanovich.

Warnier, J-P. 2006. 'The transfer of young people's working ethos from the Grassfields to the Atlantic Coast'. *Social Anthropology*. 14(1): 93-98. European Association of Social Anthropologists.

Winter, B.1994. 'Women, the Law, and Cultural Relativism in France: The Case of Excision'. *Signs* 19(4): 939-74.

Wisner, B. 1988. *Power and Needs in Africa- basic Human Needs and development Policies*. London: Earth Scan Publications.

Wolf, R. 1982. *Europe and the People Without History*. California: University of California Press.

—. 'Distinguished Lecture: Facing Power-Old Insights, New Questions. *American Anthropologist* (NS), 92(3):586-96.

—. *Envisioning Power: Ideologies of dominance and Crisis*. Berkeley: University of California Press.

—. 2001. *Pathways of Power. Building Anthropology of the Modern World*. California. University of California Press.

World Conference on Women: The Beijing Declaration and the Platform for Action on Women and Health. December, 1995. *Population and Development Review*, Vol. 21(4): 907-913.

World Bank. 1999. Sub-Saharan Africa: From Crisis to Sustainable Growth. A Long Term Perspective Study, p. 66. Washington, DC: World Bank.

Whitehead, J, Demirdireck, H. 2004.Sexual encounters, migration and the desire in post-socialist context(s).*Focaal*,Volume 43(13):1-13.Berghahn Journals.

World Health Organization. 1989. The Reproductive Health of Adolescents: A Strategy for Action. Joint WHO/UNFPA/UNICEF Statement. Geneva: WHO.

— WHO, UNICEF, UNFPA.1997. Female Genital mutilation. A Joint WHO/UNICEF/UNFPA Statement. Geneva: WHO.

—. 1998. Female Genital Mutilation. Draft from WHO Technical Working Group Meeting on Female Genital Mutilation, Geneva, July 18 P. 1.

—. 2005. Female Circumcision-Statement of WHO Position and Activities. Geneva: WHO.

—.WHO. 2008. Eliminating female Genital mutilation. An Interagency Statement. Geneva, World Health Organization.

Yelibi, S,D, Seri, V.M, Paola,V, Claudio, T. and C, Andrea. Nd. 'Socio-cultural Aspects of AIDS in an Urban Peripheral Area of Abidjan (Cote d'Ivoire), Unpublished Manuscript.

Yin, R. 1989. *Case Study Research. Design and Methods*, London: Sage.

—. 1994. *Case Study Research*, Second Edition, Newbury, CA: Sage.

INTERVIEW PROTOCOL ON FEMALE CIRCUMCISION AND HIV/AIDS

MEN AND WOMEN (Individual in-depth interviews and FGD sessions)

Problems women face in this society.
Appropriate women's behaviour in this society.
What does it mean to be a woman/ man?
Women's activities in the community.
Food items that women are not supposed to eat. Why?
Prohibitions related to pregnancy.
Do women continue to sleep with their husbands when they are pregnant?
Do they sleep with their husbands when they are breastfeeding? Why?
Rituals in which women take part in.
Rituals in which women do not take part in and why?
Rituals in which men do not take part in and why?
Groups that are specifically male / female.
Rituals performed when a child is born.
Education of girl children in the past and at present.
Qualities of a good housewife.
What does Female Genital Mutilation mean to you?
For what reasons is it practiced?
By whom and how is it practiced?
Is male circumcision a problem in this society?
How do you call an uncircumcised woman here?
Do you think those who practice FGM undergo any training? Is the training adequate?
Are there any social consequences of FGM?
Are there any medical benefits in your opinion?
What health problems do you think circumcision can resolve?
How would you react to a request to circumcise your daughter?
What will happen to a woman who is not circumcised?
What are the duties of a circumcised woman to her parents when they die?
How is an uncircumcised woman buried?
What is the difference between a circumcised woman and an uncircumcised one?

Are there any ceremonies to mark the circumcision of girls?
How does it happen?
What is a "Moninkim"? What conditions must one fulfil to become a member of the "Moninkim" cult?
What is the role of the "Moninkim" society?
What is a "social Moninkim"?
Do "social Moninkims" have the same role with "Moninkims"?
What is said about women who have no children?
What are the causes of infertility?
How is infertility cured here?
What do people say about this practice? And how do you react?
What do you think about those preaching against FC?
How do you feel women in other places can avoid FC?
How can government help in the eradication of FC?
Have you ever slept with an uncircumcised woman/man?
What were your experiences?
Do you think circumcision is good for women?
What are some of the problems women face because of their circumcision status?
Would you like your child to get married to an uncircumcised woman?
What would happen if circumcision of women is abolished?
Who are the people campaigning against FC?
What were you told by those who came here campaigning against FC?
What do you think about what they said?
In what language did they talk to you people?
What questions did you ask them and what did they say?
At approximately what age did you know a man/woman?
Did you know a man before or after your circumcision?
Do you still enjoy intercourse after your circumcision?
Have you ever had any difficulties during intercourse?
How do you feel when you are having intercourse with a circumcised girl?
Would you like to get married to an uncircumcised woman/man?
Would you like your daughter to be circumcised? Why?
What sexual problems do you think circumcised women have?
What problems related to sex do you think uncircumcised women have?
Have you ever had problems during intercourse with an uncircumcised woman?
What were these problems?
Do you think HIV/AIDS can be transmitted through circumcision?
In your opinion, what is the solution to the problem of female circumcision?

STAKEHOLDERS: NGOS, POLITICAL AND COMMUNITY LEADERS

What practices/institutions with regards to women in this society do you not like?
Which ones do you like?
What types of reproductive health practices do women in this community practice?
Are there any customs prohibiting women from consuming certain food items? Which are these food items and why?
How do you explain changes in adolescent sexual behaviour over time in this community?
Why is it that the government of Cameroon has no specific law against FC?
What is your party's position with regards to FC?
Why was a private member bill against FC tabled by the opposition SDF party defeated in parliament during the June 2004 session?
What is the activities/ programme of action of your NGO in this community?
What strategies do you use in the field against FC?
Which other NGOs are campaigning against FC?
What can you say about their campaign strategies?
What is the difference between your campaign strategy and those of other NGOs working against FGC in this community?
With which local and international NGOs do you collaborate?
In what domains do you collaborate with them?
What is the basis of this collaboration?
What is the people's reaction to your sensitization activities?
What do local community leaders think about your activities?
Do they collaborate with you? How?
Why are the people unwilling to abandon the practice of FC despite your campaigns?
Why is it that although FC was a precondition for membership of the "Moninkim" society, this is no longer the case but FC has continued?
What changes have taken place in the practice of FC over time in this community?
What do people here say about uncircumcised women?
What do they say about HIV/AIDS and circumcision?
Is male circumcision a problem in this community?
Why are some "Moninkims" called "social Moninkims"?
Who are those who want female circumcision to continue? Why?
What are their arguments?

How are uncircumcised women treated in this community? When they die?
What is said about uncircumcised women?
What is said about infertile women? How are they treated?
What are some of your achievements with regards to the fight against FC?
What obstacles do you face?

MONINKIM MEMBERS (Both circumcised and uncircumcised)
What problems do women in this society face?
How are women supposed to behave in this society?
When you say somebody is a woman, what does it mean?
When you say somebody is a man, what does that mean?
What activities do women here engage in?
Are there any food items that women are not supposed to eat? Why?
What activities must a pregnant woman not indulge in?
What types of clothes/ bangles must she not wear?
Do women continue to sleep with their husbands when they are pregnant?
Do they sleep with their husbands when they are breastfeeding? Why?
Which rituals in this society do women take part in?
Which rituals in this society can women not take part in and why?
Which rituals can men not take part in and why?
Are there any groups here that are specifically male ? female?
Which rituals are performed when a child is born?
Are there any rituals to mark the piercing of her ears?
How do you bring up your girl children here?
What is female circumcision?
How is female circumcision done?
Why are women circumcised?
By who?
What are the consequences of refusing to be circumcised?
How did you become a member of this organization?
What are your activities as members of the Moninkim cult?
How is this organization organized?
Is everybody equal in terms of status and role?
What are the various roles within this organization?
Tell me something about the history of the Moninkim cult.
Have there been changes in terms of the criteria for membership over time? Why, How?
What challcnges are you people facing as members of this group?
How do you perceive today's upbringing of female children?

What is the difference between today's upbringing of female children and the way it was done in the past?
What can you say about the sexual behaviour of the youths?
How was sexual activities regulated in the past?
Is such a regulation still necessary today in the wake of the HIV/AIDS pandemic?
What do you think are the causes of HIV/AIDS here in the village?
Are there any practices here that you think can facilitate the transmission of the HIV/AIDS virus? Which are they?
Is there a relationship between HIV?AIDS and female circumcision?
Are there any customs and practices that have negative effects on the well-being and health of women and children in this community? Which are they?
What can be done to change these practices?
How is a Moninkim buried?
Is there a difference between the burial of a circumcised woman and that of an uncircumcised woman?
How are infertile women treated in this community?
What is said about them?
What aspects of the Moninkim cult do you think should be changed and Why?
What is the solution to the problem of Female circumcision?
What do people say about Female circumcision?
Is Female circumcision good for women?
Who are these people campaigning against Female circumcision?
What do they say about this ritual?
What do you think about what they say?
What is the relationship of the Moninkim with various groups campaigning against the ritual procedures?
Why is there no law against Female circumcision in Cameroon?
What will be your reaction if a law is passed against this ritual practice?

MEDICAL PERSONNEL, TRADITIONAL HEALERS, TRADITIONAL BIRTH ATTENDANTS

What health problems do women in this society face?
Which ones do they consult you for?
What about female circumcision?
What does Female Genital Mutilation mean to you?
For what reasons is it practiced?
By whom and how is it practiced?
Is male circumcision a problem in this society?

How do you call an uncircumcised woman here?
Do you think those who practice FC undergo any training? Is the training adequate?
Are there any social consequences of FC?
What are the consequences of refusing to be circumcised?
Are there any medical benefits in your opinion?
What health problems do you think circumcision can resolve?
How would you react to a request to circumcise your daughter?
What will happen to a woman who is not circumcised?
What are the duties of a circumcised woman to her parents when they die?
How is an uncircumcised woman buried?
What is the difference between a circumcised woman and an uncircumcised one?
Are there any ceremonies to mark the circumcision of girls?
How does it happen?
What is a "Moninkim"? What conditions must one fulfill to become a member of the "Moninkim" cult?
What is the role of the "Moninkim" society?
What is a "social Moninkim"?
Do "social Moninkims" have the same role with "Moninkims"
What is said about women who have no children?
What are the causes of infertility?
How is infertility cured here?
What do people say about this practice? And how do you react?
What do you think about those preaching against FC?
How do you feel women in other places can avoid FC?
How can government help in the eradication of FC?
Do you think circumcision is good for women?
What are some of the problems women face because of their circumcision status?
Would like your child to get married to an uncircumcised woman?
What would happen if circumcision of women is abolished?
Who are the people campaigning against FC?
What were you told by those who came here campaigning against FC?
What do you think about what they said?
In what language did they talk to you people?
What questions did you ask them and what did they say?
At approximately what age did you know a man/woman?
Did you know a man before or after your circumcision?
Do you still enjoy intercourse after your circumcision?
Have you ever had any difficulties during intercourse?

How do you feel when you are having intercourse with a circumcised girl?
Would you like to get married to an uncircumcised woman/man?
Would you like your son to get married to an uncircumcised woman?
Would you like your daughter to be circumcised? Why?
What sexual problems do you think circumcised women have?
What problems related to sex do you think uncircumcised women have?
Have you ever had problems during intercourse with an uncircumcised woman?
What were these problems?
Do you think HIV/AIDS can be transmitted through circumcision? How?
In your opinion, what is the solution to female circumcision?
What activities do women here engage in?
Are there any food items that women are not supposed to eat? Why?
What activities must a pregnant woman not indulge in?
What types of clothes/ bangles must she not wear?
Do women continue to sleep with their husbands when they are pregnant?
Do they sleep with their husbands when they are breastfeeding? Why?
Which rituals in this society do women take part in?
Which rituals in this society can women not take part in and why?
Which rituals can men not take part in and why?
Are there any groups here that are specifically male ? female?
Which rituals are performed when a child is born?
Are there any rituals to mark the piercing of her ears?
How are girl children brought up here?
Are there any rituals performed when a girl is getting married?
What are the qualities of a good housewife?
Is male circumcision a problem?